A NEUROIMAGING ATLAS FOR SURGERY OF THE BRAIN

Including Radiosurgery and Stereotaxis

A NEUROIMAGING ATLAS FOR SURGERY OF THE BRAIN

Including Radiosurgery and Stereotaxis

Robert J. Coffey, M.D.
Consultant
Department of Neurologic Surgery
Mayo Clinic and Mayo Foundation
and
Associate Professor of Neurosurgery
Mayo Medical School
Rochester, Minnesota

Douglas A. Nichols, M.D.
Consultant
Department of Diagnostic Radiology
Mayo Clinic and Mayo Foundation
and
Associate Professor of Radiology
Mayo Medical School
Rochester, Minnesota

Illustrations and Graphics by
Michael A. King, M.F.A.
Visual Information Services
Mayo Clinic
Rochester, Minnesota

Lippincott - Raven
PUBLISHERS
Philadelphia • New York

Acquisitions Editor: Elizabeth Greenspan
Manufacturing Manager: Dennis Teston
Associate Managing Editor: Kathleen Bubbeo
Production Services: Colophon
Cover Designer: David Levy
Indexer: Beta Computer Indexing
Compositor: Maryland Composition
Printer: Kingsport

Printed in the United States of America

9 8 7 6 5 4 3 2 1

Library of Congress Cataloging-in-Publication Data

Coffey, Robert J.
A neuroimaging atlas for surgery of the brain : including radiosurgery and stereotaxis / Robert J. Coffey, Douglas A. Nichols : illustrations and graphics by Michael A. King.
p. cm.
Includes bibliogrpahical references and index.
ISBN 0-397-51766-1
1. Brain—Surgery—Atlases. 2. Brain—Imaging—Atlases. 3. Radiosurgery—Atlases. 4. Stereoencephalotomy—Atlases. I. Nichols, Douglas A. II. Title.
[DNLM: 1. Brain Diseases—diagnosis—atlases. 2. Brain Diseases—surgery—atlases. 3. Diagnostic Imaging—atlases. 4. Radiosurgery—methods—atlases. 5. Stereotaxic Techniques—atlases. WL 17 C674n 1997]
RD594.C633 1997
617.4′81059—DC21
DNLM/DLC
for Library of Congress 97-10983
CIP

Care has been taken to confirm the accuracy of the information presented and to describe generally accepted practices. However, the authors, editors, and publisher are not responsible for errors or omissions or for any consequences from application of the information in this book and make no warranty, express or implied, with respect to the contents of the publication.

The authors, editors, and publisher have exerted every effort to ensure that drug selection and dosage set forth in this text are in accordance with current recommendations and practice at the time of publication. However, in view of ongoing research, changes in government regulations, and the constant flow of information relating to drug therapy and drug reactions, the reader is urged to check the package insert for each drug for any change in indications and dosage and for added warnings and precautions. This is particularly important when the recommended agent is a new or infrequently employed drug.

Some drugs and medical devices presented in this publication have Food and Drug Administration (FDA) clearance for limited use in restricted research settings. It is the responsibility of the health care provider to ascertain the FDA status of each drug or device planned for use in their clinical practice.

Contents

Preface

During the late 1970s, one of the authors (R.J.C.) was inspired by the lecture and motion picture presentations of the late Irving S. Cooper. As one of the most prolific practitioners of functional neurosurgery in this country (or as he liked to call it, "physiologic neurosurgery"), Dr. Cooper revealed in dramatic fashion how neurosurgical intervention could relieve involuntary movement disorders by inflicting an appropriate lesion within the thalamus, basal ganglia, or their connecting pathways. In the 1960s, functional neurosurgical procedures that involved either stereotactic or conventional open techniques to treat movement disorders, pain, and psychiatric illness were standard fare in academic centers, residency training programs, and general neurosurgical practice. By 1980, after more than a dozen years had elapsed since the introduction of L-dopa for Parkinson's disease, stereotactic surgery for movement disorders had reached its nadir.

Meanwhile, the introduction of computed tomography (CT) and the rapid evolution of successive generations of CT scanners provided the first reliable in vivo images of the brain itself. Inevitably, investigators at various centers in the United States, Europe, and Asia applied CT technology to redesigned, imaging-compatible stereotactic instruments. All at once neurosurgeons could correlate traditional functional stereotactic targets with actual images of the brain. In the mid-1980s, just as CT appeared to have reached the limits of imaging resolution, the introduction of magnetic resonance imaging (MRI) provided even more realistic images of the brain and surrounding structures. Lingering concerns regarding potential stereotactic coordinate discrepancies between CT and MRI notwithstanding, the ability of MRI techniques to acquire and display images directly in the axial, coronal, sagittal, and oblique planes has been a boon to stereotactic imaging and surgical planning.

A number of workers have developed computerized versions of published stereotactic brain atlases to correlate with or superimpose upon CT, MRI, or traditional ventriculographic images of normal brains with the object of modernizing functional stereotactic operations. Over the past 15 years, considerable finesse also has been applied to anatomic stereotaxis for the diagnosis (biopsy) and therapy (brachytherapy, image-guided resection, and radiosurgery) of intracranial mass lesions. At present, the availability of ever more sophisticated, portable, inexpensive, and user-friendly computers has made frame-based as well as frameless stereotactic methodology the standard of practice for intracranial surgery at many academic centers, as well as in general neurosurgical practice. In the future, refinements in functional neuroimaging using MRI, position emission tomography, electroencephalography, evoked potentials, and magnetoencephalography promise to display the correlations between neuroanatomy and neurophysiology in living patients more vividly than ever.

During several years of practice that has involved analysis of neuroimaging studies for anatomic and functional stereotactic procedures (including radiosurgery), the authors have formulated a system within which to visualize tumors and other space-occupying lesions in stereotactic space. This practice was easiest for targets in the basal ganglia, thalamus, and upper brain stem—the regions where most traditional functional stereotactic targets were situated. More recently, a review of stereotactic atlases in print by one of us (R.J.C.) showed that the brain slices depicted in atlas sections from other regions of the brain provided an excellent anatomic correlation with high-quality MRIs of such diverse pathologic entities as skull base meningiomas, cerebellopontine angle tumors, and brain stem vascular malformations. The significance of such correlations has become most obvious and important in two settings. First, the occurrence of an unexpected neurologic deficit after a stereotactic or radiosurgical procedure often could be explained in retrospect by the proximity of the intended target to a neural structure or pathway that had not been apparent or demonstrated on imaging studies beforehand. Second, the radiosurgical obliteration of deeply situated arteriovenous malformations frequently has restored the normal anatomic contours of the thalamus and brain stem on follow-up MRIs without leaving an empty space, surgical tract, or other defect in the brain. This phenomenon graphically illustrated the principle that compact arteriovenous malformations displace rather than occupy cerebral tissue.

Thus began the idea to compile a stereotactic atlas of actual case material. By applying the wealth of information present in existing stereotactic brain atlases, one could show the intrusions, displacements, and other effects upon normal anatomy caused by representative examples of lesions encountered during the practice of stereotactic surgery and radiosurgery. The rapid expansion of radiosurgery and other image-guide neurosurgical procedures provided the rationale for such an undertaking. Nowadays, many neurosurgeons—and in the case of radiosurgery or brachytherapy, radiation therapists—who have had little or no previous experience in traditional stereotaxis using a brain atlas, administer high protracted or single-fraction doses of ionizing radiation to deep, important, and/or sensitive regions of the brain. Because both the potential salutory results and serious complications of ionizing radiation occur after a latency period of months to years, the learning curve for each individual practitioner is necessarily slow. The information presented in this volume should help the current generation of stereotactic neurosurgeons, radiation oncologists, radiologists, and practitioners of radiosurgery to better understand the potential consequences of their work.

Robert J. Coffey
1-B Quaker Ridge Road
New Rochelle, New York 10804
Douglas A. Nichols

Acknowledgments

The authors express thanks to the many teachers, colleagues, technical staff members and previous workers in the field whose efforts made this volume possible. Diane M. Knight, Chantaal Lichaa, and David Smyrk from Visual Information Services and Scott Stiving from the Stereotactic Neurosurgery Research Division provided valuable assistance to the authors and artist. Angela Kollasch and Mary Sawyer deserve a special acknowledgment for typing and composing the seemingly endless drafts of the manuscript. However, the authors owe the greatest debt of gratitude to the courageous patients whose images reflect the confidence and hope that all of this work will be worthwhile.

Key to Abbreviations

Amy Amygdala
AC Anterior commissure
ACA Anterior cerebral artery
AChA Anterior choroidal artery
ACoA Anterior communicating artery
AICA Anterior inferior cerebellar artery
Aq Aqueduct of Sylvius
BC Brachium conjunctivum
BCI Brachium colliculi inferioris; brachium of inferior colliculus
BCS Brachium colliculi superioris; brachium of superior colliculus
BA Basilar artery
BP Brachium pontis
BVR Basal vein of Rosenthal
Cam Cisterna ambiens
CAm Cornu Ammonis; Ammon's horn
Cav Cavum Meckelii; Meckel's cave
Ch Chiasma opticum; optic chiasm
Ci Cingulum, or cingulate gyrus
CC Corpus callosum
CCQ Cisterna corpora quadrigemini; quadrigeminal plate cistern
CF Columna fornicis; column of fornix
CGl Corpus geniculatum laterale; lateral geniculate body
CGm Corpus geniculatum mediale; medial geniculate body
ChP Choroid plexus
Cip Cisterna interpenduncularis; interpenduncular cistern
CisM Cisterna magna
Cl Claustrum
CL Corpus Luysii; subthalamic nucleus
CM Nucleus centrum medianum thalami; centromedian nucleus of thalamus
cm Corpora mammillare; mammillary body(ies)
CmHb Commisura habenularis; habenular commissure
CN Cranial nerve
(n)CN or **CN(n)** Cranial nerve nucleus
- **CN I** Olfactory tract
- **CN II** Optic nerve
- **CN III** Oculomotor nerve
- **CN IV** Trochlear nerve
- **CN V** Trigeminal nerve
  - **V1** Ophthalmic division
  - **V2** Maxillary division
  - **V3** Mandibular division
  - **Vl** Lemniscus trigemini; trigeminothalamic tract
  - **Vme** Mesencephalic trigeminal nucleus
  - **Vpr** Principal sensory trigeminal nucleus
  - **Vst** Trigeminal spinal tract
- **CN VI** Abducens nerve
- **CN VII** Facial nerve
- **CN VIII** Vestibulocochlear nerve
  - **VIIIcd** Dorsal cochlear nucleus
  - **VIIIcv** Ventral cochlear nucleus
  - **VIIIv** Vestibular nuclei
- **CN IX** Glossopharyngeal nerve
- **CN X** Vagus nerve
- **CN XI** Spinal accessory nerve
- **CN XII** Hypoglossal nerve

Coe Locus coeruleus
COI Colliculus inferioris; inferior colliculus
COS Colliculus superioris; superior colliculus
CP Commisura posterior; posterior commissure
CPE Capsula externa; external capsule
CPEx Capsula extremis; extreme capsule
CPIA Capsula interna, anterior; anterior limb of internal capsule
CPIP Capsula interna, posterior; posterior limb of internal capsule
CPIg Capsula interna, genu; genu of internal capsule
CR Corona radiata

CT	Commissura tecti; tectal commissure, commissure of the superior colliculi
Cu	Cuneus; cuneate gyrus
Cul	Culmen of cerebellar vermis
CVI	Cisterna velum interpositum
DBC	Decussation of brachium conjunctivum
DCD	Dorsal cochlear decussation
DM	Nucleus dorsalis medialis thalami; dorsomedial nucleus of thalamus
DS	Diaphragma sellae
Dt	Dentate nucleus of cerebellum
DTT	Dorsal trigeminal tract
Eb	Emboliform nucleus of cerebellum
F	Fornix
Fa	Fastigial nucleus of cerebellum
FAR	Fasciculus arcuatus; arcuate fasciculus
FH	Fissura horizontalis; horizontal fissure of cerebellum
FCh	Fissura choroidea; choroidal fissure
Fl	Flocculus of cerebellum
FLs	Fasciculus longitudinalis superioris; superior longitudinal fasciculus
FM	Foramen of Monro
FMa	Forceps major of corpus callosum
FMi	Forceps minor of corpus callosum
FOF	Fasciculus occipito-frontalis; fronto-occipital fasciculus
FoL	Foramen of Luschka
Fu	Fusiform nucleus of cerebellum
FUnc	Fasciculus uncinatus; uncinate fasciculus
GAn	Gyrus angularis; angular gyrus
Gb	Globose nucleus of cerebellum
GCC	Genu of corpus callosum
GF	Gyrus fusiformis; fusiform gyrus
GFa	Gyrus fasciolaris; fasciolar gyrus
GFi	Gyrus frontalis inferioris; inferior frontal gyrus
GFm	Gyrus frontalis medius; middle frontal gyrus
GFmd	Gyrus frontalis medialis; medial frontal gyrus
GFs	Gyrus frontalis superioris; superior frontal gyrus
GH	Gyrus hippocampalis; hippocampal gyrus
Gl	Globose nucleus of cerebellum
GL	Gyrus lingualis; lingual gyrus
GOi	Gyrus occipitalis inferior; inferior occipital gyrus
GOm	Gyrus occipitalis medius; middle occipital gyrus
GOr	Gyrus orbitalis; orbital gyrus
GOs	Gyrus occipitalis superioris; superior occipital gyrus
GOTm	Gyrus occipitotemporalis; medial occipitotemporal gyrus
GPe	Globus pallidus externus
GPi	Globus pallidus internus
GPoC	Gyrus postcentralis (postcentral gyrus)
GPrC	Gyrus precentralis (precentral gyrus)
GR	Gyrus rectus
GSc	Gyrus subcallosus; subcallosal gyrus
GSm	Gyrus supramarginalis; supramarginal gyrus
GTi	Gyrus temporalis inferioris; inferior temporal gyrus
GTm	Gyrus temporalis medius; middle temporal gyrus
GTs	Gyrus temporalis superior; superior temporal gyrus
GTT	Gyrus temporalis traversii; transverse gyrus of Hescl
H	Hippocampus; hippocampal formation
Hb	Habenula
Hpth	Hypothalamus
I	Infundibulum; pituitary stalk
IAC	Internal auditory canal
ICA	Internal carotid artery
ICP	Inferior cerebellar peduncle; restiform body
ICV	Internal cerebral vein(s)
Ins	Insula
Lg	Lingula of cerebellum vermis
LC	Lobulus centralis; central lobule of cerebellar vermis
LD	Lateral dorsal nucleus of thalamus; nucleus lateralis dorsalis
LL	Lemniscus lateralis; lateral lemniscus
LM	Lemniscus medialis; medial lemniscus
LP	Lateral posterior nucleus of thalamus; nucleus lateralis posterior
LPc	Lobulus paracentralis; paracentral lobule
LPi	Lobulus parietalis inferioris; inferior parietal lobule
LPs	Lobulus parietalis superioris; superior parietal lobule
LQ	Lobulus quadrangularis; quadrangular lobule of cerebellum
LSi	Lobulus semilunaris inferioris; semilunar lobule of cerebellum, inferior portion
LSs	Lobulus semilunaris superioris; semilunar lobule of cerebellum, superior portion

LV	Lateral ventricle
MCA	Middle cerebral artery
MLF	Medial longitudinal fasciculus
NA	Nucleus anterioris thalami; anterior nucleus of thalamus
NAc	Nucleus accumbens
n(CN)	Cranial nerve nucleus (Roman numeral I—XII)
NC	Nucleus caudatus; caudate nucleus
ND	Nodulus of cerebellum
NLP	Nucleus lateralis pontis
NP	Nuclei pontis (medial group)
NR	Nucleus ruber; red nucleus
Oli	Olive
P	Pulvinar
PAG	Periaqueductal gray matter
PChA	Posterior choroidal artery(ies)
PCu	Precuneus
Pu	Putamen
PCA	Posterior cerebral artery
PCoA	Posterior communicating artery
PICA	Posterior inferior cerebellar artery
Pes	Pes pontis
Pr	Pyramis of cerebellar vermis
Prf	Pyriform lobule of cerebellum
Pyr	Pyramidal (corticospinal) tract; pyramid of medulla
RA	Radiatio acoustica; acoustic radiation
RO	Radiatio optica; optic radiation
SC	Sulcus cingulatus; cingulate sulcus
SCa	Sulcus calcarinus; calcarine sulcus
SCm	Sulcus callosomarginalis; callosomarginal sulcus
SCmr	Sulcus cingulatus, ramus marginalis
SCR	Sulcus centralis of Rolando; central (Rolandic) sulcus
SFs	Sulcus frontalis superior; superior frontal sulcus
Sig	Sigmoid sinus
SMT	Striae medullaris thalami
SMV	Superior medullary velum of IV ventricle
SN	Substantia nigra
SOV	Superior ophthalmic vein
SP	Septum pellucidum
SPO	Sulcus parieto-occipitalis; parieto-occipital sulcus
SPoC	Sulcus postcentralis; postcentral sulcus
SPL	Splenium of corpus callosum
SR	Superior rectus muscle
StM	Stria medullaris of IV ventricle
STT	Spinothalamic tract
SV	Septal vein
Syl	Sylvian fissure
Tc	Tectum of midbrain and rhombencephalon
Tg	Tegmentum of midbrain
Th	Thalamus
Tfp	Tractus fronto-pontinus; fronto-pontine tract
To	Tonsil of cerebellum
Ts	Tractus solitarius; solitary tract
Tspc d	Tractus spinocerebellaris dorsalis; dorsal spinocerebellar tract
Tspc v	Tractus spinocerebellaris ventralis; ventral spinocerebellar tract
TSV	Thalamostriate vein
Ttc	Tractus tegmentalis centralis; central tegmental tract
Ttppo	Tractus temporo-parieto-pontinus; temporo-parieto-pontine tract
Ttsp	Tractus tectospinalis; tectospinal tract
TO	Tractus opticus; optic tract
Tu	Tuber cinereum of hypotalamus
Unc	Uncus
Uv	Uvula of cerebellar vermis
VAr	Vertebral artery
V	Vermis (of cerebellum)
VA	Ventral anterior nucleus of thalamus; nucleus ventralis anterior thalami
VPL	Ventral posterior lateral nucleus of thalamus; nucleus ventralis caudalis externus thalami
VPM	Ventral posterior medial nucleus of thalamus; nucleus ventralis caudalis internus thalami
VG	Vein of Galen
Vim	Nucleus ventralis intermedius thalami; ventral intermediate nucleus of thalamus
VL	Nucleus ventralis lateralis thalami; ventral lateral nucleus of thalamus
IIIv	Third ventricle
IVv	Fourth ventricle
IVv Slr	Fourth ventricle, superior-lateral recess

Chapter 1

Introduction

STEREOTACTIC AND DIAGNOSTIC IMAGING: METHODS OF CORRELATION WITH TRADITIONAL STEREOTACTIC ATLASES

Whereas all neurosurgeons, neurologists, and most other clinicians who care for patients with neurologic disease are familiar with modern cross-sectional neuroimaging techniques (computed tomography [CT] and magnetic resonance imaging [MRI]), traditional stereotactic atlases were designed to be compatible with the older indirect imaging techniques of positive-contrast or air ventriculography (1,3–5,7–9,11–14,17,19). In most stereotactic brain atlases the coordinates and locations for structures in the vicinity of the third ventricle are given as absolute or proportional distances relative to the intercommissural line and midsagittal plane. Serious discrepancies arise when one attempts to correlate modern diagnostic cross-sectional images with traditional atlas illustrations because the former are almost never parallel to the intercommissural line in the axial plane, nor are they orthogonal to the intercommissural line in the coronal plane (15,16). Application of a stereotactic head frame, even when an effort is made to place the base ring parallel to the Frankfort (infraorbitomeatal) line, usually does little to ameliorate the situation. Axial images obtained parallel to the stereotactic frame frequently deviate from the intercommissural plane by 20° or more. Deliberately tilting the CT gantry or acquiring oblique MRIs to compensate for the discrepancy can add troublesome complexity to coordinate and trajectory calculations and can give the surgeon a false sense of security. Likewise, coronal MRIs obtained perpendicular to the stereotactic base ring deviate from the corresponding frontal plane of traditional stereotactic atlas sections by the same number of degrees as do the horizontal sections. In practice, the situation is even more idiosyncratic because the headframe often must be shifted to accommodate a preexisting bone flap, skull defect, shunt device, or other anatomic variant. So, although the various series of cross-sectional images (axial, coronal, sagittal) that are obtained in an individual patient at a single session are internally consistent with each other, the image planes may vary considerably from those of other patients and/or the illustrations of traditional atlas sections (2,6,10,18).

Fortunately, the fact that the targets for anatomic stereotactic procedures (including radiosurgery) are visible provides a solution for this apparent dilemma. Any visible target or immediately adjacent structure that is assigned a set of coordinates corresponding to the three stereotactic axes (X = right/left, Y = anterior/posterior, Z = superior/inferior) retains the same anatomic relationships and coordinates in space regardless of the plane of stereotactic imaging (Fig. 1-1). The example in Fig. 1-2 illustrates this principle using stereotactic axial and coronal images (defined as parallel and perpendicular to the stereotactic headframe, respectively) of a cerebellopontine angle tumor. The axial image (Fig. 1-2A) is at horizontal level Z, and the coronal image (Fig. 1-2B) is at frontal level Y. The coronal image corresponds to an orthogonal plane passing through the axial image along the line marked Y. In fact, as illustrated in the three-dimensional composite image (Fig. 1-2C), lines Y and Z are really the same line, defined as the intersection of the two imaging planes. The point (labeled "t") at the tumor–brain stem interface, located along the Y/Z coordinate lines, has exactly the same X, Y, Z stereotactic coordinates—whether derived from the axial image or the coronal one. Intuitively, point t can be defined equally well on any other oblique imaging plane that passes through the same axis. Readers will recognize this phenomenon as the principle upon which present-day arc-centered and focal-point stereotactic devices operate—including the Leksell Gamma Unit and noncoplanar-arc linear accelerator radiosurgical devices. Once the target has been centered within the arc (or helmet, or gantry), the target point can be reached along an infinite number of radii defined by rotation of the arc along its axis and/or by traversing the stereotactic probe, radiation beam, or line of sight along the circumference of the arc.

In the present example and throughout this book the case has been simplified whenever possible by using the three imaging planes that correspond to the major X, Y, and Z stereotactic axes. So, for the purpose of anatomic correlation, a horizontal or coronal atlas section that corresponds to Y_t or Z_t in the example above provides accurate information regarding the neural structures present at and near point t. The atlas also suggests in which direction and by what distance adjacent structures might be displaced by a tumor or mass.

The process of correlating angiographic images with the anatomic information provided by a stereotactic atlas is simplified considerably by taking the intermediate step of matching the region of interest on the angiographic image with an appropriately-selected cross-sectional MRI. Ideally, both the angiographic study and the MRI scan should be performed during the same imaging session with the patient's head fixed in a stereotactic frame. Unlike MRI (or CT) cross sections, each of which displays the two-dimensional surface of a slice through the brain, angiographic images project vascular structures coursing through three-dimensional space onto a two-dimensional film or video screen surface. Depending upon the x-ray target-to-film distance, and the location of the target relative to the center of the x-ray beam, angiographic images may introduce a variety of magnification and parallax factors. These can be controlled, quantified, and normalized under stereotactic conditions where all relevant spatial relationships are known. Thus, one could imagine the stereotactic angiographic picture of an arteriovenous malformation (AVM) nidus as a stack of semitransparent cross-sectional slices: in the sagittal plane for the lateral (Y,Z) projection, and in the coronal plane for the frontal (anteroposterior [AP] or posteroanterior [PA]) (X,Z) projection (Fig. 1-3). In addition, axial MRI slices through any Z coordinate level correlate precisely with the shared superior/inferior dimension of both angiographic projections. The combination of two orthogonal stereotactic angiographic views with one or more MRI series provides a satisfactory method to define the three-dimensional contours of an AVM and its relationship to surrounding cerebral structures. Anatomic correlation with stereotactic atlas data then proceeds in exactly the same manner as in the case of tumors.

The case illustrated here shows PA and lateral angiographic views of an AVM accompanied by reconstructed coronal, sagittal, and the original axial MRIs through the nidus at the X, Y, and Z levels indicated on Fig. 1-3. Any point within the nidus or, more importantly, any structure at the margin of the nidus can be correlated between the angiograms and MRIs and then with appropriate illustrations from a conventional stereotactic atlas. The reader should bear in mind that each MRI or planar atlas section shows only a single selected slice (of many) through the AVM.

CASE MATERIAL AND ORGANIZATION

This work was built on a foundation laid by authors of several traditional stereotactic atlases of the human brain (1,3–5,7–9,11–14,17,19). We owe the greatest debt to Professor Jean Talairach and his collaborators over the past several decades (13–15). Although Talairach's work is available in this country, for a variety of sociological and cultural reasons his work has not been accessible to most American-trained neurosurgeons. Among his other achievements, Talairach developed a method to localize lesions seen on diagnostic imaging studies within functional stereotactic space. The present volume takes the next logical step: to present a catalogue of intracranial space-occupying lesions encountered in the practice of stereotactic surgery and radiosurgery and to supply pertinent functional and anatomical correlations in an easy-to-use format.

The case material presented in this volume represents a sampler of patients treated at the Mayo Clinic between 1990 and 1995. Almost every case includes one or more MRIs performed with a stereotactic headframe in place. The angiograms of AVMs all were performed using a stereotactic frame for radiosurgical planning purposes. Cases were selected for their illustrative and anatomic value. No implication was intended regarding whether stereotactic localization was useful or necessary, or whether the cases treated using radiosurgery could have been handled another way. Although all radiosurgical cases at the authors institution were treated using the Leksell Gamma Unit (Gamma Knife, Elekta Instruments, Atlanta, GA), the authors do not make any claims or inferences whatsoever regarding the suitability of other radiosurgical instruments to treat similar lesions. Likewise, the authors have avoided any but the most general statements regarding radiosurgical dose planning or stereotactic trajectory selection. Those issues continue to be debated and discussed in other textbooks, journal articles, and symposia. Rather, the information presented in this volume was intended to be of a more general, enduring, and noncontroversial nature.

In each case, the images were selected to provide a useful correlation with anatomic information from one or more stereotactic atlases. Readers who have a basic understanding of neuroanatomy but who are unaccustomed to viewing multiplanar imaging studies and those who are unfamiliar with traditional functional stereotactic localization terminology based on the intercommissural line should find this atlas most useful and will want to study this chapter carefully. Those more accustomed to viewing stereotactic imaging studies may wish only to peruse it. In either case, readers are urged to study the figures and sample cases as a preview of what the rest of this volume has in store.

The first section of this chapter explains how the variety of images used for radiosurgical and operative planning (and in some cases, conventional diagnostic images) were analyzed and manipulated to provide a useful correlation with the information contained in stereotactic brain atlases. The ''meat'' of this book is contained in Chapters 2 through 4, wherein extra-axial and skull-base tumors, intra-axial tumors, and vascular malformations are presented in that order. The figures for tumor cases are reproduced at approximately 1.5× magnification to permit the identification and labeling of small structures and pathways, yet to preserve as much image resolution as possible. To this end, each figure in Chapters 2 and 3 is presented first as a raw, unlabeled MRI accompanied by a labeled, retouched version for convenient comparison. Extra-axial tumors are presented first owing to the relative simplicity and familiarity of anatomical relationships involved in lesions that, by definition, make contact with or displace the brain from the outside-in. Skull base tumors are included together with the simpler extra-axial tumors because of the somewhat arbitrary distinction between "borderline" cases. In general, tumors that arise over the cerebral convexity, anterior cranial fossa, falx, and/or tentorium are considered extra-axial. Those that involve the cranial nerves (especially V–XII) or their foramina, the sphenoid bone, petrous bone, and/or the clivus are designated as skull base lesions. The difficulty in categorizing borderline cases arises when one surface of a tumor presents in an easily accessible arachnoid cistern or cerebral fissure, whereas another component of the tumor involves the deep venous sinuses or cranial base. Cases of tumor "recurrence," or persistent tumor residue after resection of the more accessible portions of the lesion, are identified for the reader throughout Chapter 2. Intra-axial tumors are presented next in Chapter 3. Although metastases are presumed to displace brain structures, primary glial tumors at least partially occupy or infiltrate the illustrated structures as well as displace them. Because of this additional degree of anatomic uncertainty, the authors wished readers to become more accustomed to the relatively straightforward pathologic anatomy of extra-axial tumors beforehand.

Intracerebral AVMs are presented in Chapter 4. The additional complexity involved in angiographic correlation with cerebral anatomy for AVMs, as well as the wealth of important neuroanatomic structures surrounding the malformations selected for inclusion in this chapter, makes it more appropriate for presentation at the end of the book. In order to illustrate the global anatomical picture for AVM cases, most of the figures are approximately life-size (not magnified). Thus, the anatomical relationship of feeding arteries and draining veins to areas of known neural function can be shown over larger regions of the brain. Also, because of the greater number and larger format of the AVM figures, unlabeled images were not included in Chapter 4.

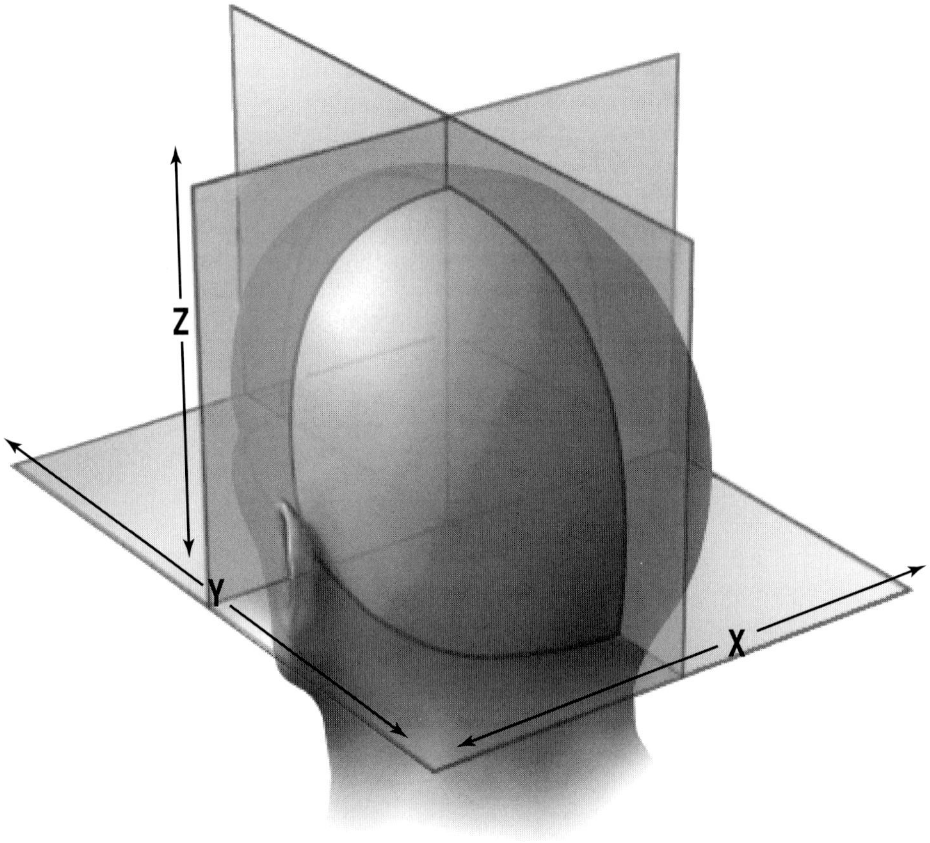

FIG. 1-1. Artist's drawing of the human head showing the three principal stereotactic axes (X = right/left, Y = anterior/posterior, Z = superior/inferior) and their three corresponding imaging planes. The axial or horizontal plane is at superoinferior level Z and contains points having various XY coordinate values; the coronal or frontal plane is at anteroposterior level Y and contains points having different XZ values; and the sagittal or lateral plane is at right/left level X and contains points having different YZ coordinate values. Although these three primary imaging/viewing planes are always orthogonal to each other, their orientation with respect to an individual patient's head may vary considerably from one case to another depending on placement of the stereotactic headframe and/or positioning during the imaging procedures.

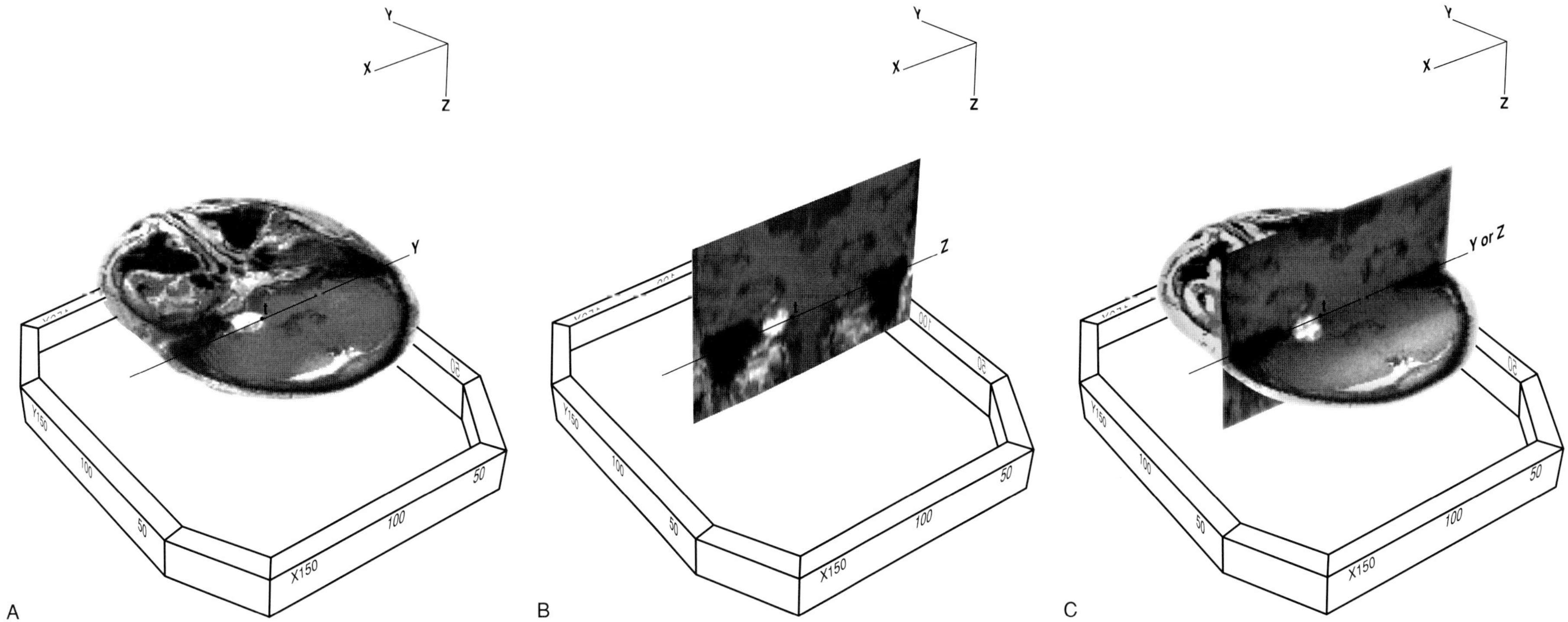

FIG. 1-2. Stereotactic T_1-weighted contrast-enhanced MRIs of a left-sided cerebellopontine angle tumor viewed in perspective and showing the outline of the Leksell model G stereotactic headframe and coordinate system. Note that the patient's right and left correspond to the same viewer's orientation as in Fig. 1-1. The axial image (**A**) appears suspended in space at superoinferior level Z. Line Y in **A** corresponds to the Y coordinate level of the coronal image in **B**. Because the two imaging planes intersect at a right angle along a single line, lines Y and Z represent exactly the same line that had been projected onto different planes (**C**). Point t at the tumor–brain stem interface is located at coordinates X_t, Y_t, and Z_t regardless of the imaging plane from which it is derived or upon which it is viewed.

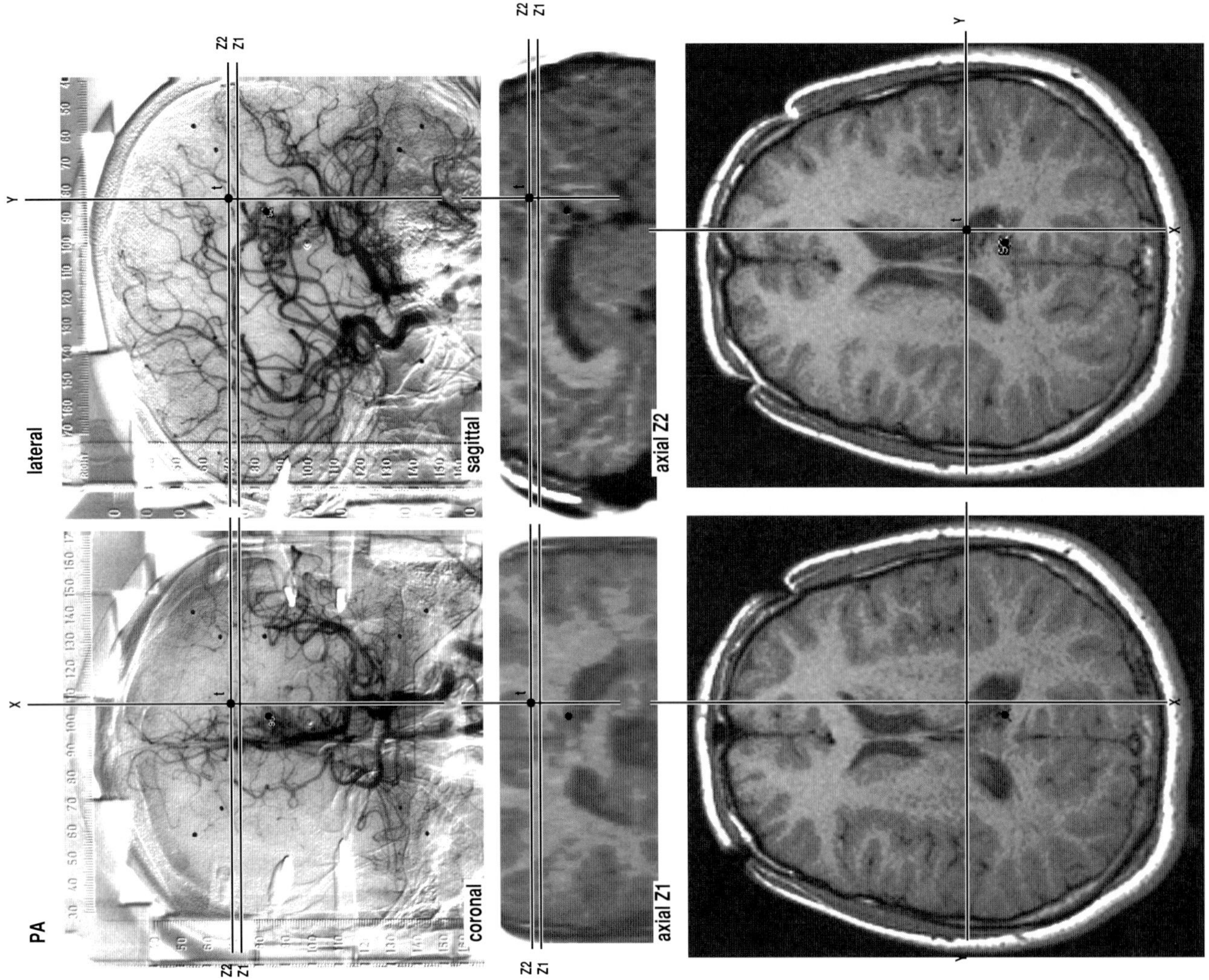
lateral
sagittal
axial Z2
PA
coronal
axial Z1
X
Y
Z2
Z1

FIG. 1-3. Composite illustration of stereotactic imaging studies of an AVM: posteroanterior (*upper left*) and lateral (*upper right*) angiographic projection films; reconstructed coronal (*middle left*) and sagittal (*middle right*) MRIs at planes Y and X, respectively; and axial MR images at levels Z_1 and Z_2 (*lower left and lower right*, respectively). Note that point t has stereotactic coordinates X_t, Y_t, and Z_2 and that it appears on all of the images except the axial MRI at level Z_1. This is because the plane of Z_1 is located 3 mm inferior to point t.

Chapter 2

Extra-axial and Skull Base Tumors

The extra-axial and skull base tumors illustrated in this chapter include histologically benign meningiomas, cranial nerve schwannomas, and low-grade (but histologically malignant) chemodectomas and chordomas. They are presented in anatomical sequence from the anterior, frontal, and superficial regions of the cranium through the course of the venous sinuses and dural folds toward the deeper and less accessible reaches of the cranial base. In this manner the reader can become accustomed to the authors' style, method, and terminology in relatively straightforward cases before tackling the more difficult ones.

The authors selected small and medium-sized tumors with well-demarcated margins in order to emphasize the relevant anatomical relationships clearly. In this sense the catalogue of tumors is a representative rather than a comprehensive one. Therefore, although the clinical decision-making algorithms, radiosurgical dosimetry, or conventional surgical strategy may differ according to tumor type, the neural structures at risk should remain relatively constant for each tumor locale illustrated in the following pages.

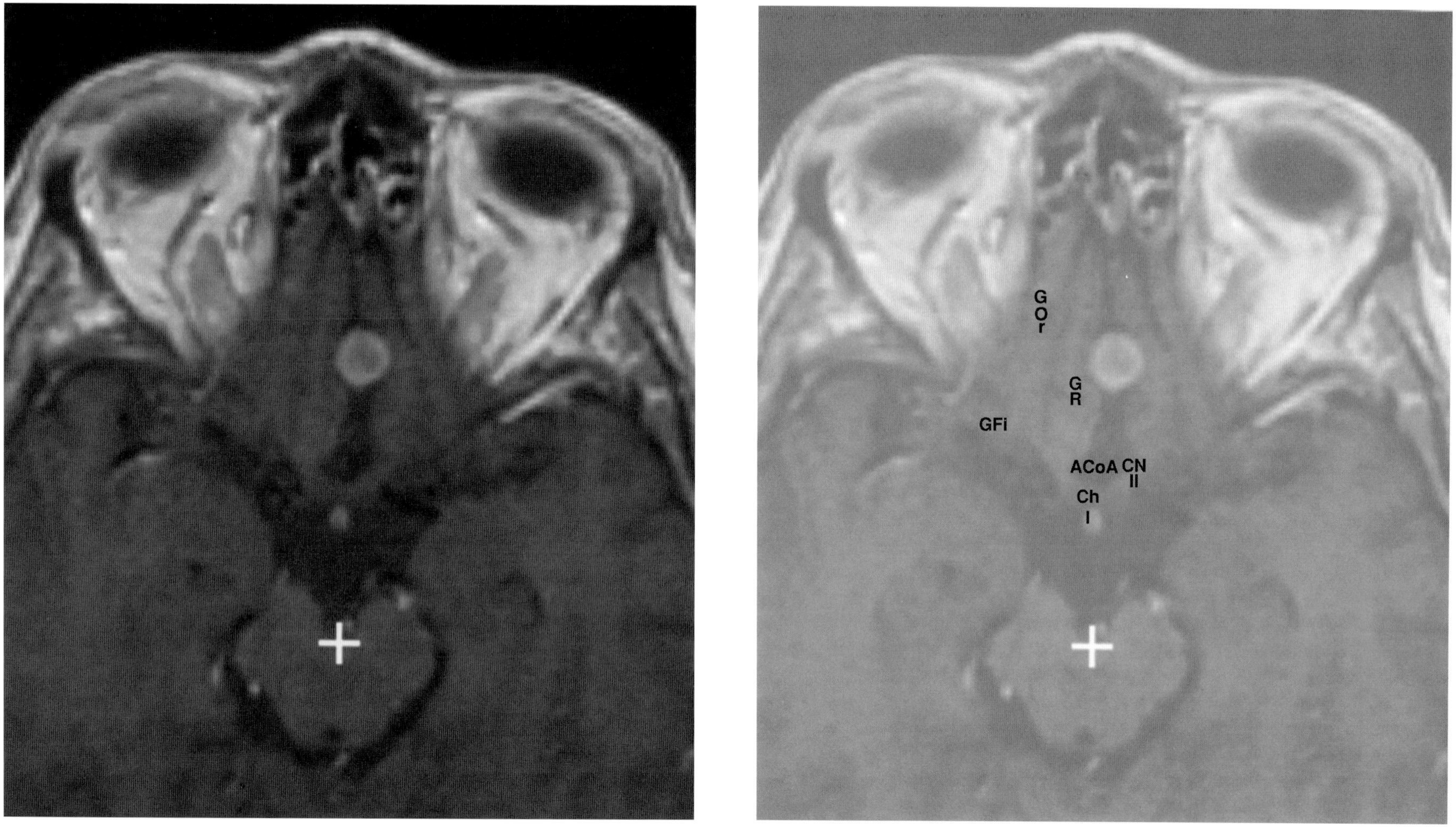

FIG. 2-1.

FIG. 2-1. Tiny olfactory groove meningioma (8.5 mm diameter) in the same patient as shown in Fig. 2-4; T_1-weighted contrast-enhanced stereotactic axial MRI. The tumor sits on the floor of the anterior cranial fossa within the anterior interhemispheric fissure and between the left and right gyrus rectus (GR). The olfactory tracts on either side run on the undersurface of the sulcus between the gyrus rectus and orbital gyrus (GOr), just outside of the plane of section. The optic chiasm (Ch), optic nerves (II), and pituitary stalk (I) lie 6 to 12 mm posterior to the tumor. The anterior communicating artery complex (ACoA) lies just superior to the optic chiasm.

FIG. 2-2. Anterior clinoid/tuberculum sellae meningioma, T_1-weighted, contrast-enhanced stereotactic axial (**A**) and coronal (**B**) MRIs. The axial level of **A** is located 9.5 mm inferior to the crosshair cursor seen in **B** and shows the superior tumor margin. The coronal plane of **B** is located 20 mm anterior to the crosshair cursor seen in **A** and shows the posterior tumor margin, just ahead of the optic chiasm (Ch) and optic nerve (CN II) junction. The left optic nerve appears to pass around the tumor superiorly, just outside the plane of section.

The anterior cerebral artery (ACA)/anterior communicating artery complex lies medial to the tumor within the chasmatic and interhemispheric cisterns. The anterior half of the superior tumor margin elevates the gyrus rectus (GR) and just touches the medial border of the contralateral gyrus rectus, and the ipsilateral orbital (GOr) and inferior frontal (GFi) gyri.

The inferior tumor margin appears to partially encase the internal carotid artery (ICA) as the vessel emerges from beneath the anterior clinoid process. Although the optic chiasm, left optic nerve, internal carotid artery, and ophthalmic artery would be at risk during microsurgical removal of this tumor, the optic apparatus would be of primary concern during radiosurgical treatment of the tumor. The lack of any cerebrospinal fluid–containing space at the posterior tumor margin would limit the radiation dose in that region. *(Figure continued on following pages.)*

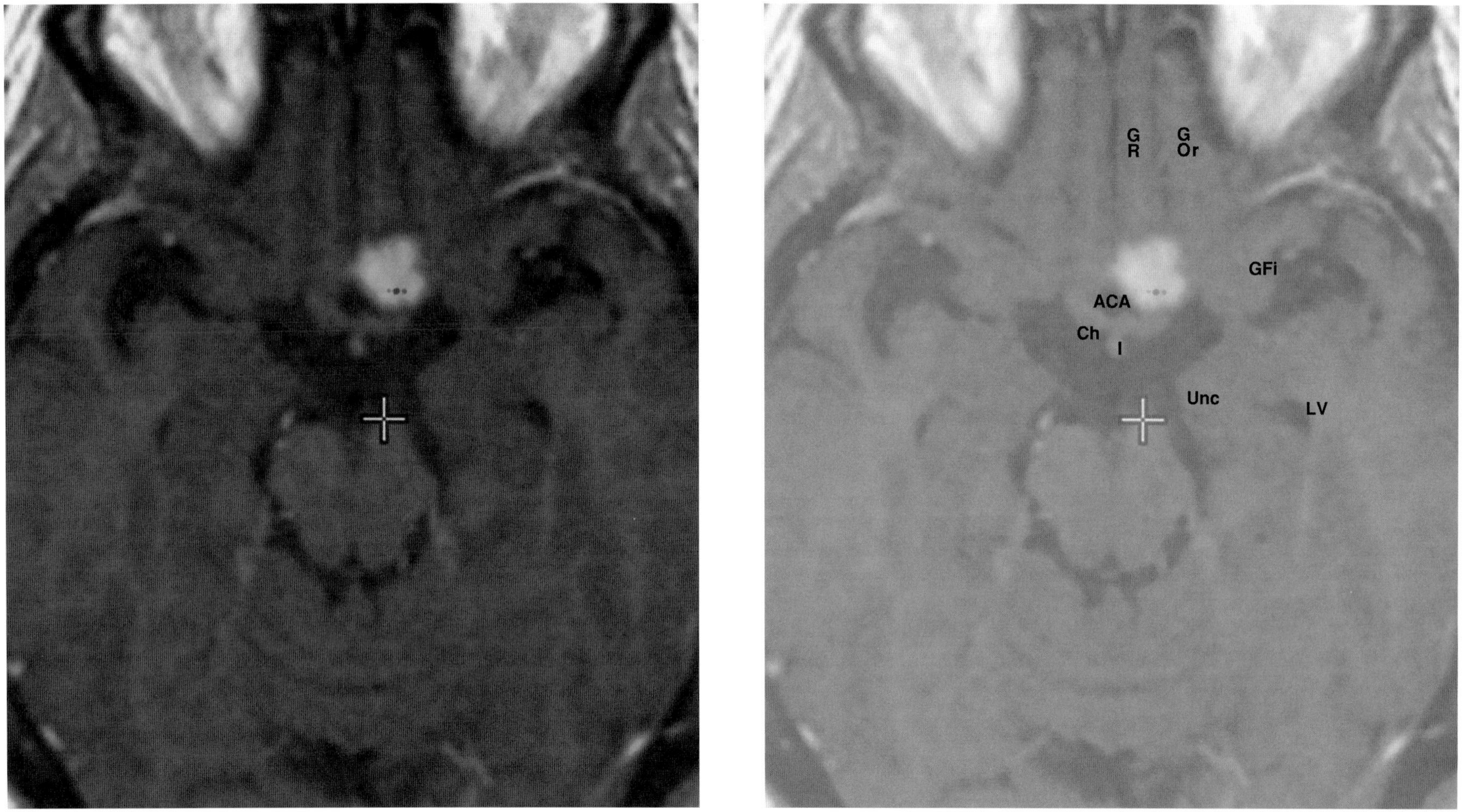

FIG. 2-2A.

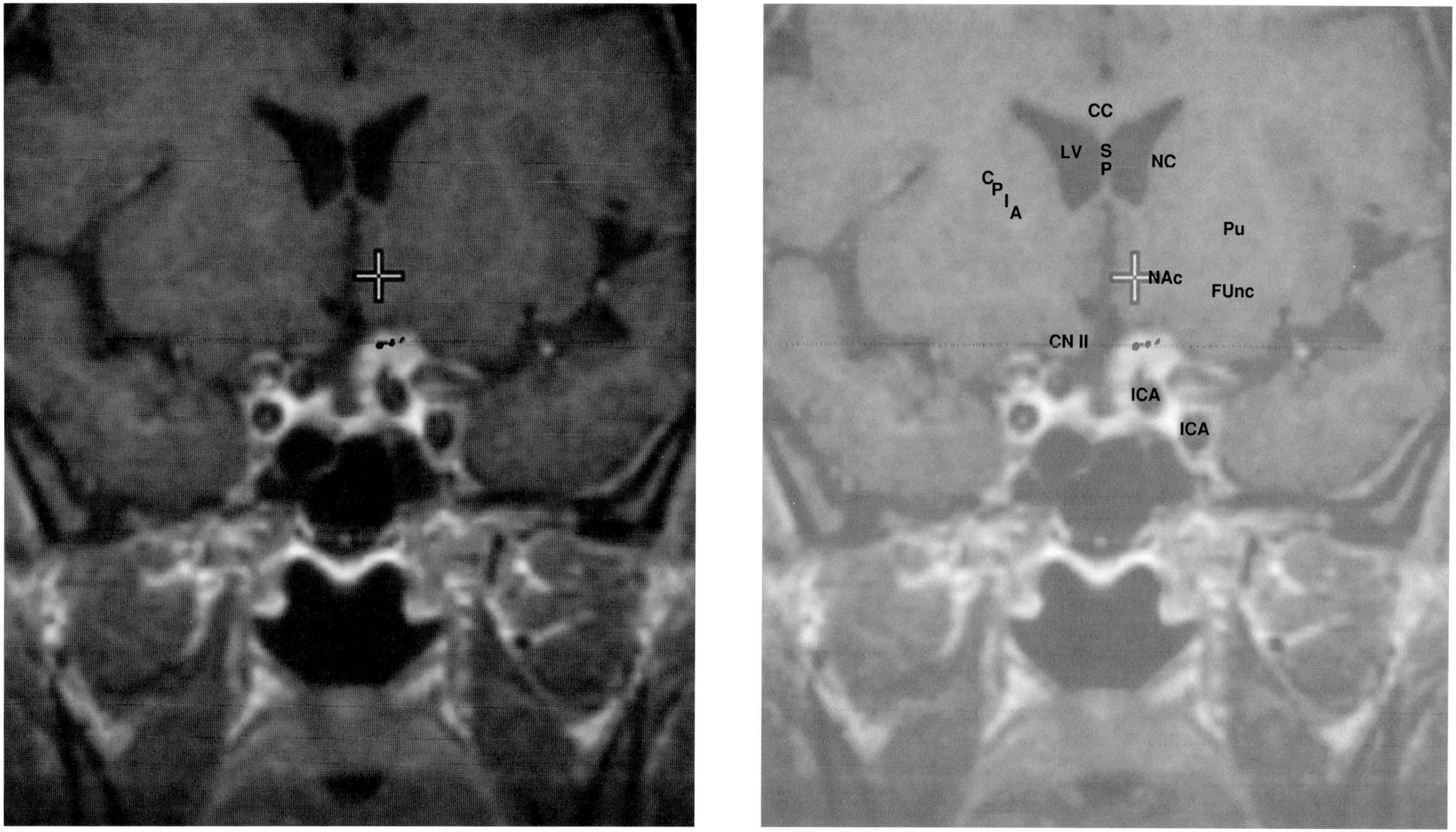

FIG. 2-2B.

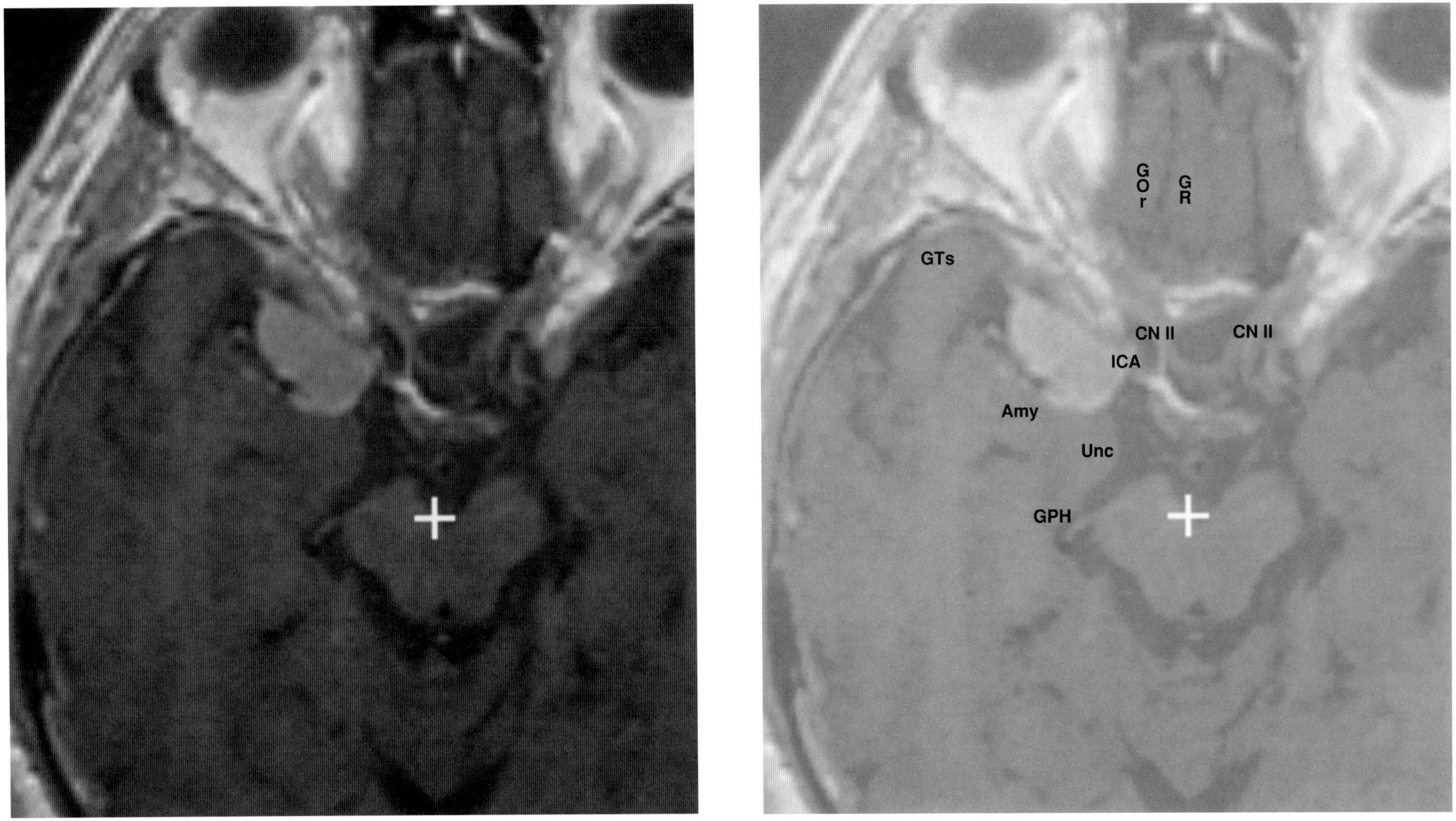

FIG. 2-3A.

FIG. 2-3. Right-sided meningioma of the anterior clinoid process (possibly radiation induced) 17 years after trans-sphenoidal surgery and fractionated external beam radiation therapy for a pituitary adenoma. T_1-weighted, contrast-enhanced stereotactic axial MRIs separated by 6 mm from inferior to superior (**A and B**) and stereotactic coronal image through the center of the tumor (**C**). The axial levels of **A** and **B** are located 6.5 mm and 12.5 mm, respectively, superior to the crosshair cursor seen in **C**. The coronal level of image **C**, in turn, is located 23 mm anterior to the crosshair cursor displayed on each axial image.

The tumor arises from the superolateral edge of the anterior clinoid process, superior and anterior to the cavernous sinus. The most anterior portion of the cavernous segment of the internal carotid artery (ICA) runs inferior to the base of the tumor (**C**), while the clinoidal and cisternal segments of the internal carotid artery touch the medial tumor margin (**A and C**). The right optic nerve (CN II) runs just medial to the internal carotid artery; the optic chiasm (Ch) lies medial and posterior to the optic nerves (**A and C**), and the optic tracts (TO) lie dorsal, posterior, and lateral to the chiasm (**B**). Postoperative changes after trans-sphenoidal surgery have caused the optic apparatus to sag within the suprasellar space in this case.

The anterior tumor margin abuts the gyrus rectus (GR), orbital gyrus (GOr), inferior frontal gyrus (GFi), and superior temporal gyrus (GTs), respectively, from medial to lateral. The lateral and posterior tumor margins displace the uncus of the temporal lobe (Unc) posteriorly, whereas the superior tumor margin lies within the medial anterior portion of the sylvian fissure. The putamen (Pu), globus pallidus (GPe, GPi), anterior limb of the internal capsule (Cpia), external capsule (Cpe), and lateral projection of the anterior commissure (AC) all lie superior to the tumor in the coronal view (**C**). *(Figure continued on following pages.)*

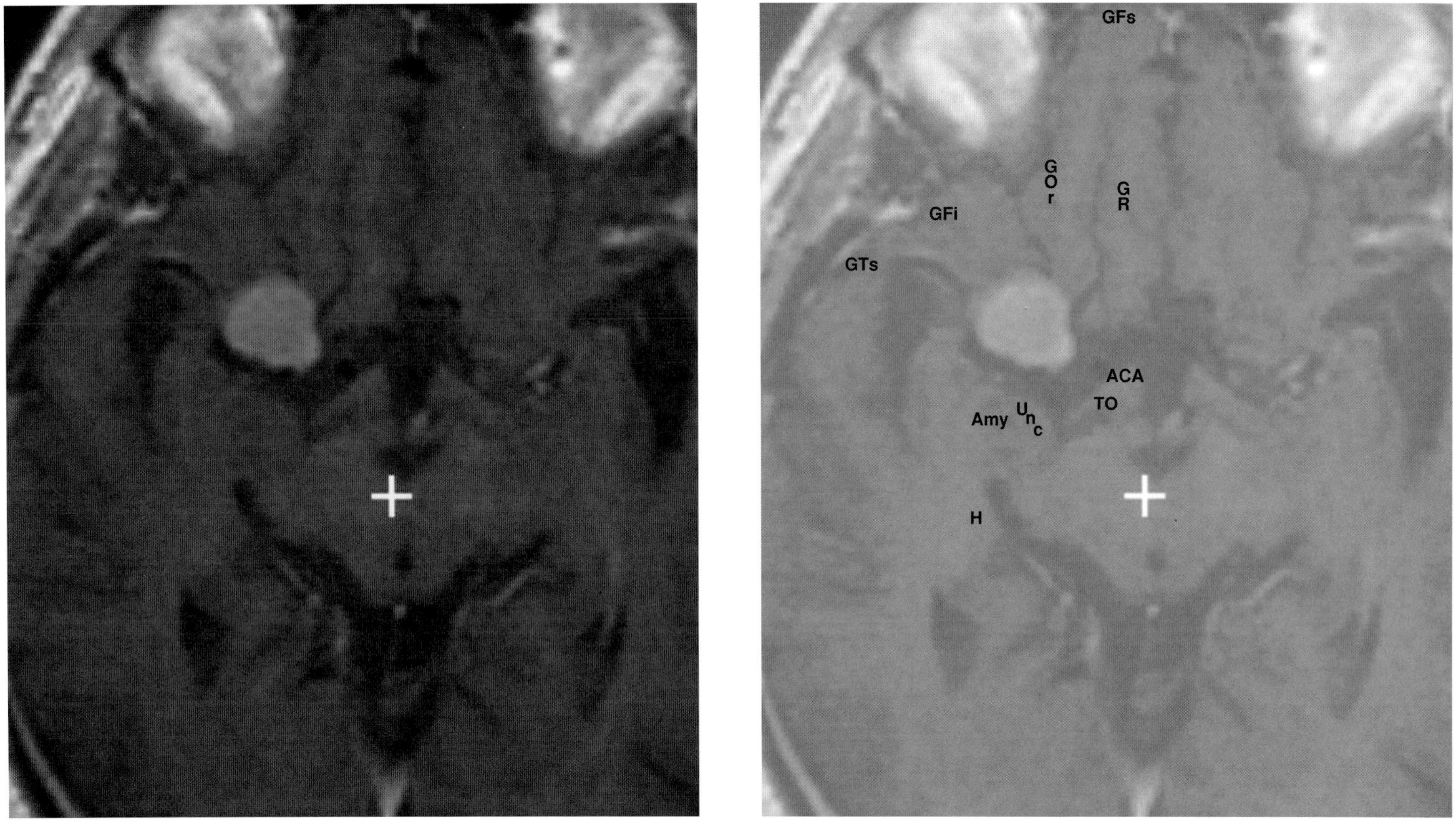

FIG. 2-3B.

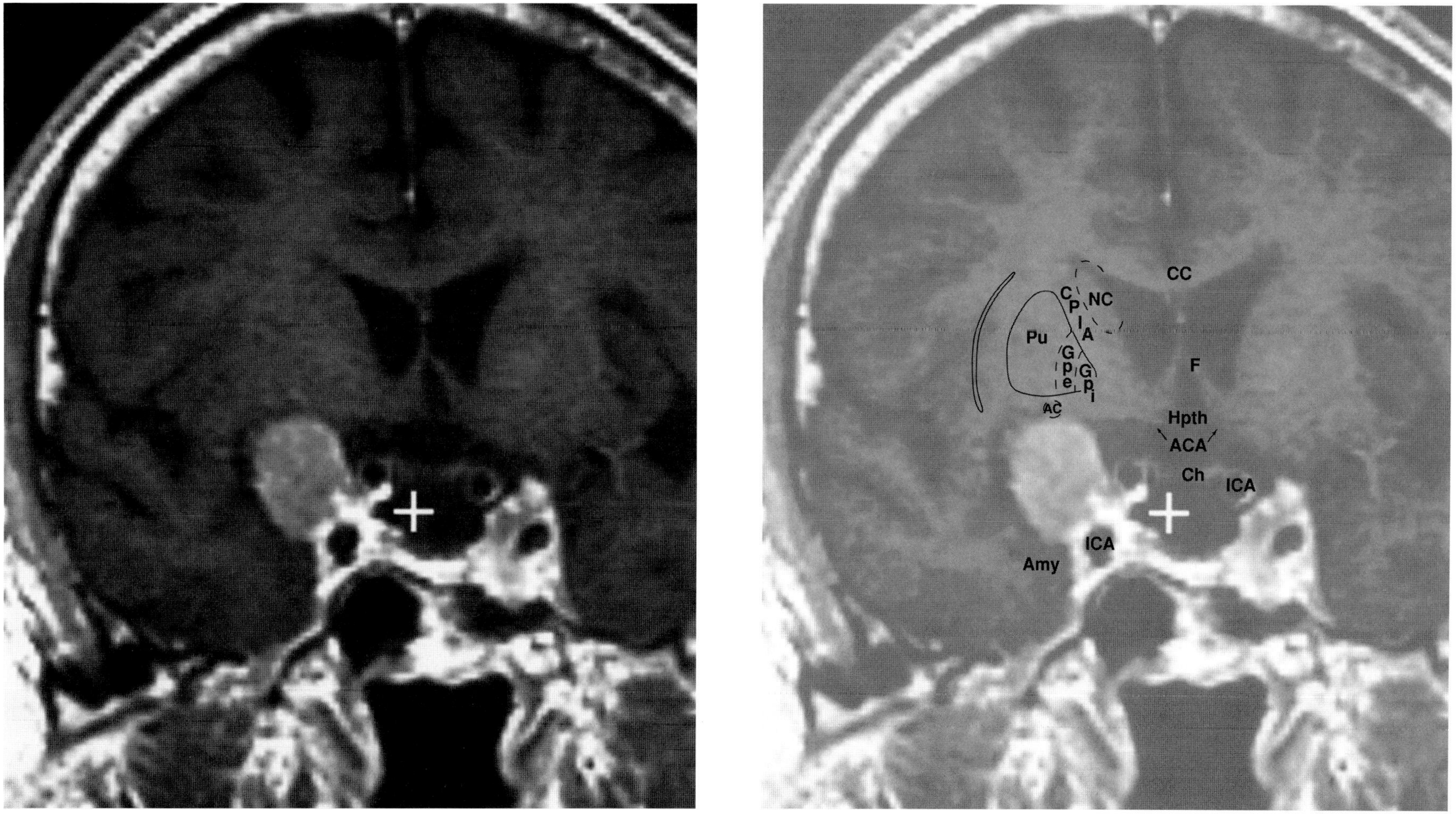

FIG. 2-3C.

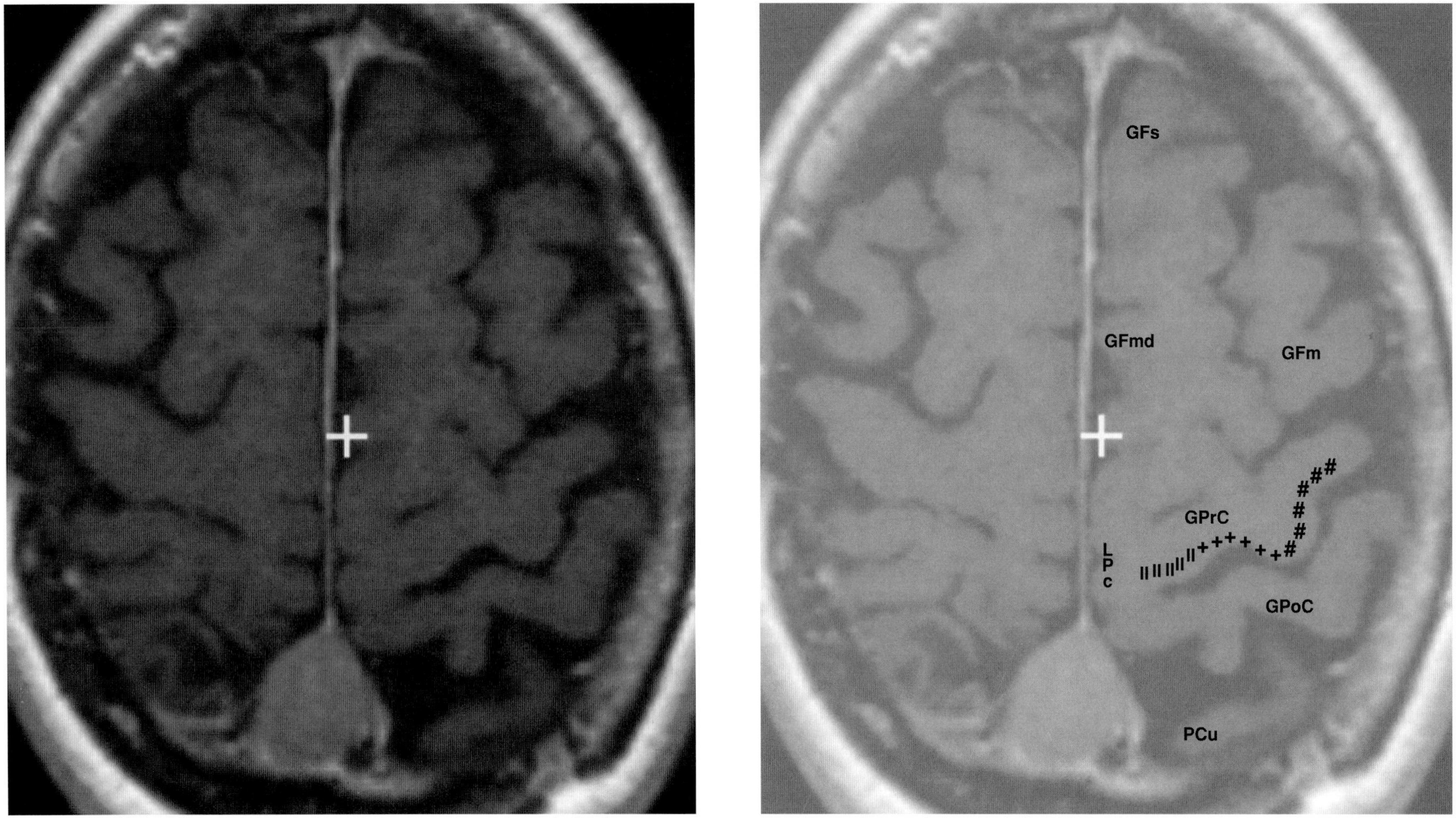

FIG. 2-4A.

FIG. 2-4. Recurrent sagittal sinus and posterior falx meningioma, T_1-weighted, contrast-enhanced stereotactic axial MRIs (**A and B**) separated by 3 mm from inferior to superior, respectively. The tumor fills and expands the superior sagittal sinus (SSS) and nearly occludes the lumen (compare with normal-appearing SSS at the frontal edge of each image). The lateral tumor margin displaces the paracentral lobule (LPc) and precuneus (PCu) away from the falx on each side. Pyramidal neurons of Brodmann's area 4, the primary somatomotor area—in this case, corresponding to the lower extremity and trunk—are closest to the tumor. The portions of area 4 that control the upper extremity, face, and pharynx are located more laterally and farther away from the tumor. (Subdivisions of precentral gyrus: ///, leg and trunk; + + +, upper extremity; ###, face and pharynx.) The corresponding sensory organization of Brodmann's areas 3, 1, and 2 also is present in the postcentral gyrus (GPoC). The enlarged cerebrospinal fluid space between the precuneus and the tumor, especially on the left side, is the result of prior surgery. *(Figure continued on following page.)*

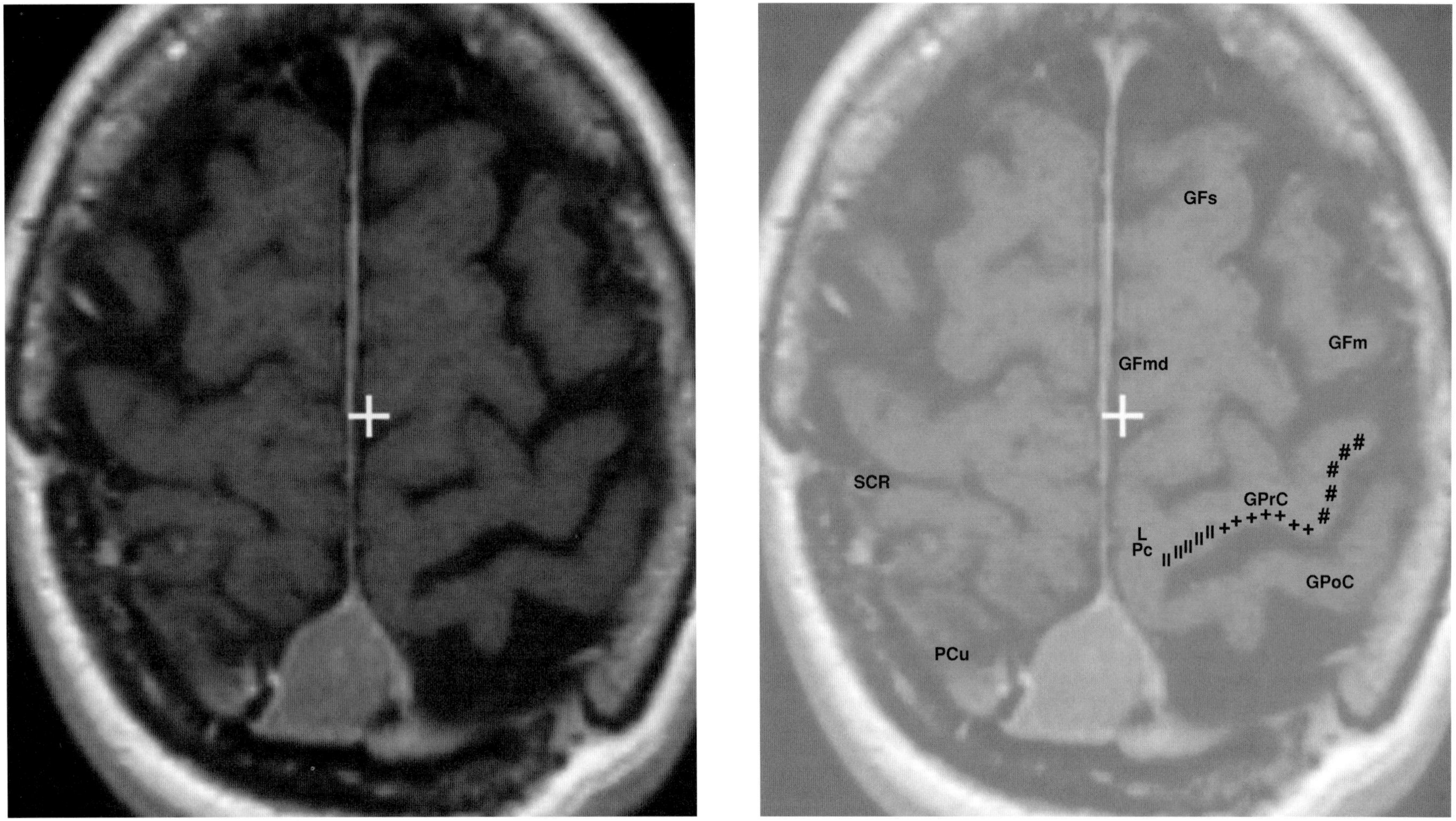

FIG. 2-4B.

FIG. 2-5. Small (approximately 12 mm diameter) tentorial meningioma, T_1-weighted, contrast-enhanced stereotactic axial (**A**) and coronal (**B**) MRIs. The tumor arises from the superior medial edge of the tentorium on the right side. In the axial plane (**A**) at the level of the optic chiasm (Ch) and inferior colliculi (COI), the medial edge of the tumor projects into the ambient cistern (Cam). In both the axial and coronal planes, the temporo-parieto-pontine tract (Ttppo) is illustrated coursing through the caudal mid-brain medial to the center of the tumor. The corticospinal tract (Pyr) runs medial and ventral to the temporo-parieto-pontine tract. The spinothalamic tract (STT), lateral lemniscus (LL), and brachium of the inferior colliculus (BCI) lie adjacent to the dorsomedial tumor margin, separated from the tumor by the narrowed ambient cistern. Fibers of the trochlear nerve (CN IV) run through the tectum of the rhombencephalon near the mid-line to exit the brain stem and course through the ambient cistern medial to the tumor.

The lateral and superior tumor margins indent and displace the hippocampal gyrus (GH), hippocampal formation (H), and adjacent cingulate bundle (Ci). The termination of the optic tract (TO) within the lateral geniculate body (CGI) lies medial to the choroid fissure, 5 mm superior to the tumor margin. *(Figure continued on following pages.)*

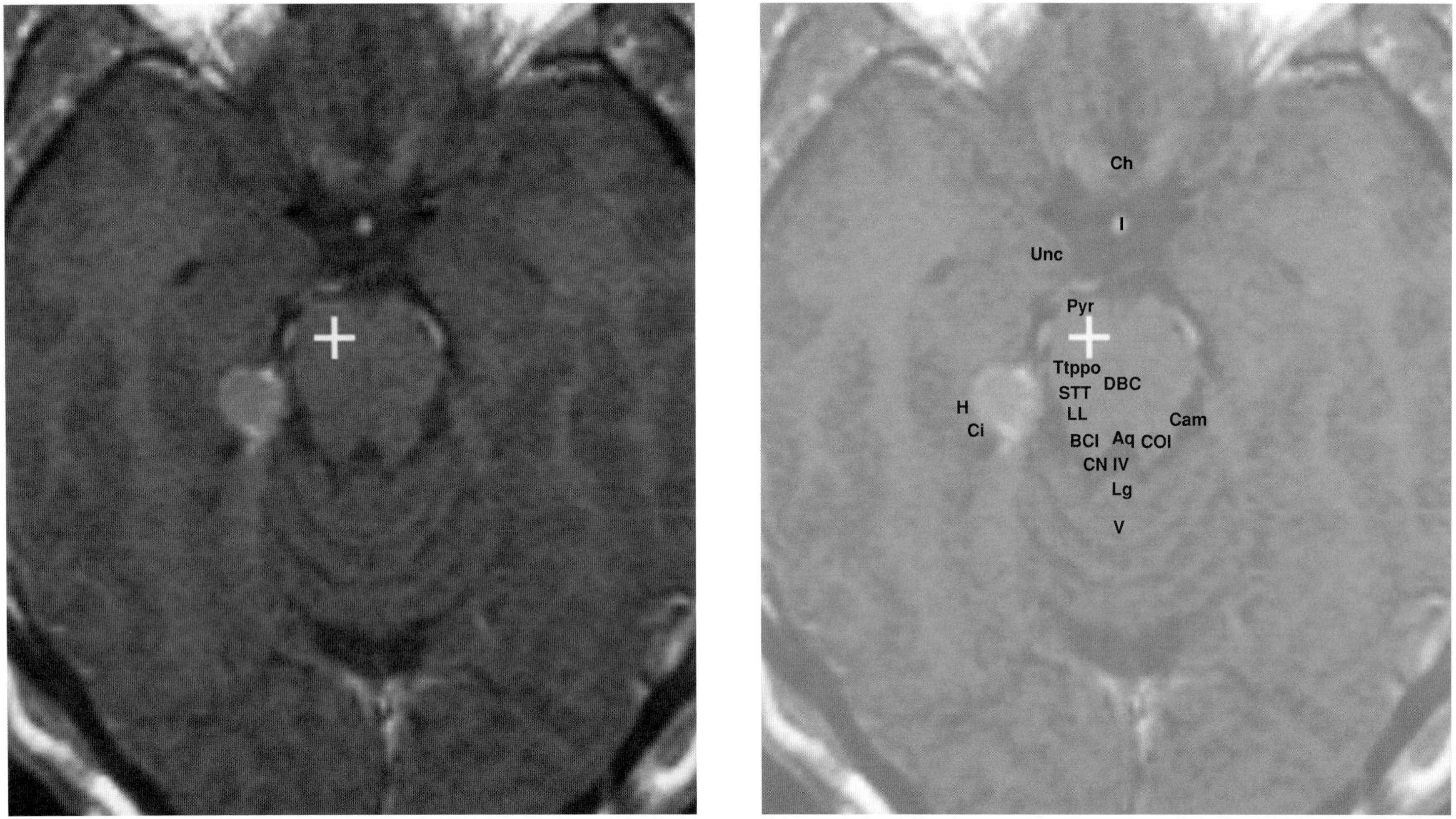

FIG. 2-5A.

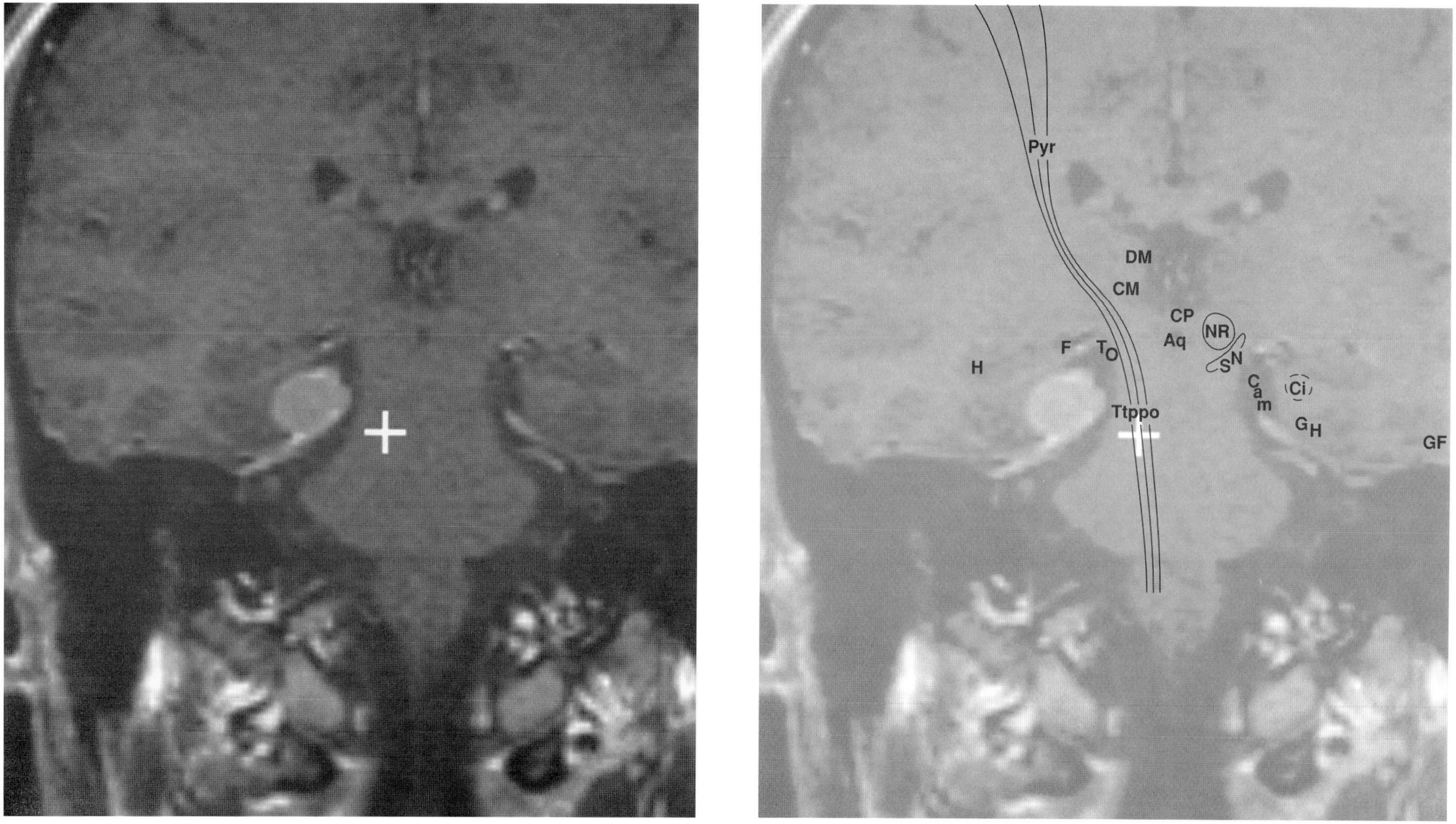

FIG. 2-5B.

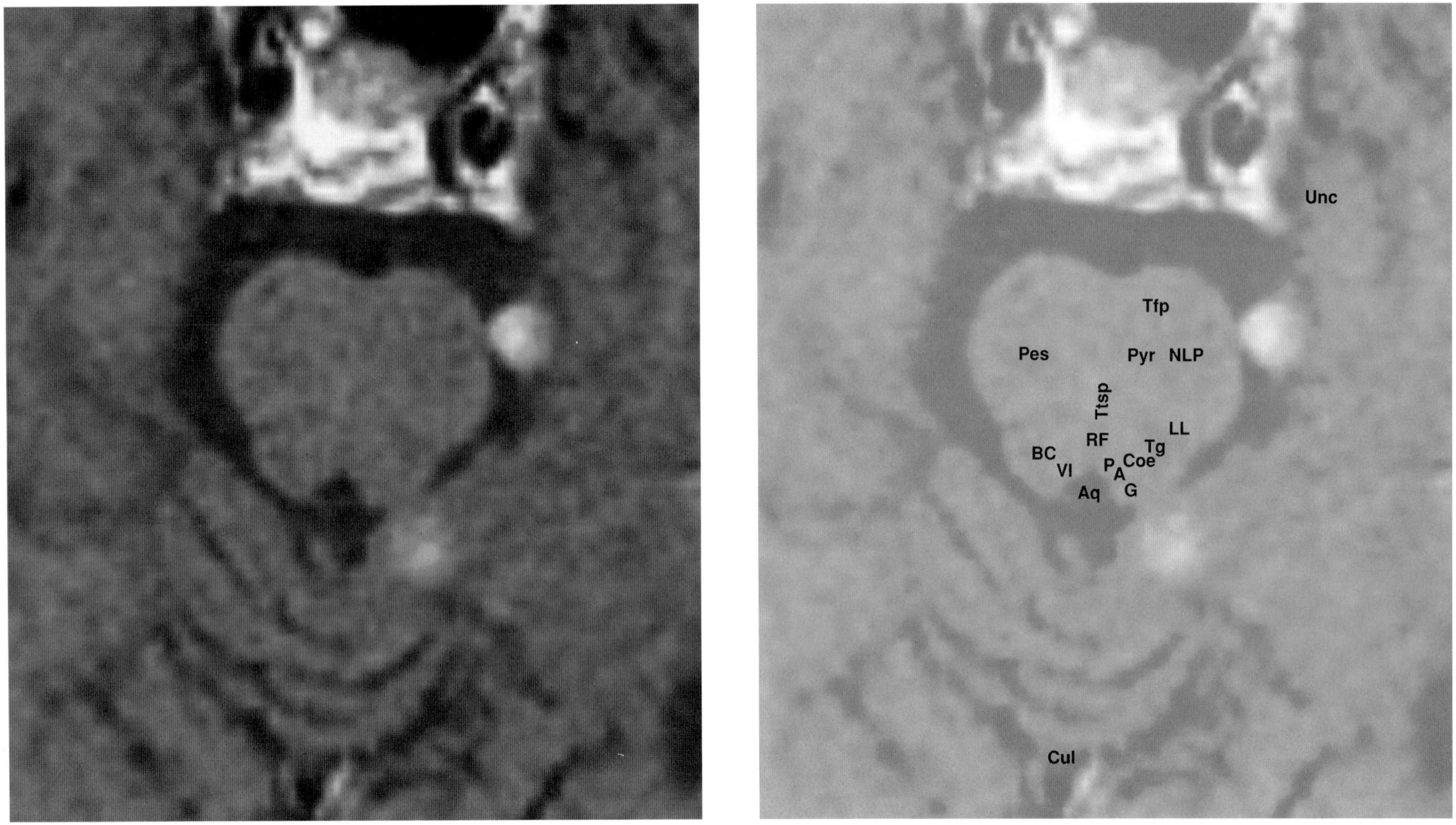

FIG. 2-6.

FIG. 2-6. Hemangiopericytoma of the meninges, T_1-weighted contrast-enhanced stereotactic axial image. The faintly-seen tumor that involves the anterior cerebellar vermis and dorsal tentorial incisura is illustrated in more detail in Fig. 2-7A and B. This tumor is attached to the medial edge of the tentorium on the left side. The lateral margin of the tumor indents the inferomedial surface of the temporal lobe just behind (dorsal to) the uncus (Unc) at its junction with the hippocampal gyrus. On its medial margin, the tumor touches the ventrolateral surface of the rostral pons (pes pontis) several millimeters above the level of the trigeminal sensory root (CN V). Neural structures and pathways at the tumor–pons interface include the fronto-pontine tract (Tfp) and the nucleus lateralis pontis (NLP).

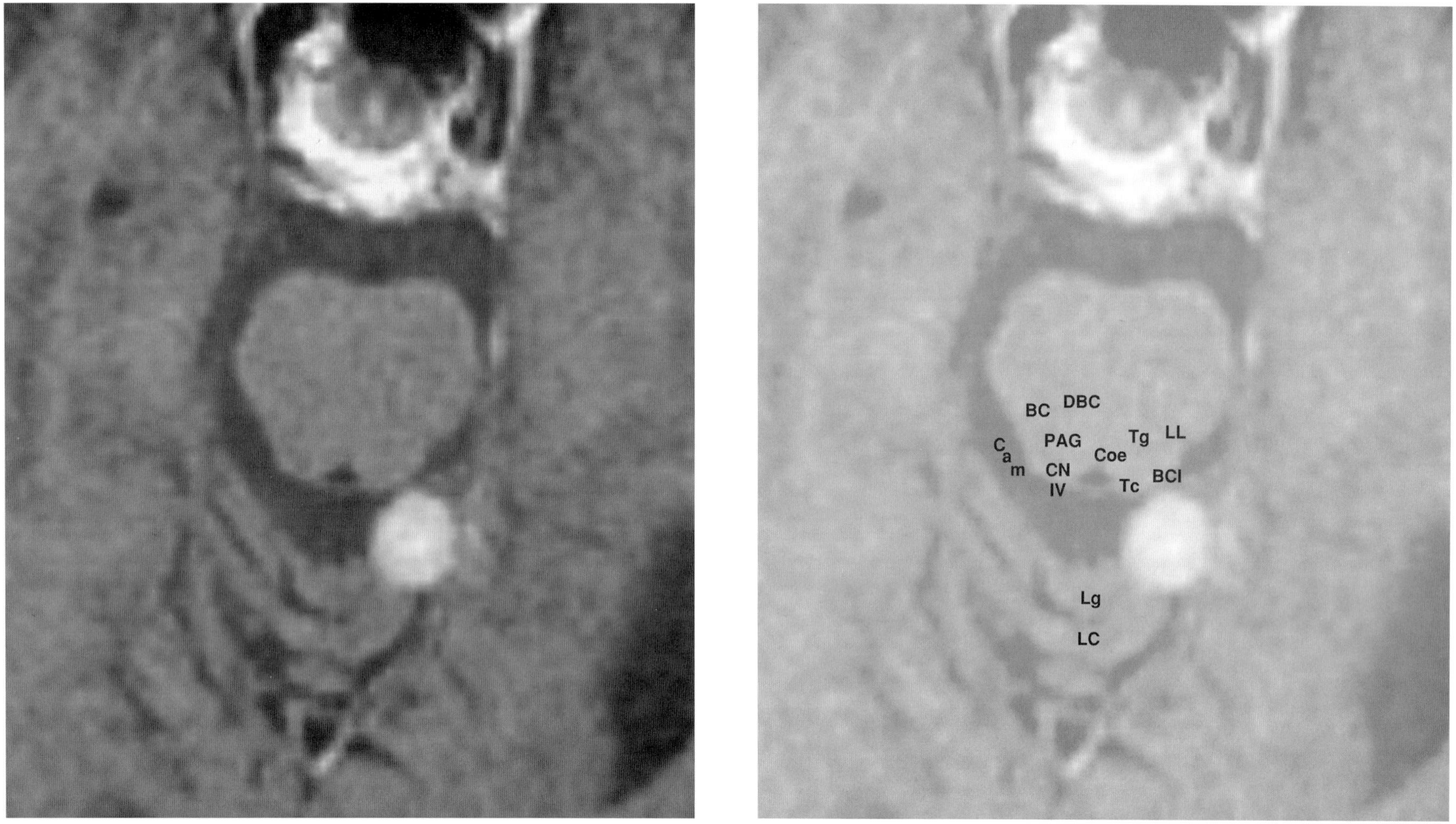

FIG. 2-7A.

FIG. 2-7. Same patient and T_1-weighted, contrast-enhanced stereotactic MRI series as shown in Fig. 2-6. Figs. 2-6 and 2-7A and B are each separated by 3 mm in the inferior-to-superior direction. **A:** The caudal/posterior edge of the more posterior meningeal hemangiopericytoma indents and displaces the anterolateral corner of the superior cerebellar vermis (lobulus centralis [LC]), whereas the lateral edge of the tumor touches the left hippocampal gyrus (GH) 24 mm behind the more anterior tumor illustrated in Fig. 2-6. **B** demonstrates the dural attachment of the tumor to the free edge of the tentorium. In both images, a narrow cerebrospinal fluid space, the cisterna ambiens (Cam), remains between the anterior edge of the tumor and the dorsal midbrain (**B**) and pontomesencephalic junction (**A**).

Important structures within the portion of the dorsal brain stem closest to the tumor illustrated here include (from medial to lateral): crossing filaments of the root of CN IV, locus coeruleus (Coe, ventral to the aqueduct of sylvius and filaments of CN IV), roof of the rhombencephalon (Tc), brachium of the inferior colliculus (BCI), and lateral lemniscus (LL). *(Figure continued on following page.)*

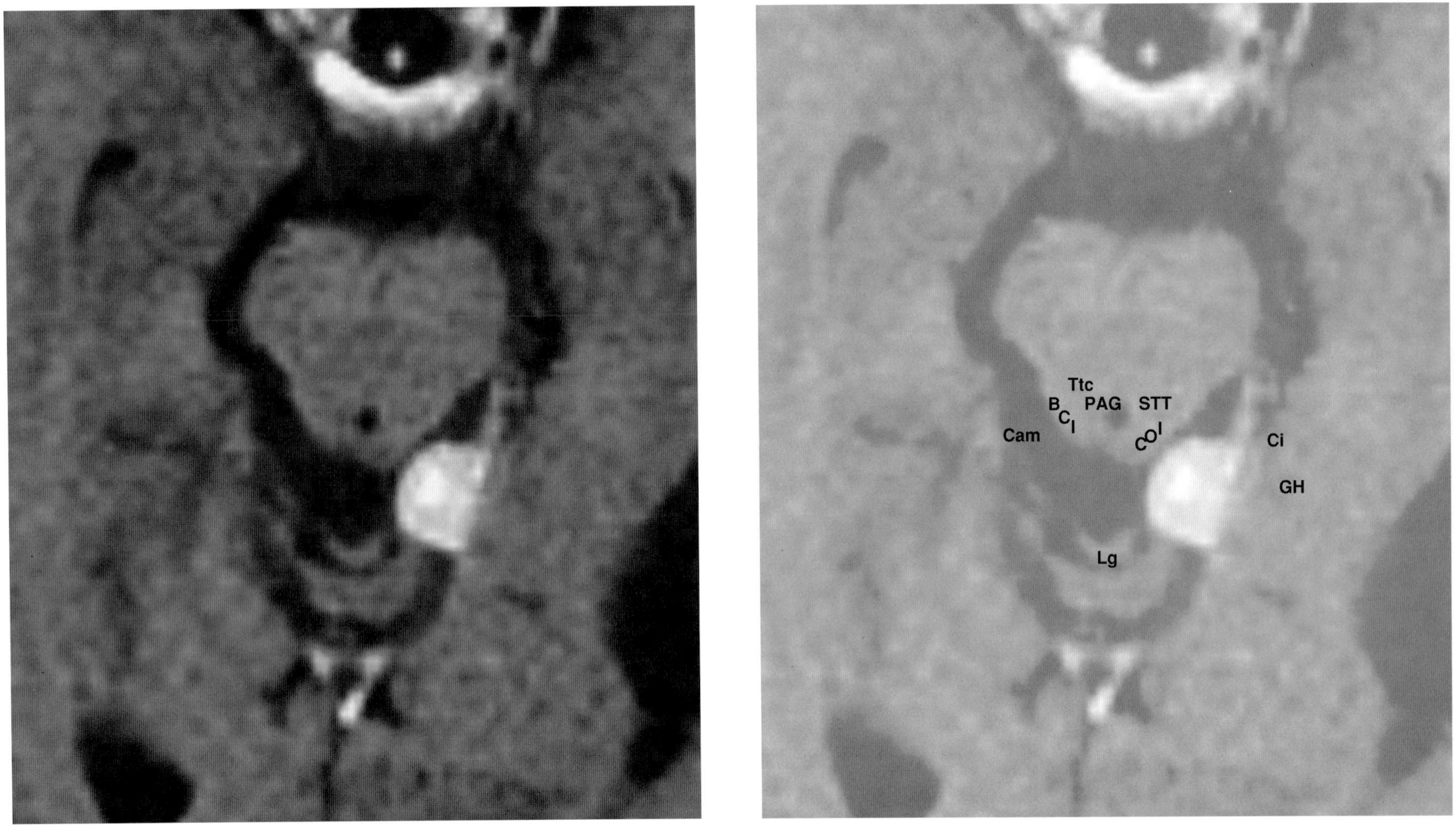

FIG. 2-7B.

FIG. 2-8. Recurrent meningioma arising from the confluence of the falx and tentorium, axial (**A**) and coronal (**B**) stereotactic T_1-weighted, contrast-enhanced images. The cursor represents the center of the stereotactic frame in each imaging plane. Line Y in **A** denotes the plane of section of the coronal image (**B**). Line Z in **B** denotes the axial level of **A**.

The posterior margin of the tumor closest to the mid-line is partly surrounded by cerebrospinal fluid of the pineal cistern. Farther laterally, the tumor abuts the body of the fornix (F). The most posterior portion of the hippocampal formations and hippocampal gyri (GH) lie more posterolaterally, away from the tumor margin. The anterior edge of the tumor enters the posterior third ventricle (IIIv) in the mid-line at the level of the habenular commissure (CmHb), where the pulvinar of the thalamus lies on either side.

In the coronal plane (**B**), the superior tumor margin indents the undersurface of the splenium of the corpus callosum (SPL). The fornices lie along the lateral tumor margin on each side, between the tumor and the atria of the lateral ventricles (LV). Inferolaterally, the most caudal and inferior portion of cingulum (Ci) courses through the plane of section between the tumor margin and the hippocampal gyrus and lateral ventricle. Note that the optic radiation (RO) and the tail of the caudate nucleus are on the lateral side of the ventricle, remote from the tumor.

The inferior tumor margin touches the dorsal mid-brain (tectum) at the level of the superior colliculi (COS) and the tectal commissure (CT) (in the mid-line). The anatomical relationships in this case suggest that injury to structures in the immediate vicinity of the tumor would more likely lead to deficits of higher cortical function (interhemispheric information transfer, memory) and/or extraocular movements than to a visual field deficit per se. *(Figure continued on following pages.)*

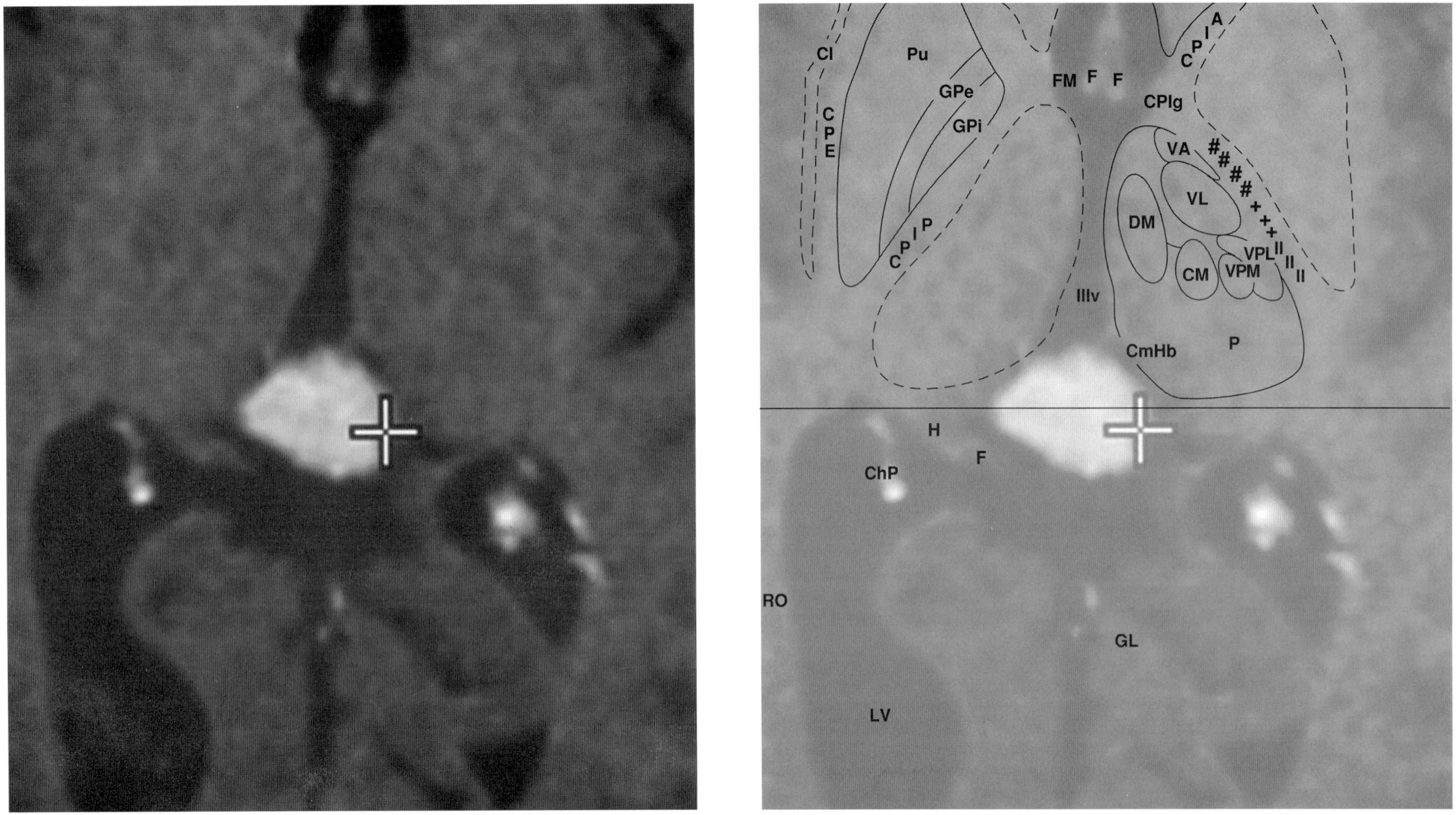
Cl
Pu
C
P
E
GPe
GPi
C
P
I
P
FM
F
F
C
P
I
A
CPlg
VA
VL
DM
CM
VPL
VPM
IIIv
CmHb
P
Y
H
F
ChP
RO
GL
LV

FIG. 2-8A.

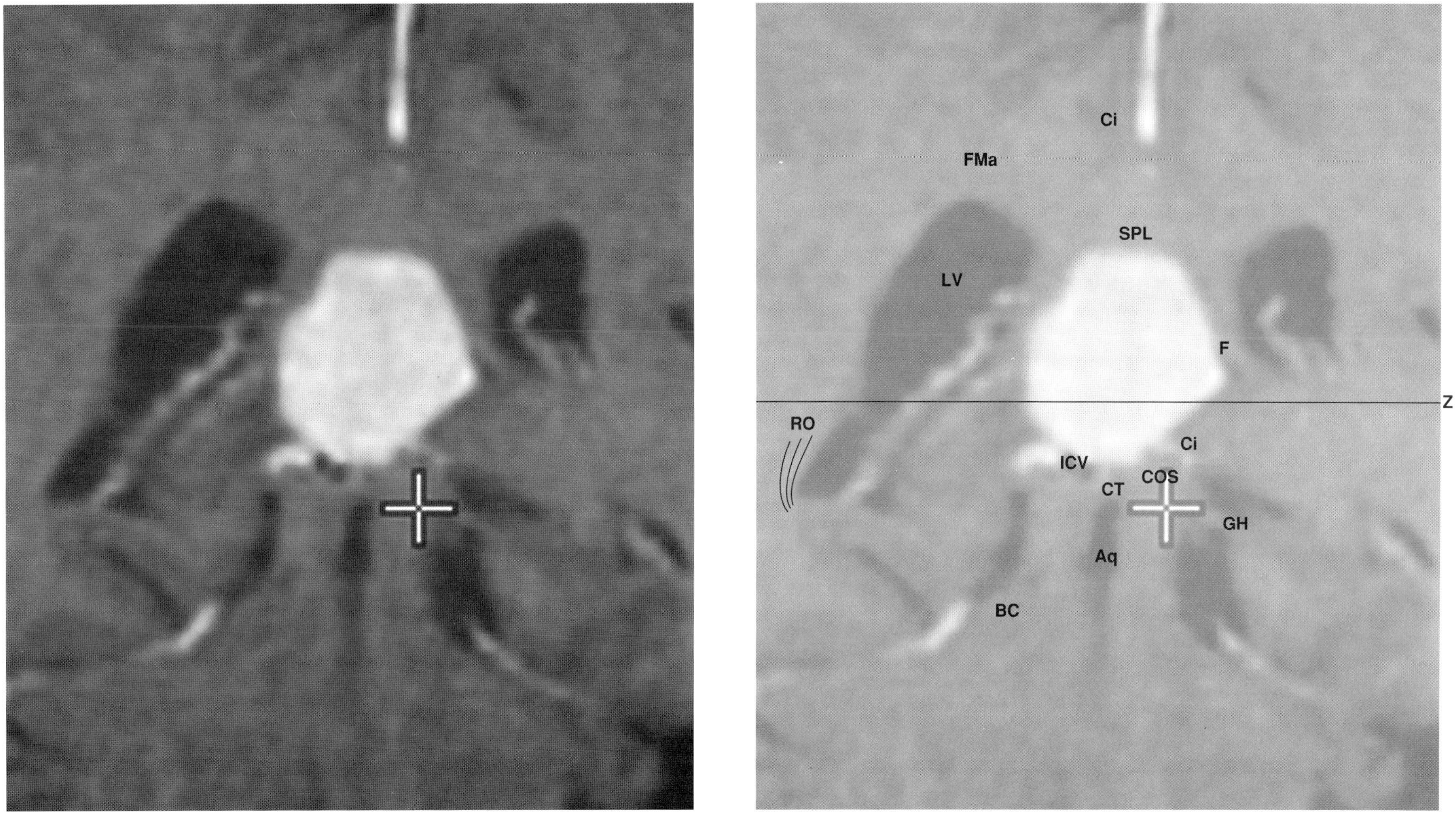

FIG. 2-8B.

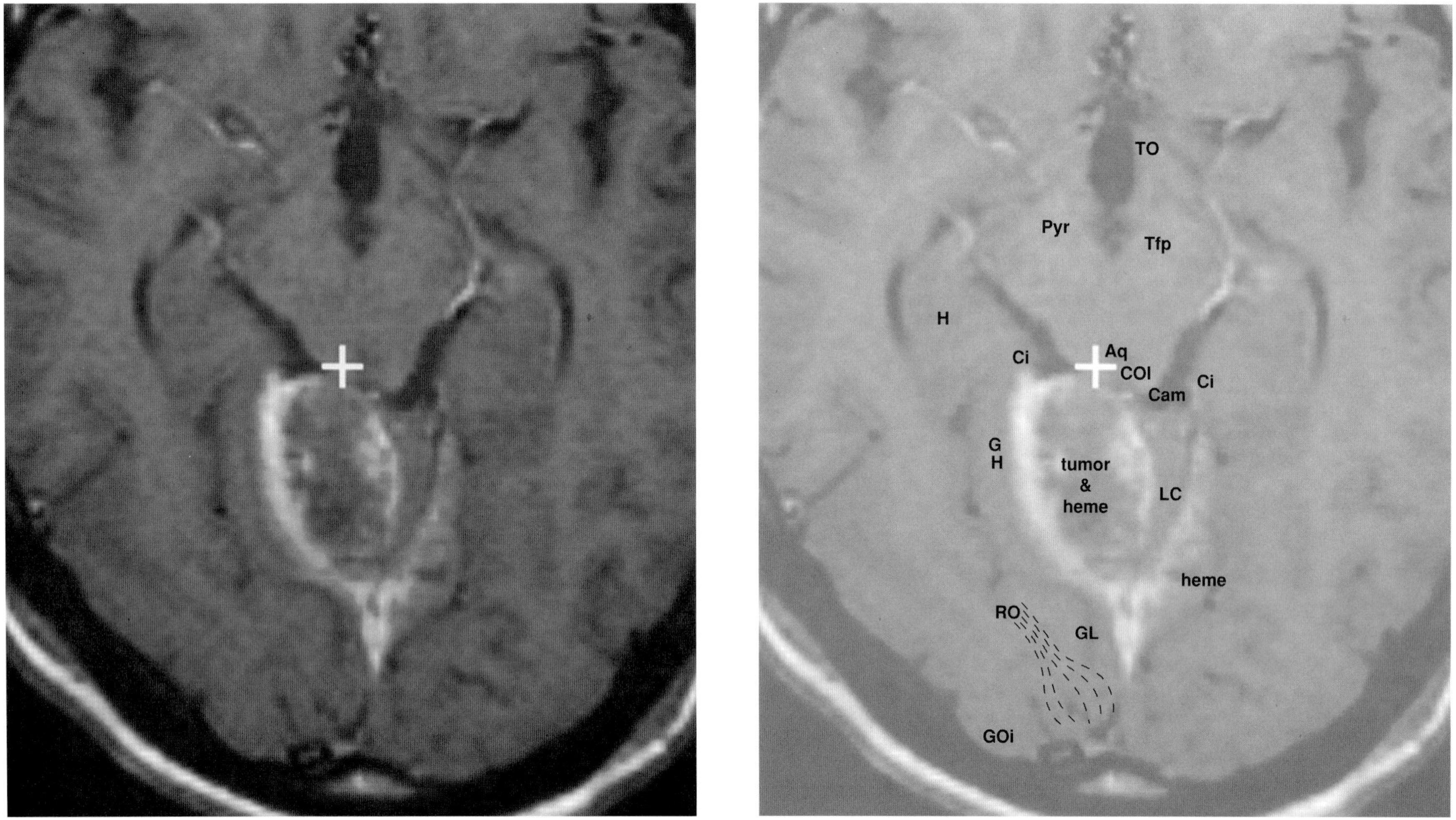

FIG. 2-9A.

FIG. 2-9. Meningeal hemangiopericytoma with subacute intratumoral hemorrhage involving the confluence of the falx and tentorium, right tentorial leaf, and pineal region; T_1-weighted, contrast-enhanced stereotactic axial MRIs separated by 12 mm from inferior to superior. **A:** The inferior margin of the hemorrhagic tumor occupies the right-hand side of the incisural notch. The central lobule (LC) of the cerebellar vermis is compressed by the medial edge of the tumor and displaced from right to left. A second, smaller focus of hemorrhage (and possibly tumor) is layered upon the left tentorial leaf. The lateral tumor margin displaces the medial edge of the hippocampal gyrus (GH) laterally, whereas the anterolateral tumor edge just touches the cingulate bundle (Ci). The anterior and anteromedial tumor edges cross the right-hand side of the ambient cistern (Cam) to compress the mid-brain tectum and displace it anteriorly at the level of the inferior colliculus (COI). The crosshair cursor, indicating the center of the stereotactic frame, overlies a portion of the right inferior colliculus and its brachium. The lateral lemniscus courses just lateral to the crosshair. The posterior tumor margin abuts the lingual gyrus (GL) just medial and anterior to the inferior edge of the optic radiation (RO).

B: Twelve millimeters superior to **A**, the heart-shaped tumor mass displaces the hippocampal and lingual gyri (GH and GL) of each hemisphere away from the falx and each other. At this axial level, the posteriorly pointing apex of the tumor lies 25 mm anterior to the optic radiations and calcarine sulcus (SCa). The cleft of the heart-shaped tumor mass, which forms its anterior border in the mid-line, abuts the junction of the internal cerebral veins (ICV) with the vein of Galen. The anterolateral tumor margin on the right side nearly reaches the cingulate bundle (Ci) as it crosses the plane of section in association with the hippocampal gyrus. The pulvinar thalami (P), fornices (F), and posterior limb of the internal capsule (CPIP) on either side all lie well anterior to the tumor.

The neurologic functions at greatest risk after radiosurgical treatment of this tumor include vision (optic radiations, visual cortex), memory (hippocampal gyri), binaural hearing and ocular reflexes (dorsal mid-brain), and postural stability (superior vermis). *(Figure continued on following page.)*

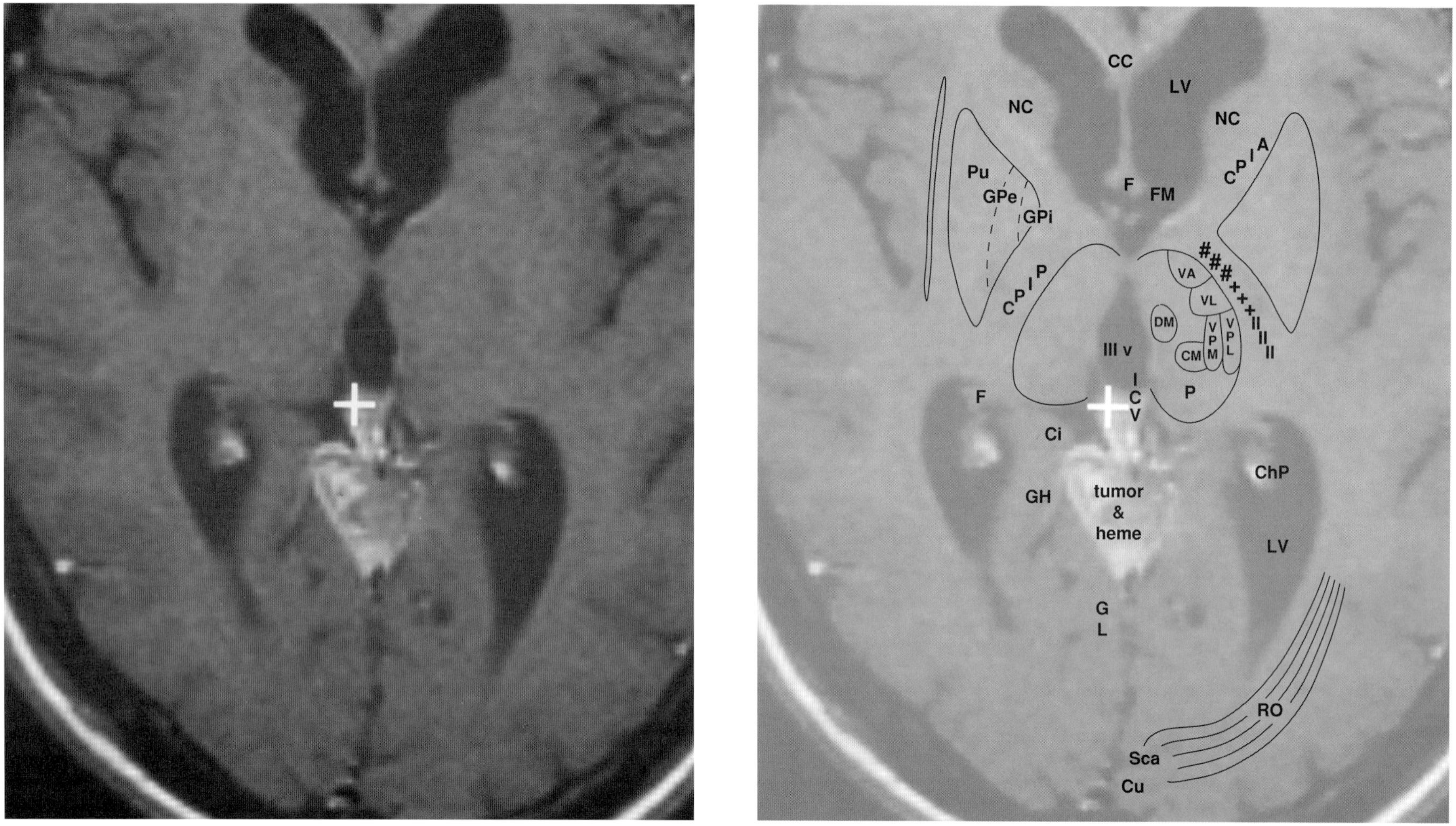
CC
LV
NC
NC
Pu
GPe
GPi
F
FM
C P I A
C P I P
VA
VL
DM
V P M
V P L
CM
III v
I C V
P
F
Ci
ChP
GH
tumor
&
heme
LV
G
L
RO
Sca
Cu

FIG. 2-9B.

FIG. 2-10. Meningioma within the left cavernous sinus, sella, suprasellar space, and medial sylvian fissure (medial sphenoid wing), T_1-weighted, contrast-enhanced stereotactic coronal MRI at the level of the optic chiasm (Ch) and infundibular stalk (Inf). The tumor fills and expands the left cavernous sinus, encases the cavernous portion of the internal carotid artery (ICA), and partially surrounds the supraclinoid carotid artery (just dorsal to the crosshair cursor that marks the stereotactic frame center in the X and Z axes). The lateral tumor margin flattens the normally convex medial margin of the temporal lobe near the most anterior extent of the amygdala (Amy). The superolateral tumor margin occupies and elevates the medial sylvian fissure (Syl) and anterior perforated substance. Fibers of the anterior commissure (AC) traverse the stem of the temporal lobe dorsal and lateral to the tumor. Medial to the carotid artery, the inferior portion of the tumor erodes into the sella and displaces the pituitary gland and stalk toward the right. The superomedial margin of the tumor almost touches the inferolateral edge of the optic chiasm. Radiosurgical treatment of this portion of the tumor would place the adjacent edge of the chiasm at risk because the radiation dose delivered to the tumor, for all practical purposes, also would be delivered to the optic apparatus at this point. *(Figure continued on following page.)*

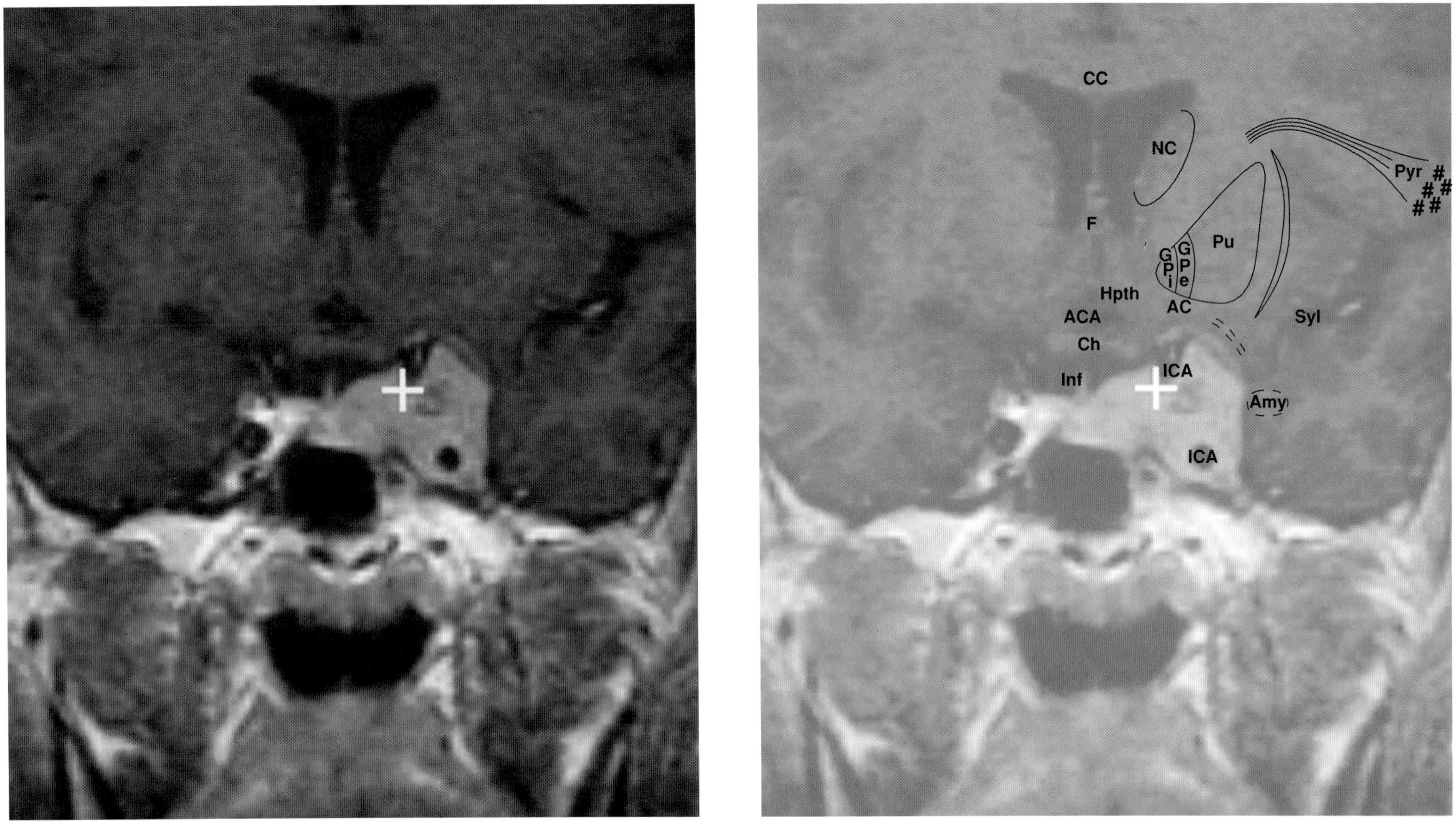

FIG. 2-10.

FIG. 2-11. Left trigeminal nerve schwannoma, recurrent after previous surgical resection. T_1-weighted, contrast-enhanced stereotactic axial MRIs separated by 3 mm from inferior to superior (**A and B**), and a stereotactic coronal MRI through the center of the tumor (**C**). Lines Z_1 and Z_2 in **C** represent the axial planes in **A** and **B**. Line Y in **A** and **B** represent the coronal plane in **C**. The tumor has an anterior component within Meckel's cave (Cav), posterolateral to the vertical segment of the internal carotid artery (ICA) within the posterior cavernous sinus (**A**). An isthmus of tumor extends through the porus trigeminus and crosses the line of insertion of the tentorium to join the larger tumor mass within the left cerebellopontine angle seen in all three figures. The cisternal segment of the right trigeminal nerve (CN V) is seen within the subarachnoid space in **B** and **C**, whereas the left nerve has been replaced completely by the tumor. Although the lateral tumor margin appears to be pressed against the parahippocampal gyrus, the tentorial edge lies between them.

Both the anterior and posterior poles of the tumor lie free within the subarachnoid space. However, in **A**, the left abducens nerve appears to traverse the prepontine cistern just anterior to the tumor (partially obscured by crosshair cursor). The medial tumor margin abuts the lateral pontine surface and indents it slightly. The brachium pontis (BP, middle cerebellar peduncle) crosses the tumor margin, beneath which lies the nucleus lateralis pontis (NLP). The pyramidal and frontopontine tracts (Pyr, Tfp) run anteromedial to the tumor, deeper within the pons. Other nuclei and tracts also lie deeper within the brain stem, away from the tumor margins. A small artery, probably the superior cerebellar artery (SCA), is trapped between the tumor and brain stem in **B** and **C**. Some of the structures potentially at risk of injury during surgery or radiosurgery of this tumor include the superior cerebellar artery, the middle cerebellar peduncle, the petrous or cavernous segments of the internal carotid artery, the left parahippocampal gyrus and underlying hippocampal formation, and the medial and lateral geniculate bodies with their corresponding auditory and optic radiations. *(Figure continued on following pages.)*

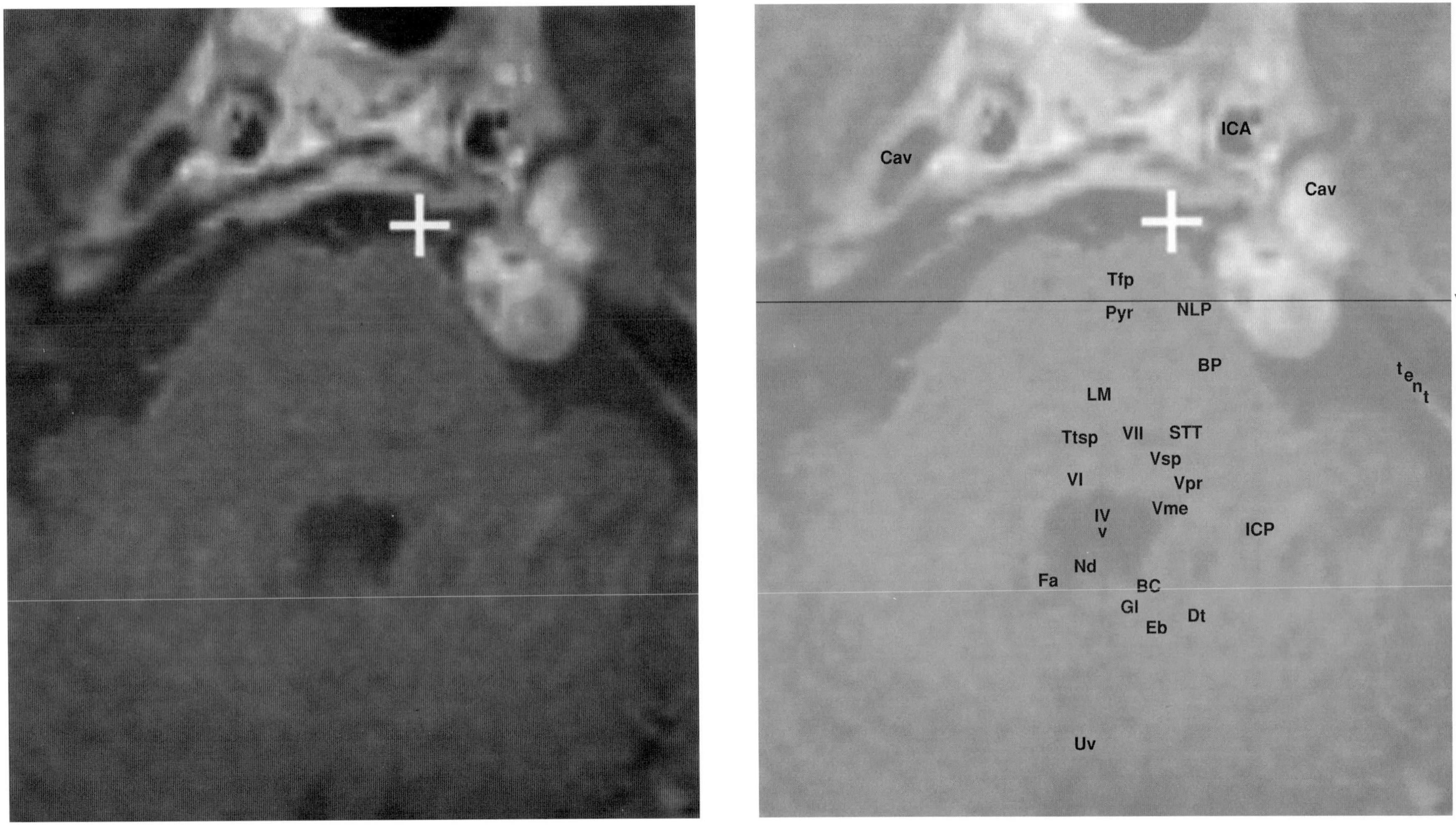
ICA
Cav
Cav
Tfp
Y
Pyr
NLP
BP
tent
LM
Ttsp
VII
STT
Vsp
VI
Vpr
IV
Vme
V
ICP
Nd
Fa
BC
Gl
Dt
Eb
Uv

FIG. 2-11A.

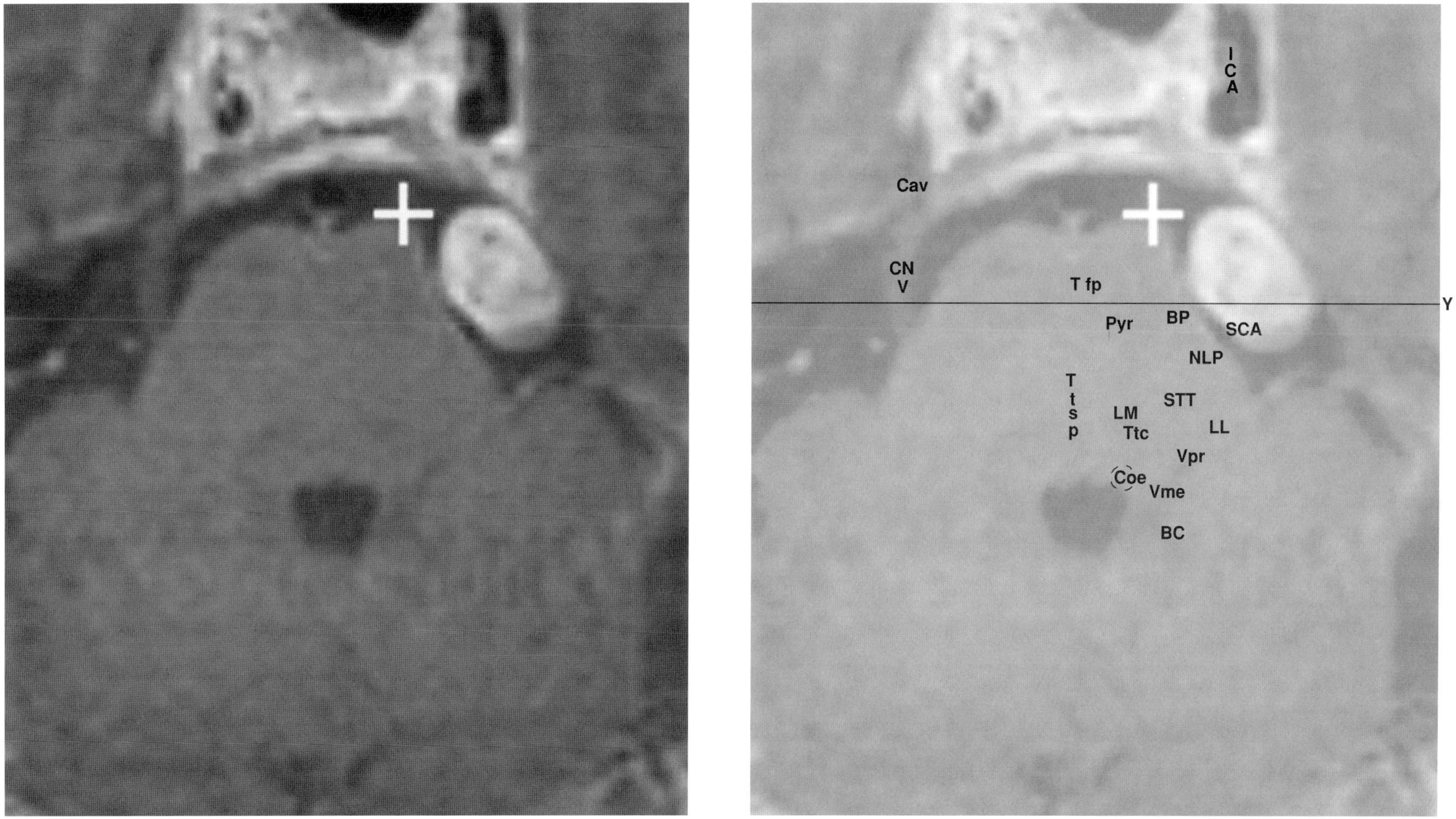

FIG. 2-11B.

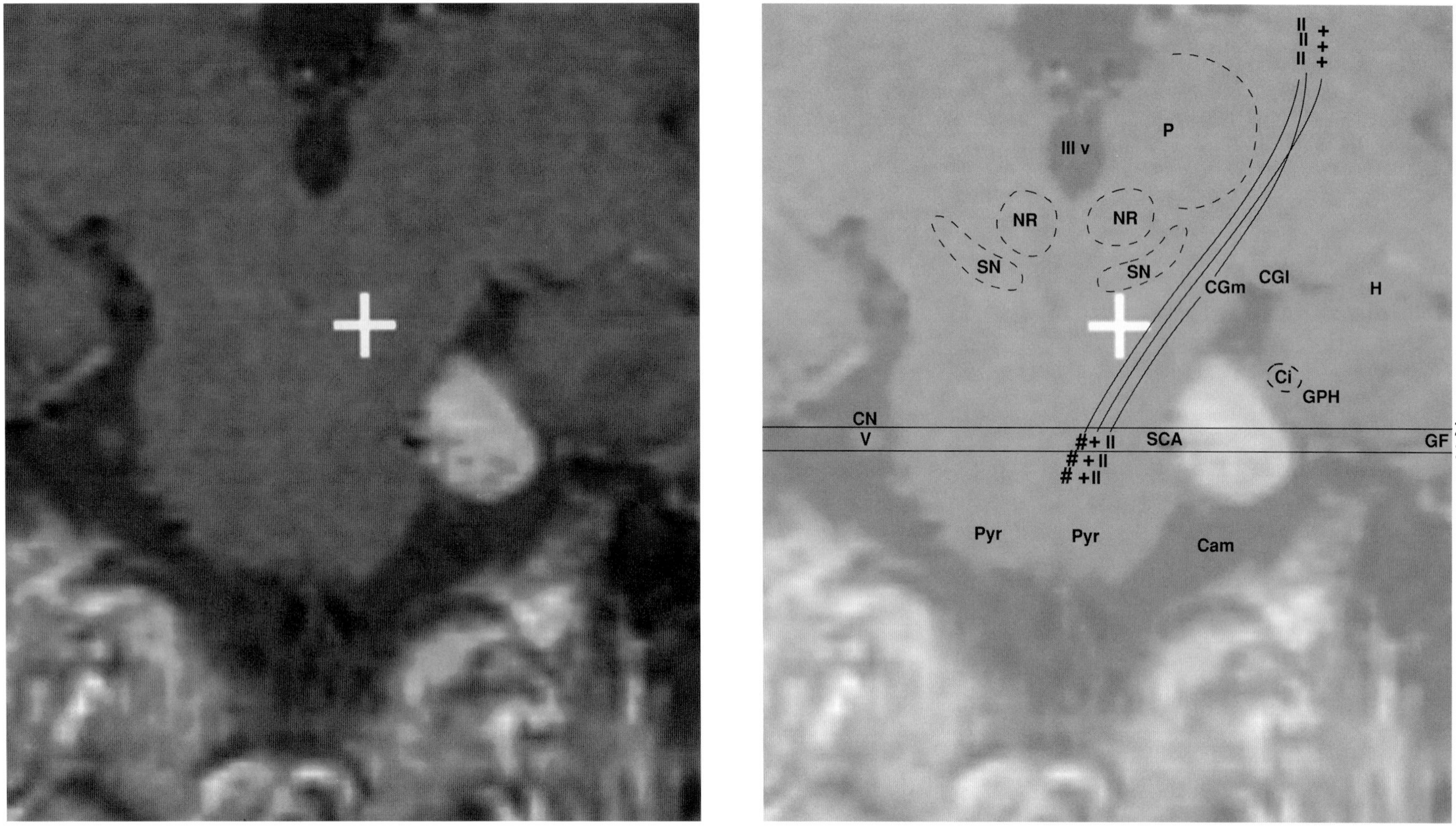

II +
II +
II +
P
III v
NR
NR
SN
SN
CGm
CGl
H
Ci
GPH
CN
V
+ II
+ II
+ II
SCA
Z2
GF
Z1
Pyr
Pyr
Cam

FIG. 2-11C.

FIG. 2-12. Acoustic neuroma, T_1-weighted, contrast-enhanced stereotactic axial MRIs (**A and B**) separated by 6 mm from inferior to superior at the level of the porus acousticus (internal auditory canal) and sensory root of the trigeminal nerve (CN V), respectively. **A:** The tumor widens the porus acousticus, where the fibers of the facial nerve (CN VII) usually are located in the anterior-superior quadrant. The posterior half of the tumor mass has separated the flocculus (Fl) of the cerebellum from the middle cerebellar peduncle (BP, brachium pontis) and pons within the cerebellopontine angle. More importantly, the entire medial surface of the tumor is in contact with the lateral pons and has compressed and displaced the more peripherally located neural structures and pathways toward the mid-line. Along the medial tumor margin, from ventral to dorsal one finds the nucleus lateralis pontis (NLP), the (descending) spinal trigeminal tract (Vst), the ventral cochlear nucleus (VIIIcv), the principal (sensory) trigeminal nucleus (Vpr), and the fibers of the brachium pontis. The next more medial tier of structures, 3 to 6 mm from the tumor–pons interface, includes the fibers of the corticospinal (Pyr, pyramidal) tract, tectospinal tract (Ttsp), dorsal cochlear decussation (DCD), medial longitudinal fasciculus (MLF), vestibular nuclei (VIIIv), and dorsal cochlear nucleus (VIIIcd). Many of these anatomical relationships continue in **B** (6 mm cephalad to **A**). Here, the cisternal portion of CN V appears at the ventral tumor–pons interface. The trigeminal mesencephalic nucleus (Vme) lies 5 mm deep to the tumor, next to the locus coeruleus (Coe), and just lateral and ventral to the displaced floor of the fourth ventricle (IVv). The foregoing anatomical relationships might help to explain the occurrence of unexpected cranial nerve deficits after radiosurgery or microsurgery for acoustic neuroma in the setting of preserved anatomical continuity of the nerves themselves (V, VII, VIII cochlear or inferior vestibular). Subtle mechanical, vascular, or radiation injury to cranial nerve nuclei or tracts within the pons (already compromised by chronic pressure effects) might be more likely to cause a clinically detectable deficit than would a similar insult to the cisternal portion of the individual nerves themselves. *(Figure continued on following pages.)*

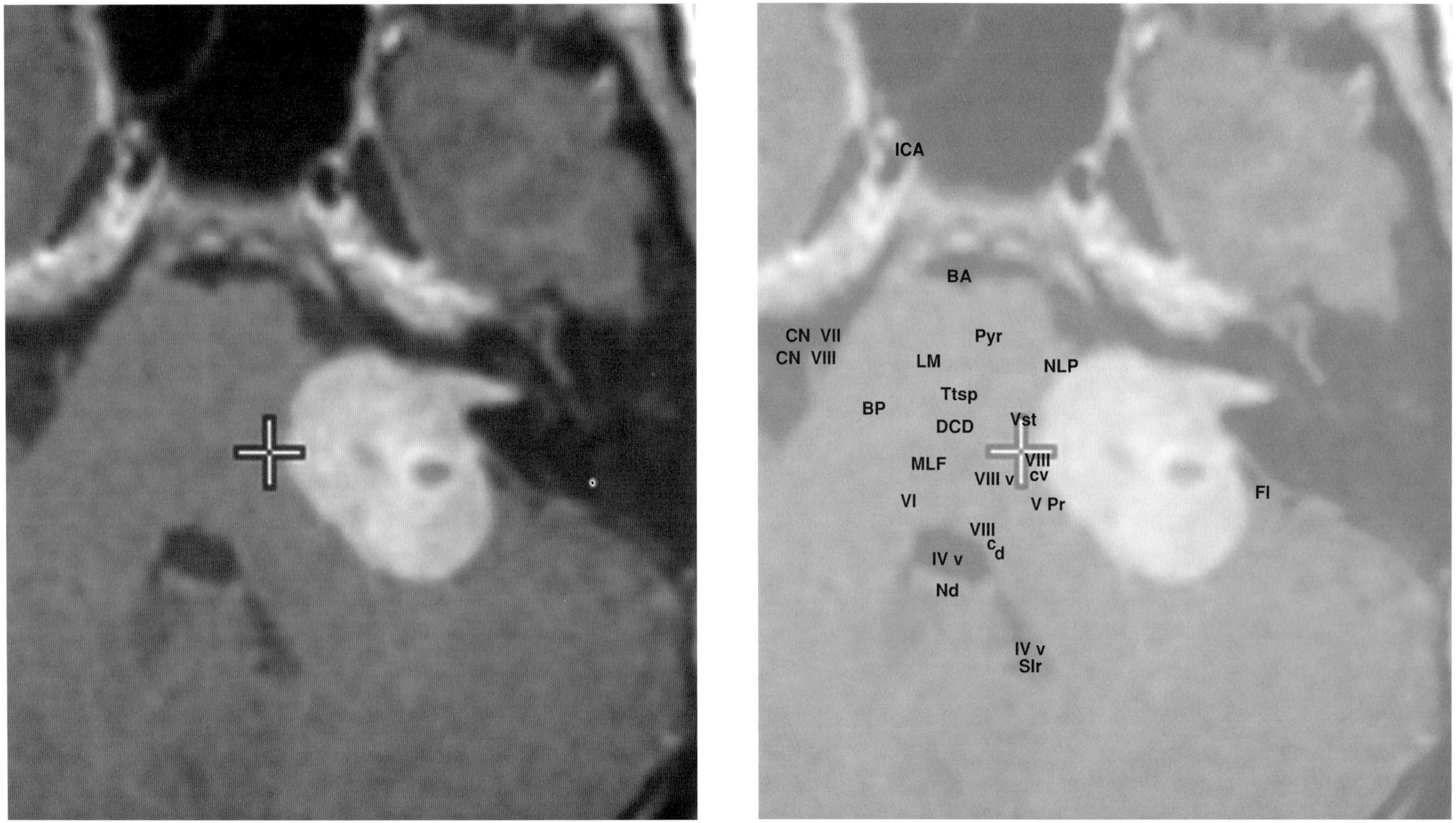
ICA
BA
CN VII
CN VIII
Pyr
LM
NLP
Ttsp
BP
Vst
DCD
MLF
VIII
VIII v
cv
VI
V Pr
Fl
VIII
c
d
IV v
Nd
IV v
Slr

FIG. 2-12A.

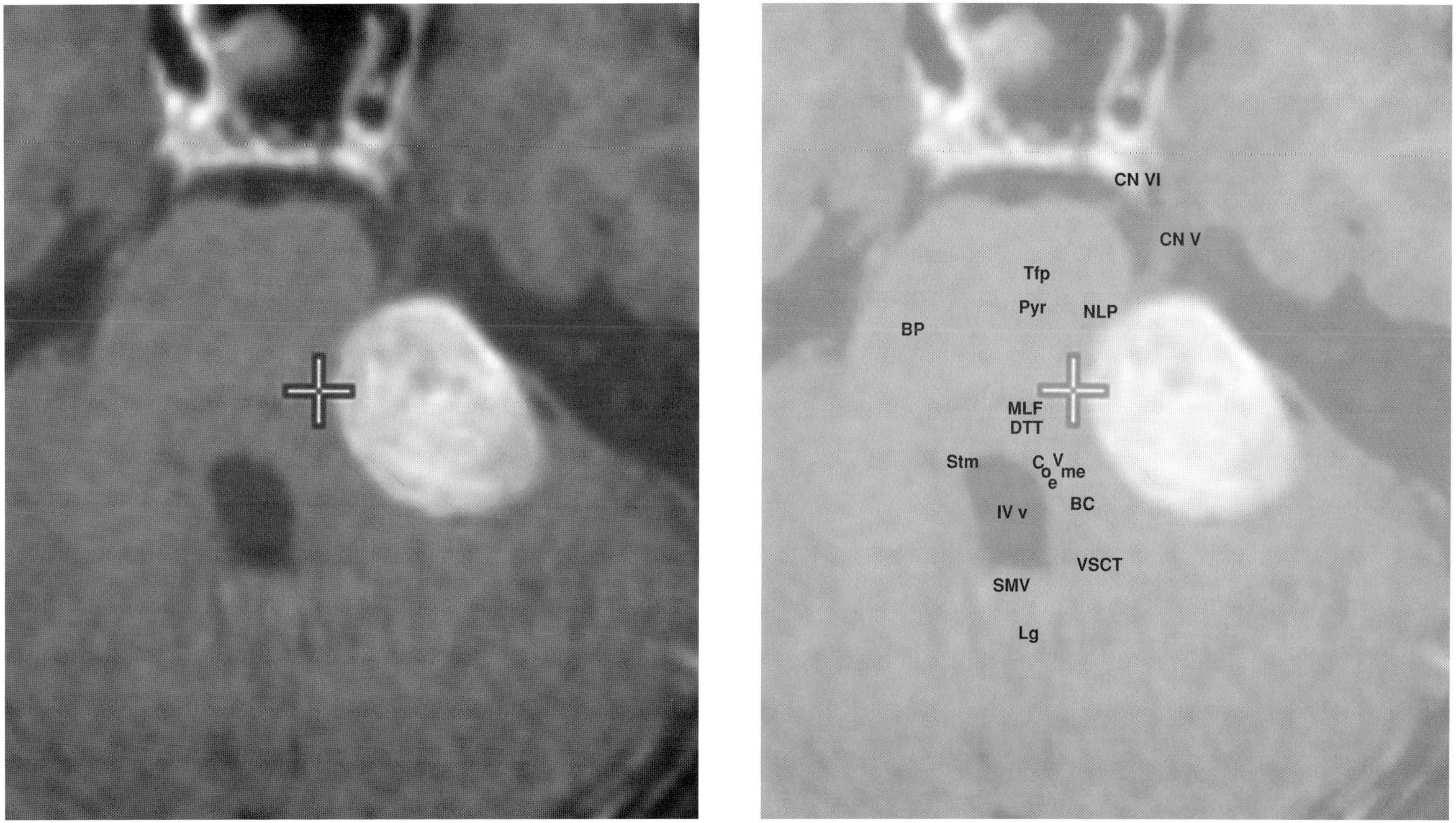

FIG. 2-12B.

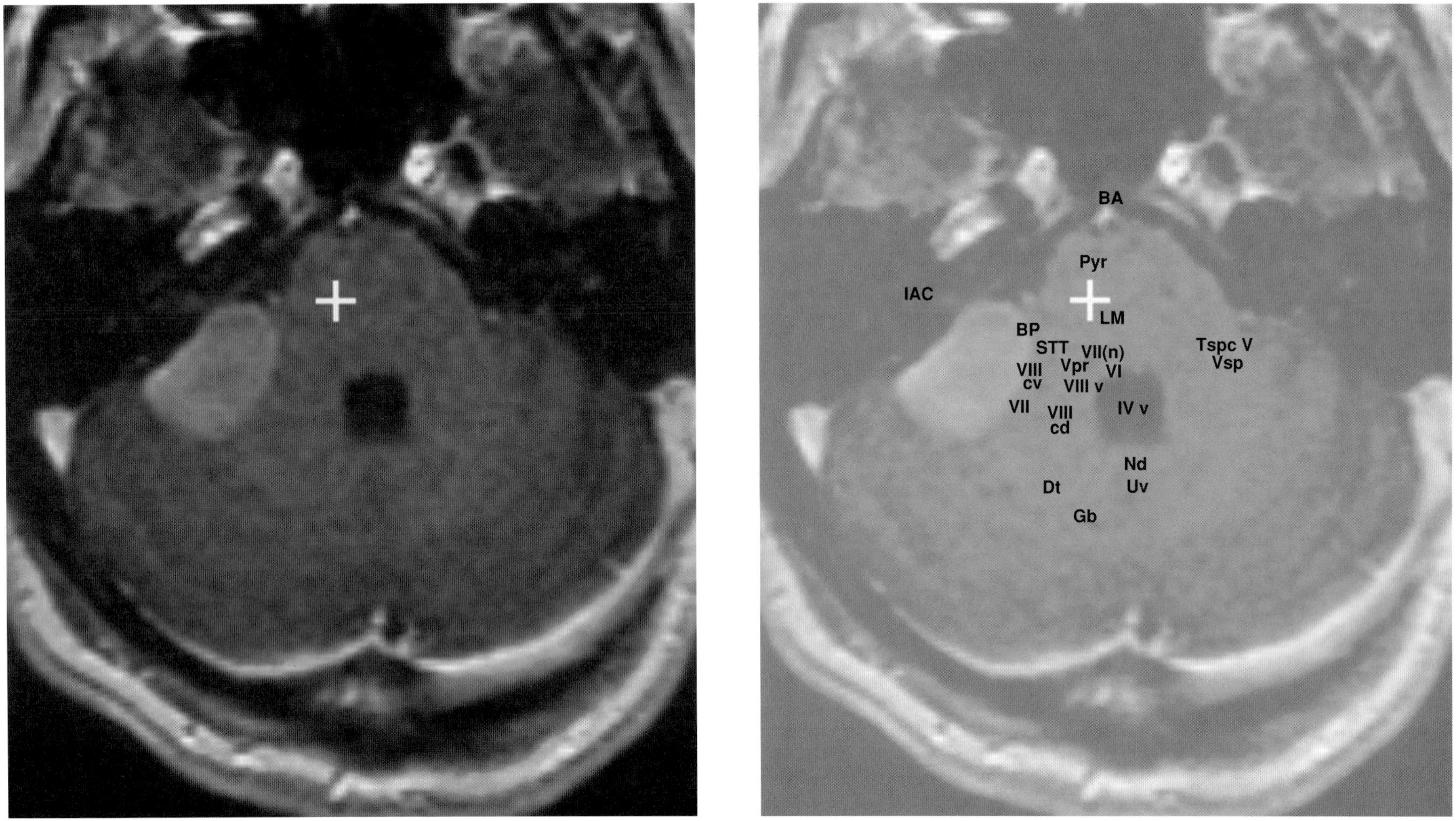
BA
Pyr
IAC
LM
BP
STT
VII(n)
Tspc V
Vsp
VIII
cv
Vpr
VI
VIII v
VII
VIII
cd
IV v
Nd
Dt
Uv
Gb

FIG. 2-13A.

FIG. 2-13. Right-sided tentorial and cerebellopontine angle meningioma in a patient with neurofibromatosis type 2 who has undergone removal of a left-sided acoustic neuroma. T_1-weighted, contrast-enhanced stereotactic axial MRIs separated by 3 mm from inferior to superior. **A** is at the level of the superior edge of the internal auditory canals (IAC). The left IAC is widened as a consequence of prior surgery. The superior attachment of the tumor to the undersurface of the tentorium on the right-hand side is outside the plane of these images. The lateral base of the tumor involves the dura covering the petrous bone between the sigmoid sinus (located 10 mm posterolaterally) and the right internal auditory canal. The anterior tumor margin extends slightly beyond the IAC, probably displacing the facial and vestibulocochlear nerve complex (CN VII and VIII) in the anterior-inferior direction. The flocculus of the cerebellum appears to be displaced medially and anteriorly against the lateral belly of the pons and brachium pontis (BP). Other neural structures that lie within the brain stem and that are displaced medially along the tumor–pons interface include (from anterior to posterior): the spinothalamic tract (STT), ventral cochlear nucleus (VIIIcv), and fibers of the facial nerve (VII). The next tier of nuclei and pathways lying more medial within the pons include the nucleus of the facial nerve [VII(n)], ventral spinocerebellar tract (T spc v), descending spinal trigeminal tract (Vsp), principal trigeminal nucleus (Vpr), nucleus of the abducens nerve (VI), vestibular nuclei (VIIIv), and dorsal cochlear nucleus (VIIIcd). The pyramidal tract (Pyr) lies well anterior and medial to the tumor, whereas the dentate and globose nuclei of the cerebellum (Dt, Gb) lie well dorsal and medial to the tumor margin.

B: At the level of the trigeminal nerve root entry zone (CN V, showing mild, abnormal enhancement 3 mm superior to **A**), the same relationships are observed more rostrally within the brain stem. Here the anterior tumor margin just touches the trigeminal nerve at its root-entry zone. More medially within the pons, the principal nucleus of CN V has given way to the mesencephalic nucleus (Vme) and trigeminal lemniscus (trigeminothalamic tract).

Neurologic functions at risk after treatment of this tumor include hearing and balance (CN VIII), facial movement (CN VII), facial sensation (CN V), and, to a lesser degree, contralateral hemibody sensation (spinothalamic tract) and ipsilateral limb coordination (ventral spinocerebellar tract and brachium pontis). *(Figure continued on following page.)*

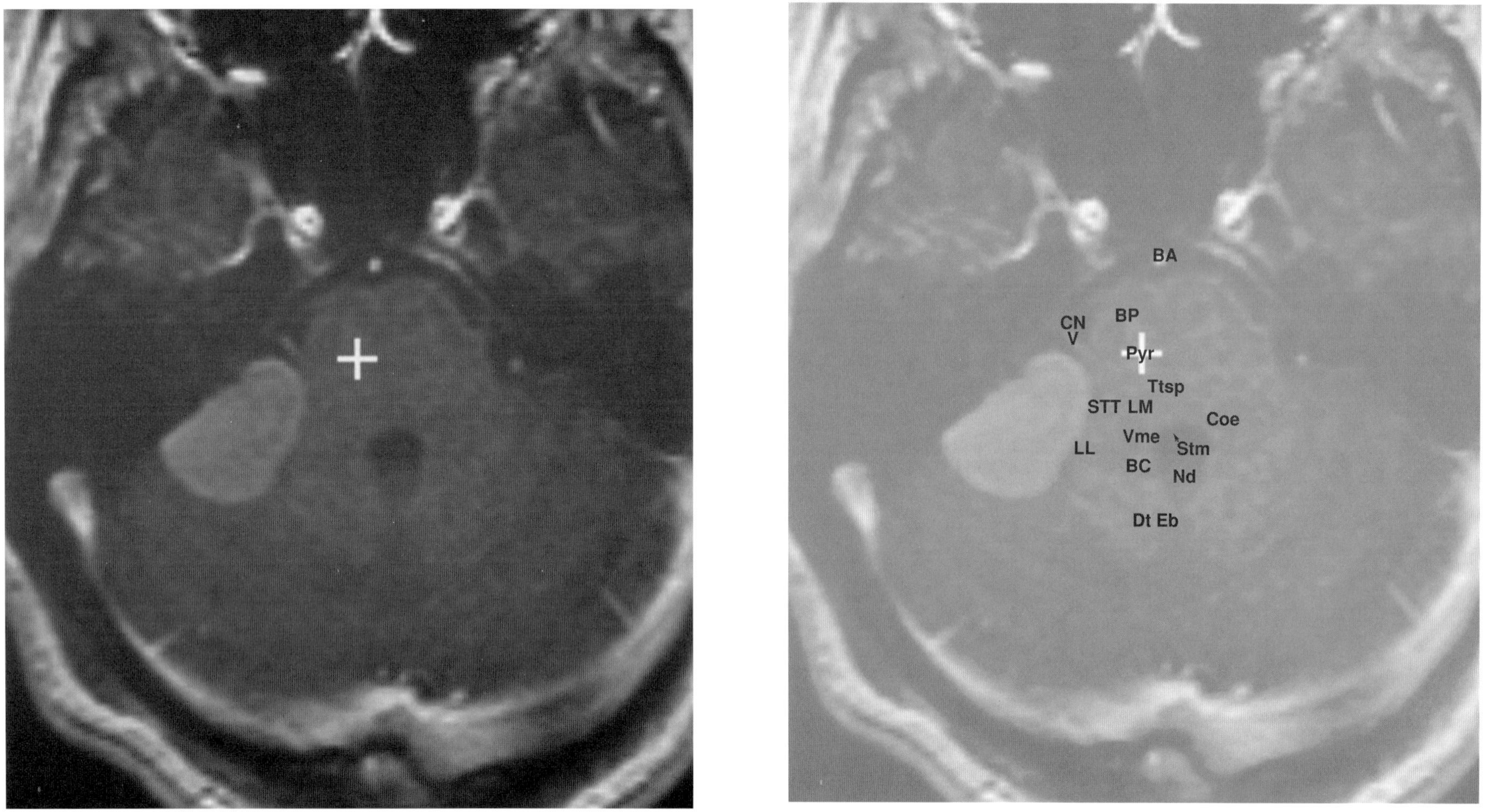

Fig. 2-13B.

FIG. 2-14. Small, left-sided, petroclival meningioma, T_1-weighted, contrast-enhanced stereotactic axial MRI. The tumor arises from the dura at the junction of the anterior-superior edge of the petrous bone with the superior clivus. The lateral, superior edge of the tumor lies along the petroclival ligament, just medial to the inferior portion of the uncus of the temporal lobe (Unc). The medial tumor margin slightly indents the ventrolateral pons on the left side. The tiny filamentous structure seen within the prepontine cistern on the contralateral (right) side may be the right abducens nerve (CN VI); the left abducens nerve probably is displaced medially and/or inferiorly by the tumor. Part of the cisternal portion of the trigeminal nerve (CN V) also may be visible on the right-hand side. It is displaced superiorly by the tumor on the left-hand side.

Because the tumor only indents the pons slightly, the frontopontine tract (Tfp) and pyramidal tract (Pyr) are not displaced. *(Figure continued on following page.)*

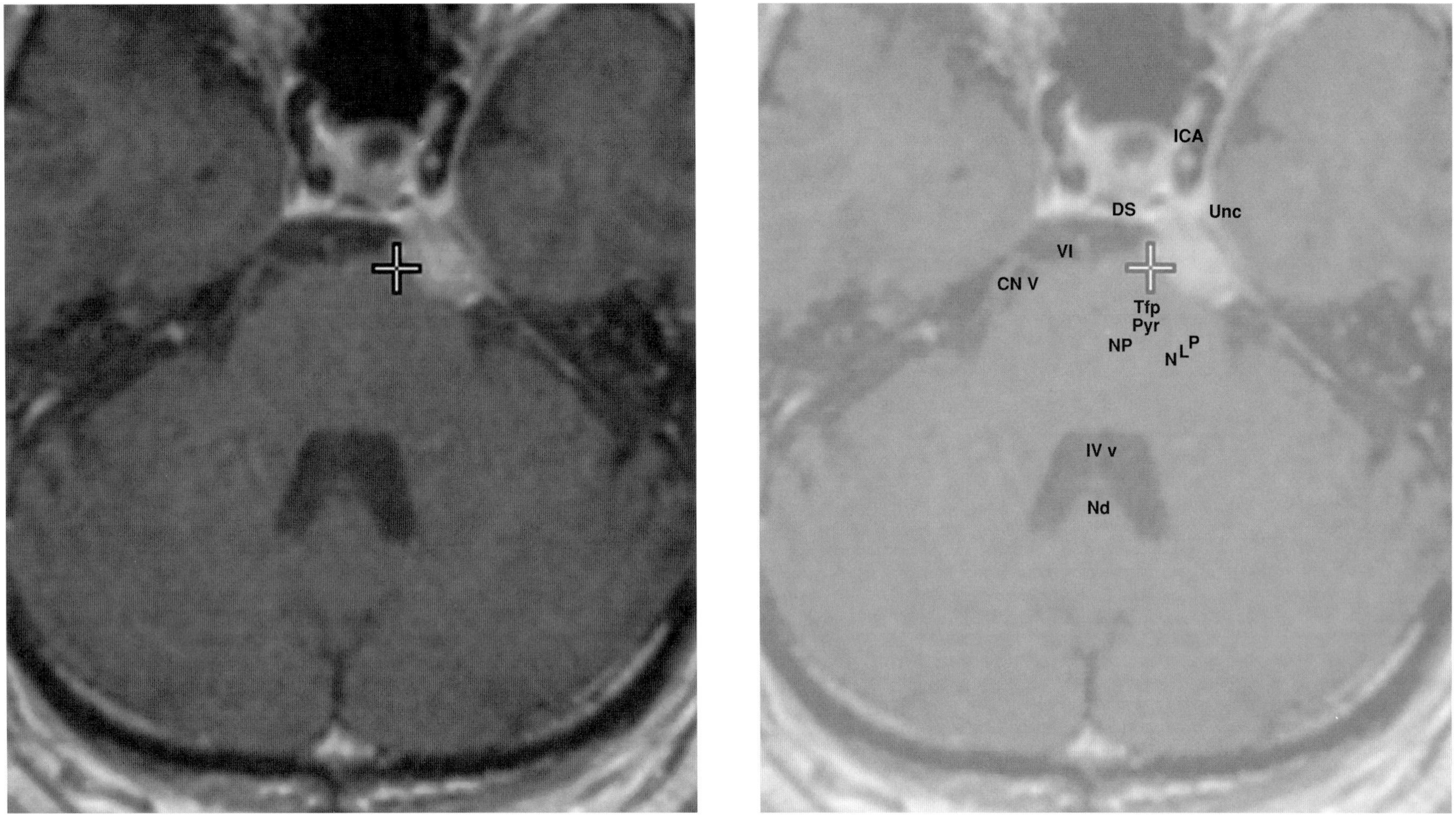

FIG. 2-14.

FIG. 2-15. Clivus chordoma, recurrence after surgical resection; T_1-weighted, contrast-enhanced stereotactic axial MRIs separated by 3 mm, inferior to superior (**A and B**). The tumor erodes and expands the clivus, leaving only a thin shell of bone anteriorly within the sphenoid sinus and obliterating the prepontine cistern posteriorly to compress and distort the belly of the pons, especially in the mid-line and on the right side. The anterolateral tumor margin extends into the posterior cavernous sinus and Meckel's cave (Cav) on the right and nearly occludes the lumen of the right internal carotid artery (ICA, vertical cavernous segment). On the left side the tumor partly encircles but does not compress the cavernous ICA.

The posterior tumor margin encases most of the basilar artery (BA) and pushes the vessel against the ventral pons just to the right of the mid-line. The frontopontine and pyramidal tracts (Tfp and Pyr) are displaced posteriorly, especially on the right side, by the bulk of the tumor. The anterior portion of the right brachium pontis (BP) also is indented and displaced backward by the tumor. The entry of both abducens nerves into the posterior cavernous sinuses through Dorello's canal on each side is encased by tumor, as are cranial nerves III, IV, V_1 and VI within the cavernous sinuses bilaterally. The posterolateral tumor margin is medial to the trigeminal root entry zone on the right and, consequently, does not reach the porus acousticus on either side. Therefore, cranial nerves caudal to VI are unaffected.

The neurologic risks associated with cranial nerve or brain stem injury from radiosurgical treatment of this tumor could include: bilateral ophthalmoplegia (CNN III, IV, VI and frontopontine tracts), bilateral orofacial numbness and masticatory muscle weakness (trigeminal sensory and motor function), and left hemiparesis (right pyramidal tract). *(Figure continued on following pages.)*

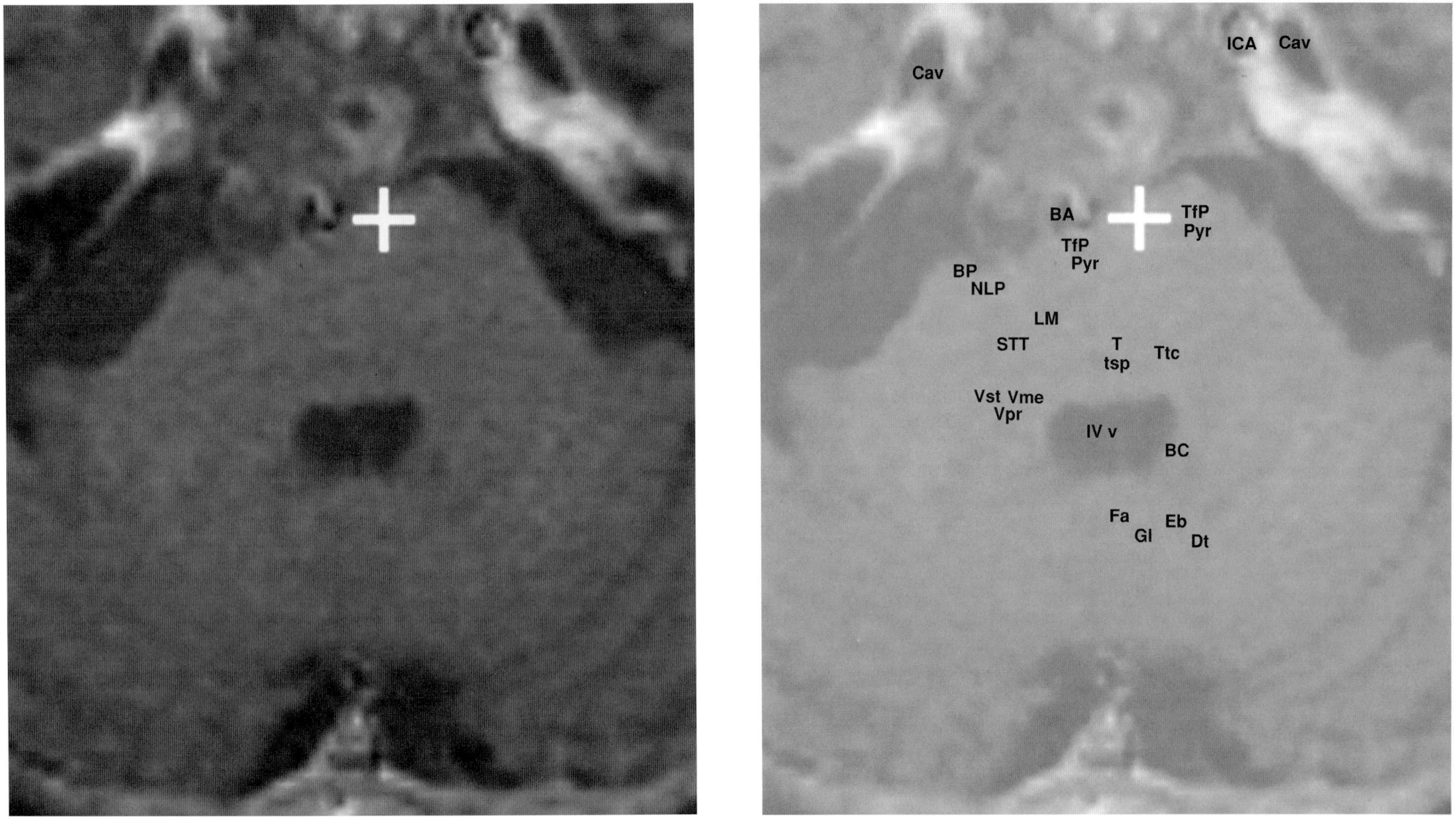
Cav
ICA
Cav
BA
TfP
Pyr
TfP
Pyr
BP
NLP
LM
STT
T
tsp
Ttc
Vst
Vme
Vpr
IV v
BC
Fa
Gl
Eb
Dt

FIG. 2-15A.

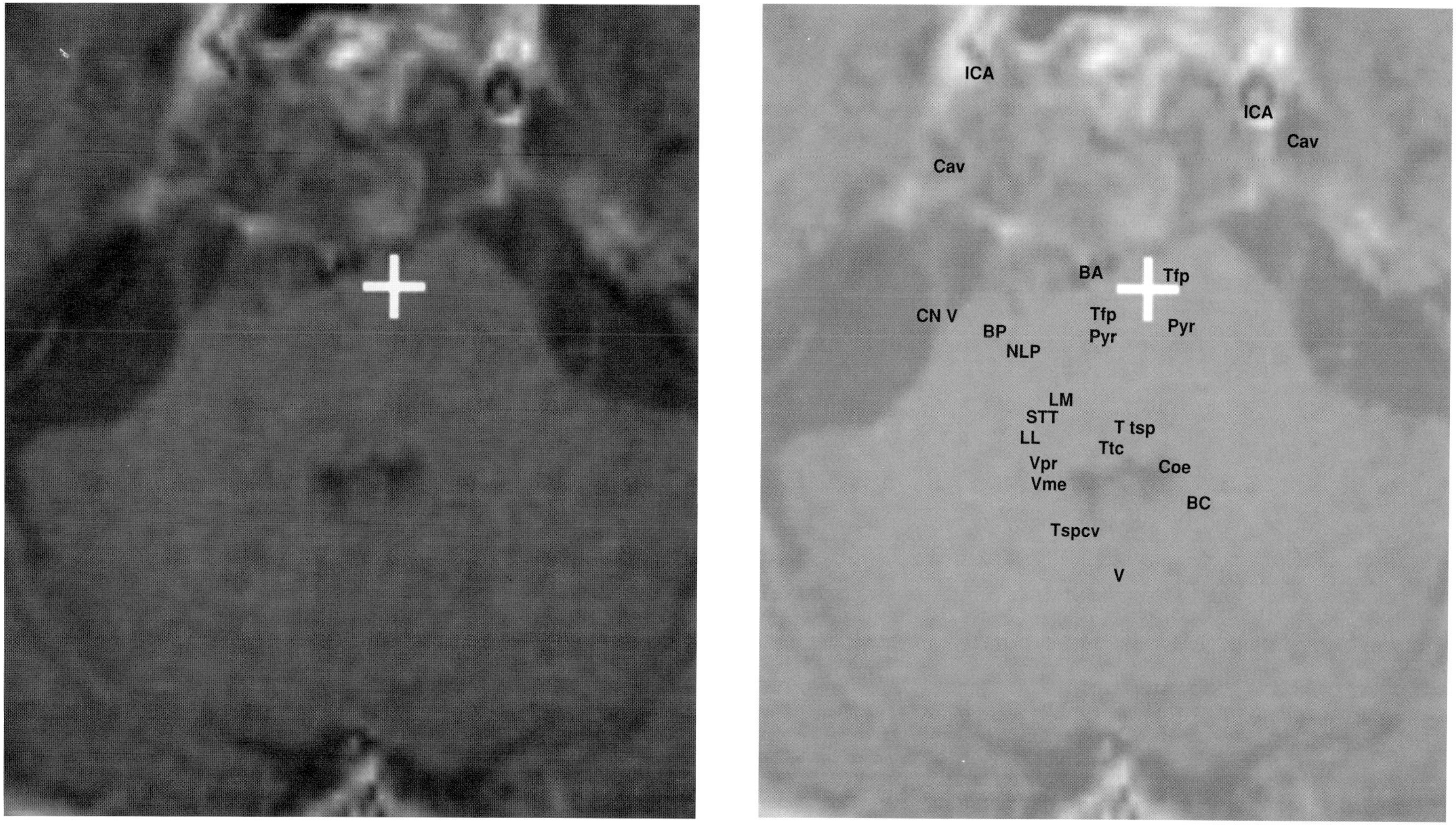
ICA
ICA
Cav
Cav
BA
Tfp
CN V
BP
Tfp
Pyr
Pyr
NLP
LM
STT
T tsp
LL
Ttc
Vpr
Coe
Vme
BC
Tspcv
V

FIG. 2-15B.

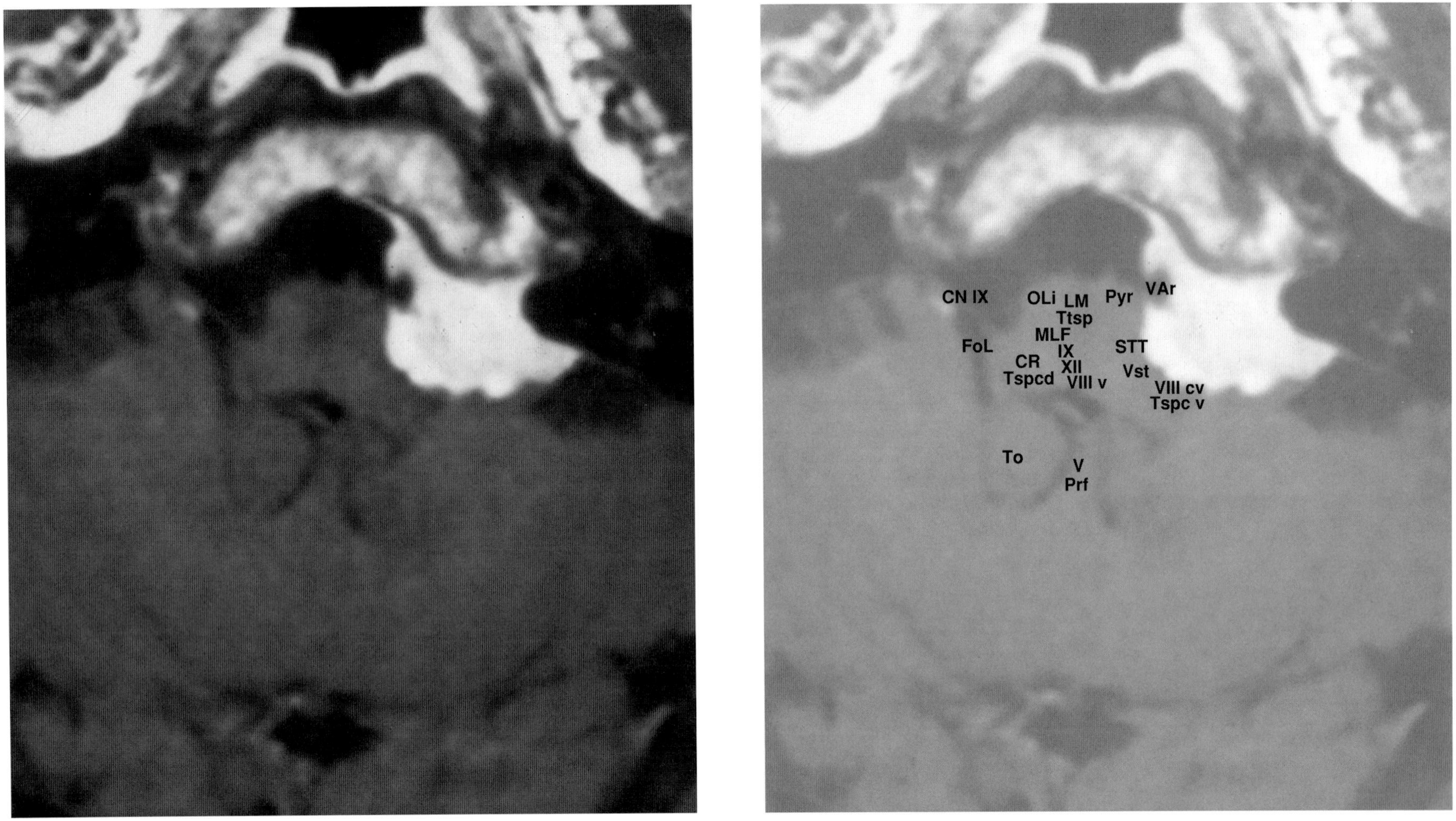
CN IX
OLi
LM
Pyr
VAr
Ttsp
MLF
FoL
IX
STT
CR
XII
Vst
Tspcd
VIII v
VIII cv
Tspc v
To
V
Prf

FIG. 2-16.

FIG. 2-16. Jugular foramen region meningioma, T_1-weighted, contrast-enhanced nonstereotactic axial image at the level of the glossopharyngeal nerve (CN IX), visible on the right side (opposite tumor). The lateral and anterior (ventral) tumor margin arises from the dura of the clivus near the mid-line and extends laterally to involve the jugular foramen and hyperostotic jugular tubercle on the left side. The tumor fills the cerebellomedullary angle cistern and appears to occlude or cap the lateral aperture of the left foramen of Luschka (FoL).

The medial tumor margin slightly displaces and rotates the medulla dorsally and to the right. Neural pathways and structures in contact with the tumor margin include (from ventral to dorsal) the pyramid (Pyr, corticospinal tract), inferior olive (Oli), spinothalamic tract (STT), glossopharyngeal nerve, and ventral cochlear nucleus (VIII cv). Deeper within the medulla, the pathways and structures include the medial lemniscus (LM); tectospinal tract (Ttsp); medial longitudinal fasciculus (MLF); restiform body (CR, inferior cerebellar peduncle); glossopharyngeal, hypoglossal, and vestibular nuclei (IX, XII, and VIIIv, respectively); and dorsal spinocerebellar tract (Tspcd). The notch along the semicircular medial tumor-ventrolateral medulla interface contains the left vertebral artery partially encased by tumor.

Neurologic functions associated with structures along the tumor–brain stem interface that potentially would be at risk during radiosurgical treatment include contralateral motor function (Pyr), limb coordination (Tspcd, Tspcv), facial sensation (Vst), and lower cranial nerve function (VIIIcv, IX, XII) plus pain and temperature sensation in the contralateral hemibody (STT).

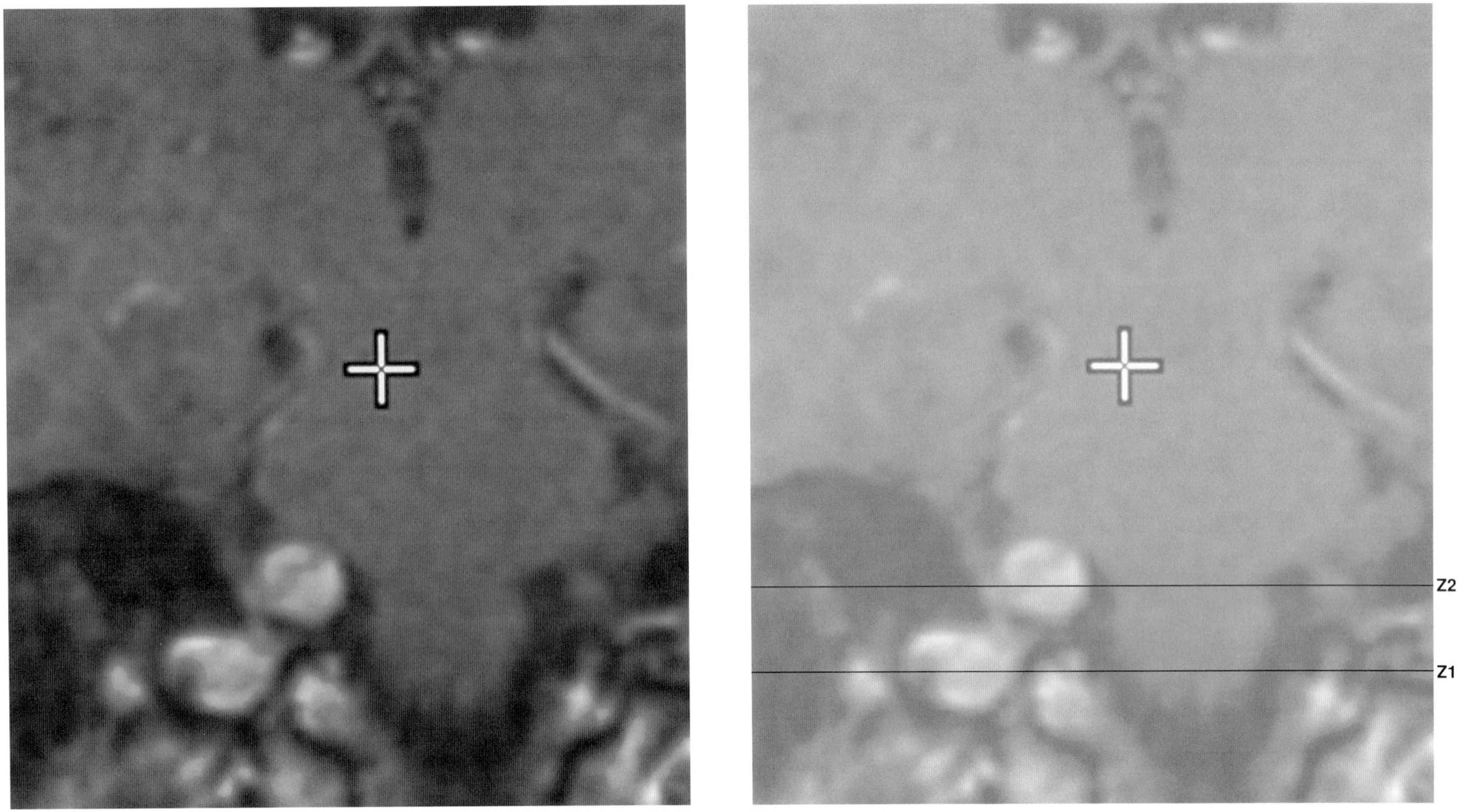

FIG. 2-17A.

FIG. 2-17. Glomus jugulare et tympanicum tumor of the right jugular foramen and cerebellomedullary angle T_1-weighted, contrast enhanced stereotactic coronal (**A**) and axial MRIs separated by 12 mm from inferior to superior (**B and C**). The tumor is bilobed, having a skull base component inferolaterally (jugular bulb and middle ear) and an intracranial component superomedially. **A** is provided for orientation and shows the axial levels of **B** and **C** (lines Z_1 and Z_2, respectively).

The inferior, skull-base portion of the tumor seen in **B** has its posterior margin just anterior to the junction of the sigmoid sinus with the jugular bulb. The anterior tumor margin nearly encircles the vertical intrapetrous segment of the right internal carotid artery (ICA). The lateral tumor margin encroaches upon the middle ear, whereas the medial margin extends superomedially in dumbell fashion through the jugular foramen into the subarachnoid space.

The intracranial tumor nodule in **C** has a narrow anterolateral isthmus that joins the two tumor components. This nodule is tucked into the aperture of the foramen of Luschka (FoL) within the angle formed by the flocculus of the cerebellum (Fl), which is displaced posterolaterally, and the lateral surface of the medulla, which is indented slightly. The ventral cochlear nucleus (VIIIcv) lies within the medulla at the point of contact with the medial tumor surface. The spinothalamic tract (STT) lies just anterior to VIIIcv, and is against the anteromedial tumor surface. The next tier of structures deeper within the medulla include the inferior olive (Oli), which lies anteromedial to the STT, the ventral spinocerebellar tract (Tspcv), which lies medial to VIIIcv, and the inferior cerebellar peduncle (ICP), which runs between the ventral and dorsal spinocerebellar tracts (Tspcv and Tspcd, respectively).

The Pyramid (Pyr), spinal trigeminal tract (Vsp), and other long tracts and cranial nerve nuclei lie well away from the tumor in this imaging plane. A narrow sliver of the belly of the pons is projected ventral to the pyramid of the medulla because of the angle between the long axis of the brain stem and the plane of imaging.

Symptoms associated with this tumor include mixed sensorineural and conductive hearing loss as well as vestibular system dysfunction (vestibulocochlear nerve, nuclei, middle ear, and flocculonodular lobe of the cerebellum). Injury to those structures as a consequence of surgery or radiosurgery could worsen the preexisting systems. In addition, damage to the spinothalamic tract, which lies superficial within the medulla, could cause contralateral hemisensory loss. Injury to the glossopharyngeal, vagal, and/or spinal accessory nerves also could occur within the jugular foramen. *(Figure continued on following pages.)*

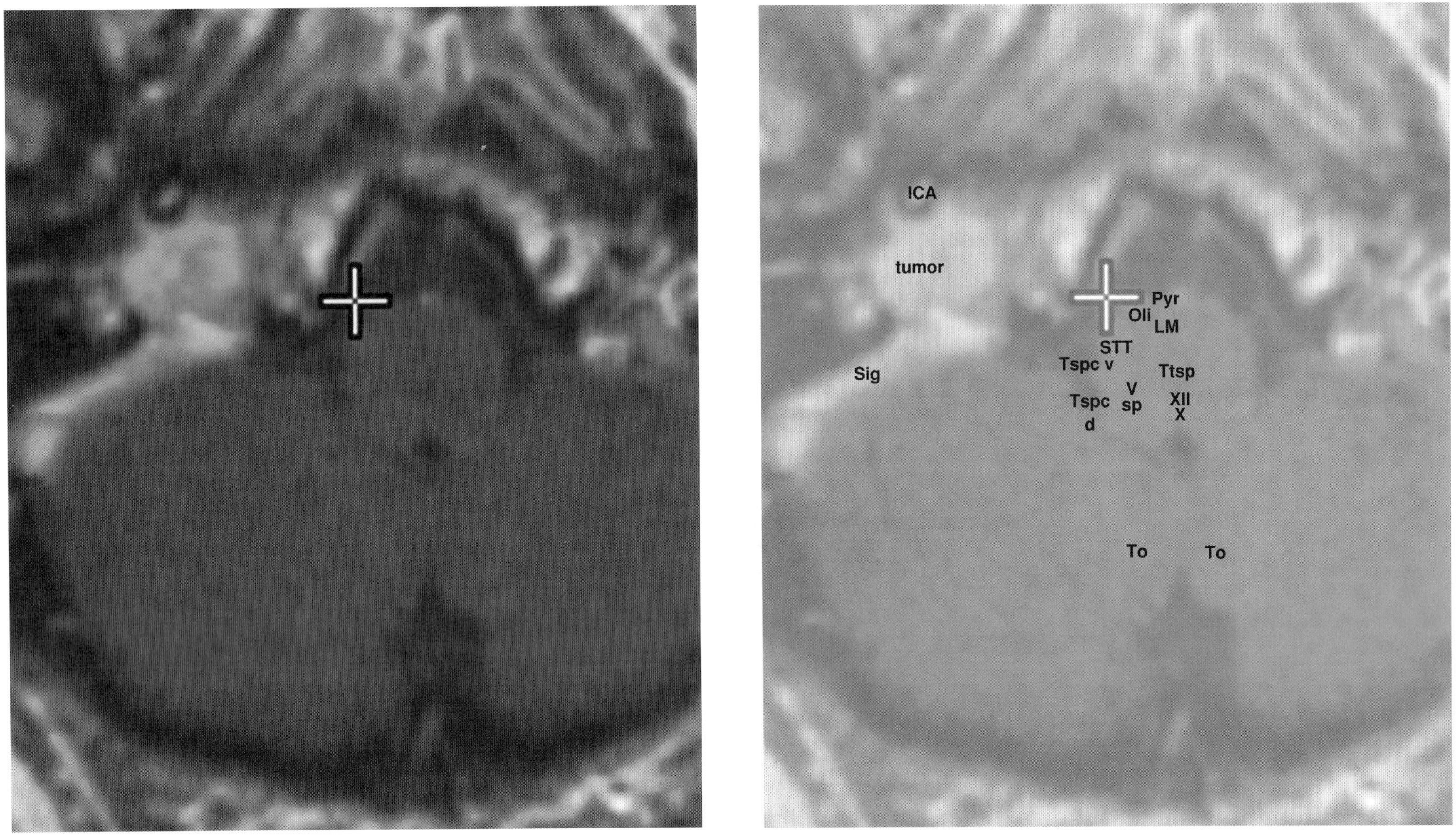

FIG. 2-17B.

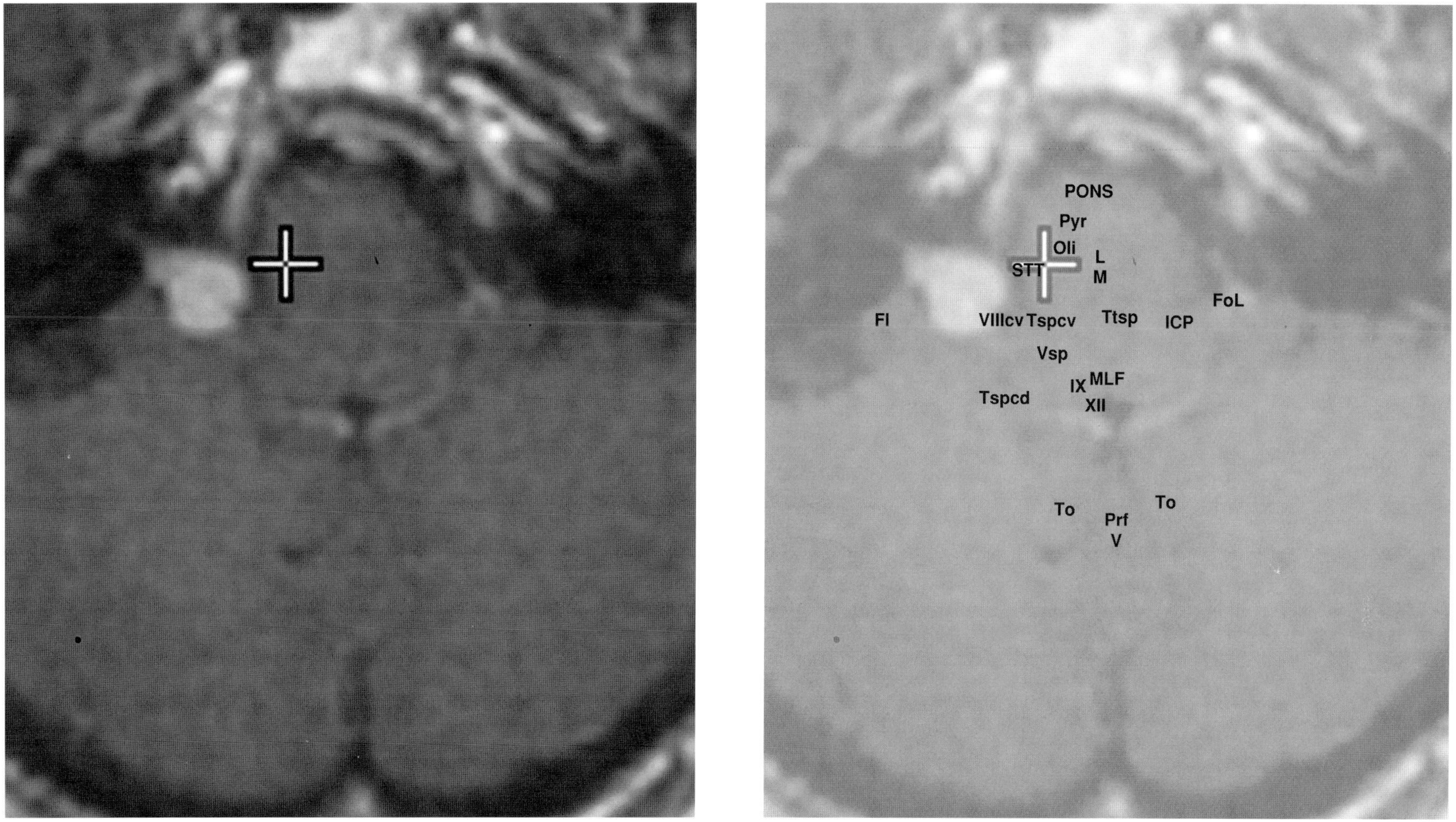
PONS
Pyr
Oli
L
STT
M
FoL
Fl
VIIIcv
Tspcv
Ttsp
ICP
Vsp
IX
MLF
Tspcd
XII
To
To
Prf
V

FIG. 2-17C.

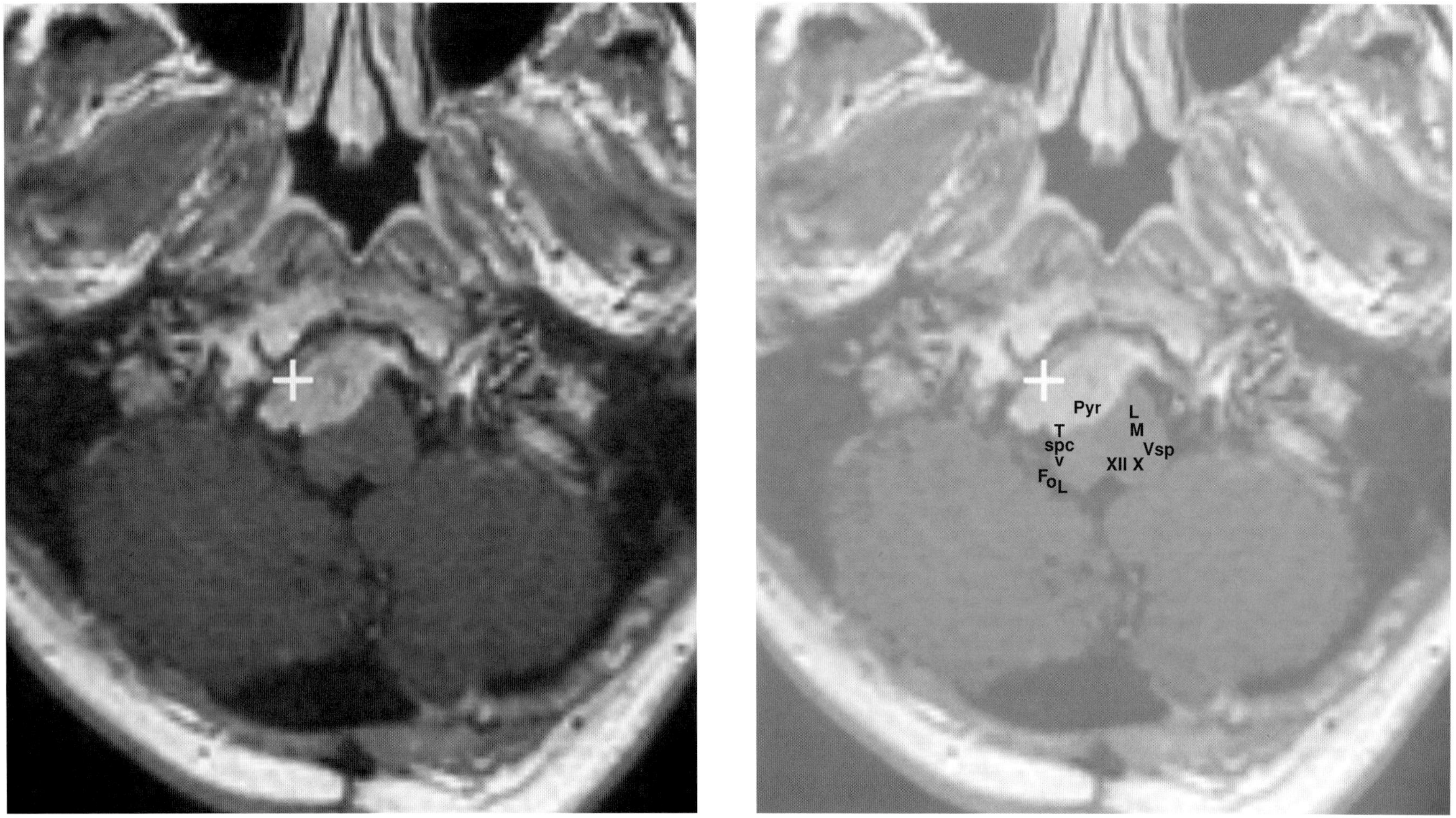

FIG. 2-18A.

FIG. 2-18. Residual (postoperative) ventrolateral foramen magnum meningioma, T_1-weighted, contrast-enhanced stereotactic axial MRIs (**A and B**) spaced 6 mm apart from inferior to superior, respectively. The tumor compresses the ventral medulla on the right side and, to a lesser extent, in the mid-line. The pyramid (Pyr, corticospinal tract) on the right side is compressed markedly in the ventral-to-dorsal direction and from right to left. The subtle bulge of the olive (Oli), visible on the left side, also has been displaced medially by the tumor on the right side. Thus, the corticospinal tract (Pyr), spinothalamic tract (STT), descending spinal trigeminal tract (Vsp), and ventral spinocerebellar tract (Tspcv) all lie at or very close to the dorsomedial tumor margin and are pushed closer together by the tumor. The medial lemniscus (LM) lies just dorsal to the tumor on either side of the mid-line. The ventral cochlear nucleus (VIIIcv) lies at the superior edge of the tumor–brain stem interface (B), whereas the vestibular nuclei (VIIIv) lie in the more dorsomedial location beneath the lateral floor of the fourth ventricle. The ventral spinocerebellar tract (Tspcv) forms part of the ventral margin of the foramen of Luschka (FoL) just lateral to the vestibular nuclei. The vagal (X) and hypoglossal (XII) nuclei also lie within the floor of the fourth ventricle on either side of the mid-line.

Because a substantial portion of this tumor is located caudal to the pyramidal decussation, injury to the medulla at the medial tumor margin could cause ipsilateral hemiparesis, limb ataxia, hemifacial sensory loss, and contralateral hemibody sensory loss (corticospinal tract, ventral spinocerebellar tract, descending spinal trigeminal tract, and spinothalamic tract, respectively). *(Figure continued on following page.)*

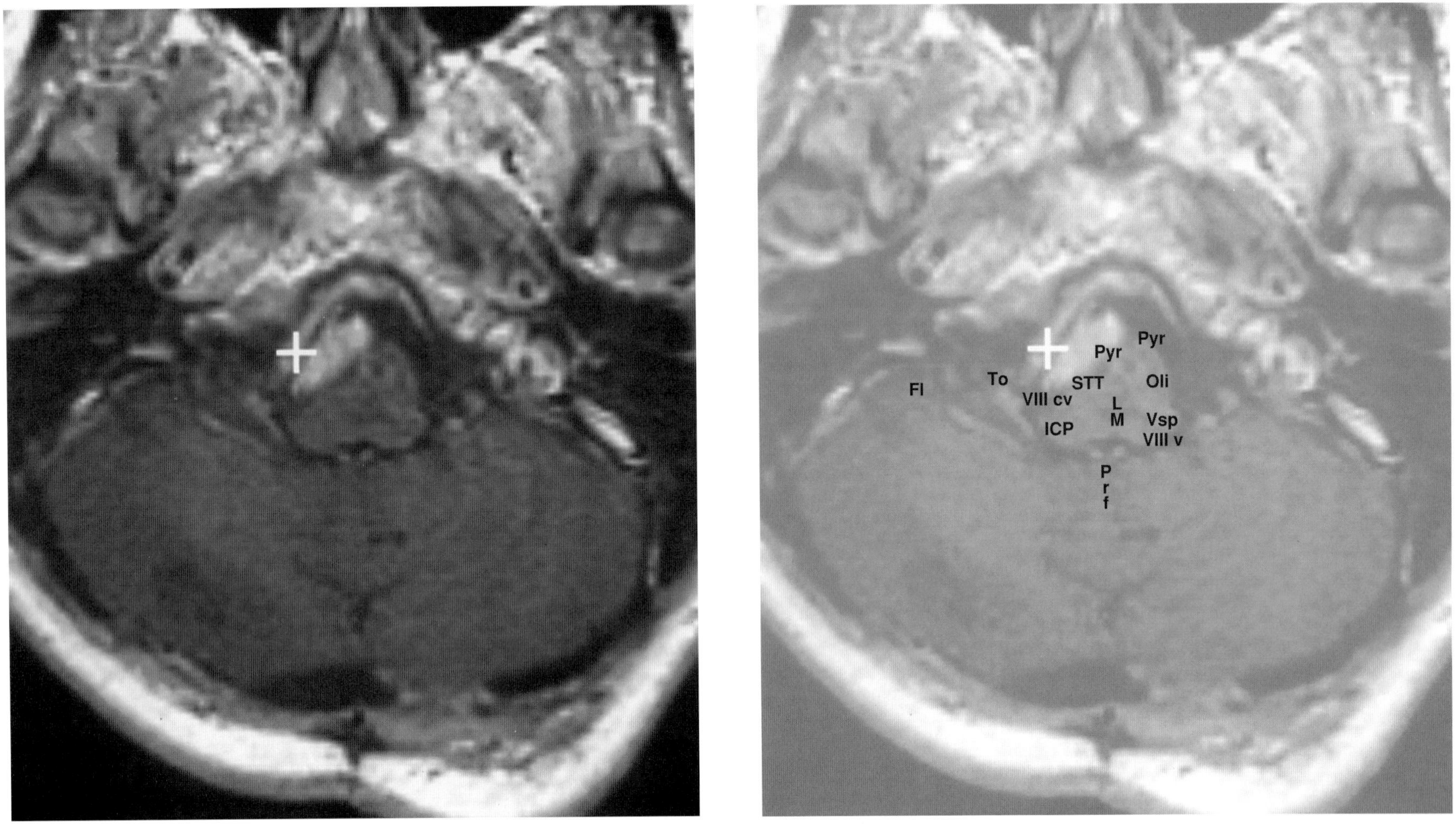

FIG. 2-18B.

Chapter 3

Intra-axial Tumors

The intra-axial tumors presented in this chapter consist predominantly of metastatic neoplasms from primary carcinomas that arose from the skin (melanoma), lung, breast and kidney. Only two examples of unusually well-circumscribed glioblastomas of the pineal region and thalamus–mid-brain junction are included. This selection of cases reflects the authors' desire to illustrate tumors that are fairly well demarcated from surrounding brain structures. In this manner the reader can recognize normal cerebral anatomy and landmarks despite the edema or mass effect generated by the tumor. In every patient the diagnosis was confirmed by previous biopsy, surgery, or the appearance of the new metastasis illustrated here after histologic confirmation of earlier brain metastasis and/or persistent systemic cancer.

As in Chapter 2, cases are presented in order beginning in the anterior frontal lobe and progressing posteriorly toward the occipito-temporal region. Next, tumors of the deep supratentorial structures are illustrated, followed by tumors of the brain stem and cerebellum. Again, the rationale is to familiarize the reader with more easily recognizable gross anatomical structures before proceeding to deeper regions of the cerebrum and brain stem, where the multiplicity of nuclei and tracts adds considerable complexity to each example.

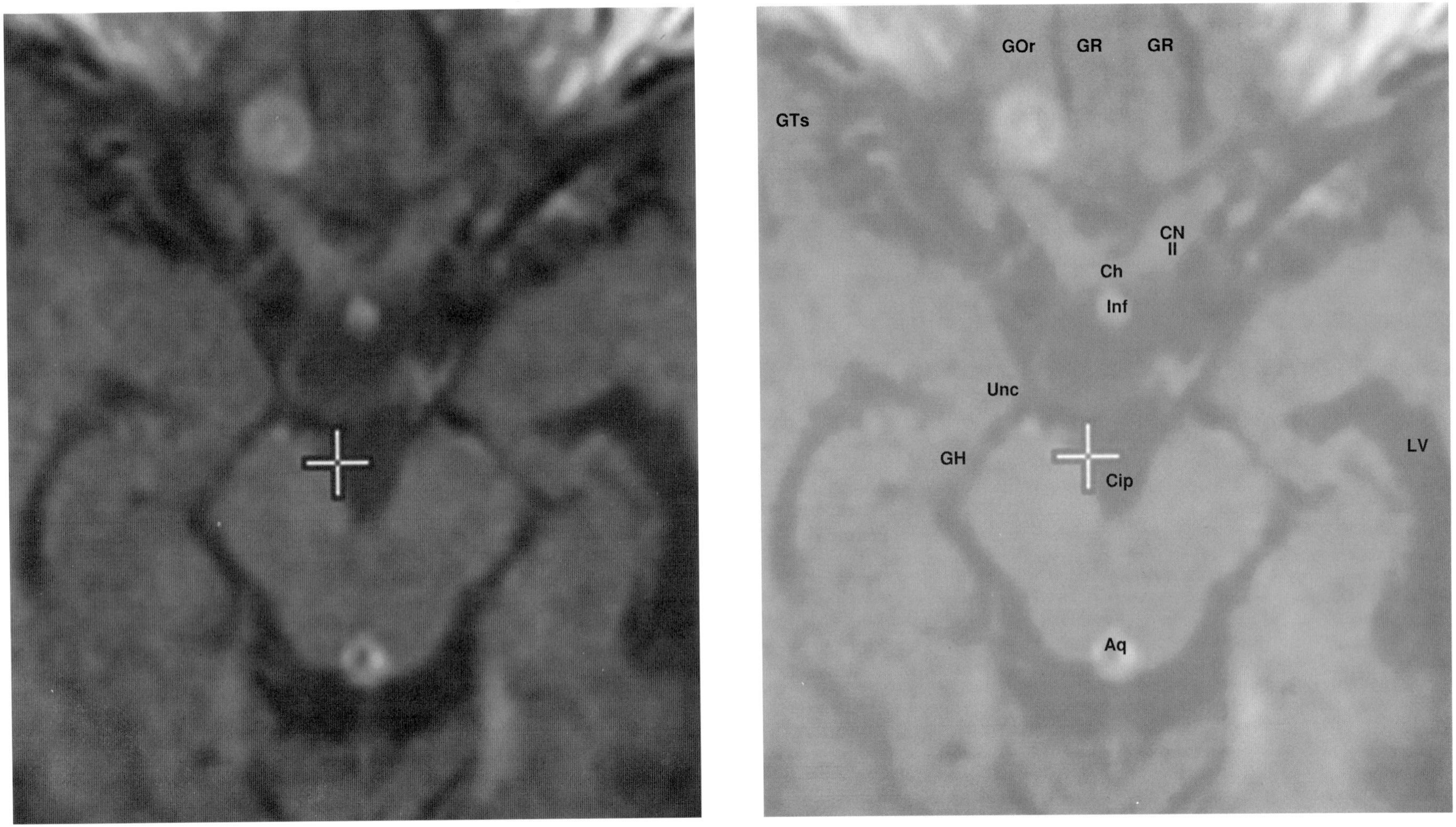

FIG. 3-1A.

FIG. 3-1. Malignant melanoma, metastatic to the right inferior frontal/subfrontal region, T_1-weighted, contrast-enhanced stereotactic axial MR images separated by 3 mm from inferior to superior. **B:** This small (7 mm) tumor lies within the gray-white junction of the orbital (GOr) and medial frontal (GFm) gyri near the floor of the anterior cranial fossa. The above-named gyri form the anterior tumor margin. The inferior frontal gyrus (GFi), gyrus rectus (GR), and subcallosal gyrus (GSc) form the lateral, medial, and posterior tumor margins, respectively. **A:** The inferior tumor margin lies almost completely within the orbital gyrus.

Although the tumor appears completely surrounded by silent areas of the brain in **B**, 3 mm inferiorly, the medial edge of right optic nerve (CNII) touches the tumor in the plane of **A**. Thus, the principal risk of radiosurgical treatment of this tumor would be right-sided visual loss. Whatever radiation dose was administered to the tumor margin would be delivered to the optic nerve as well.

Note that the high signal seen around the aqueduct of Sylvius (Aq) in **A** is artifactual flow-related enhancement at the edge of an image pack. The phenomenon is absent in **B**, located only 3 mm more superiorly. *(Figure continued on following page.)*

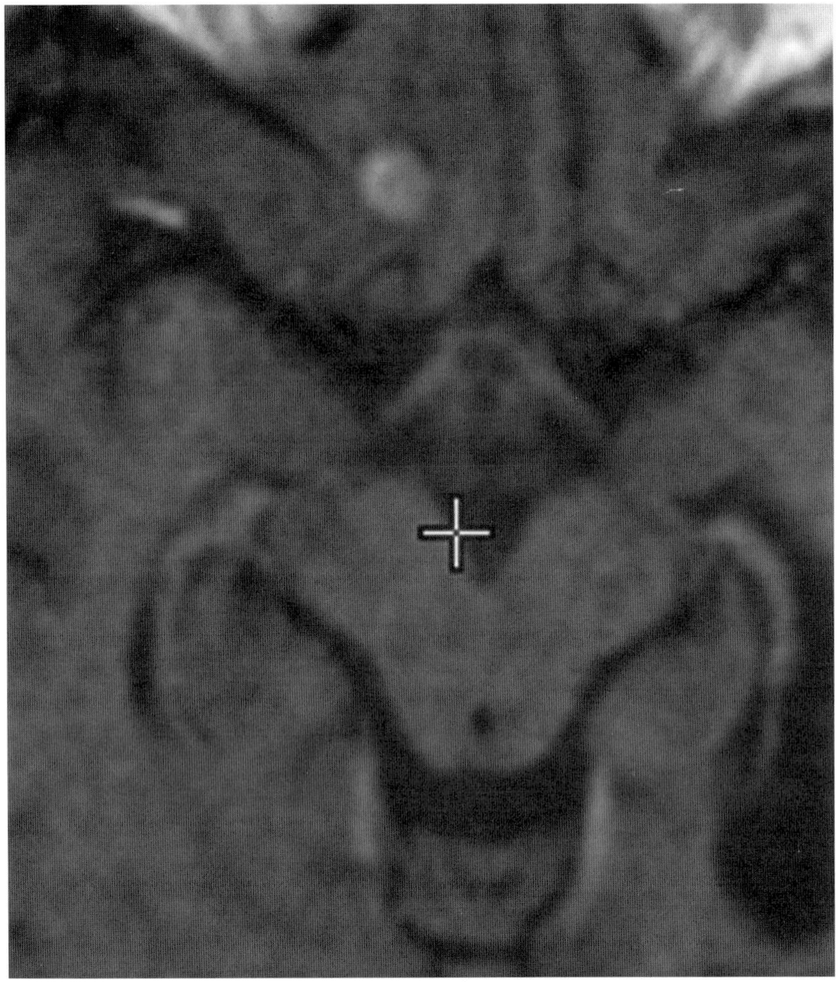

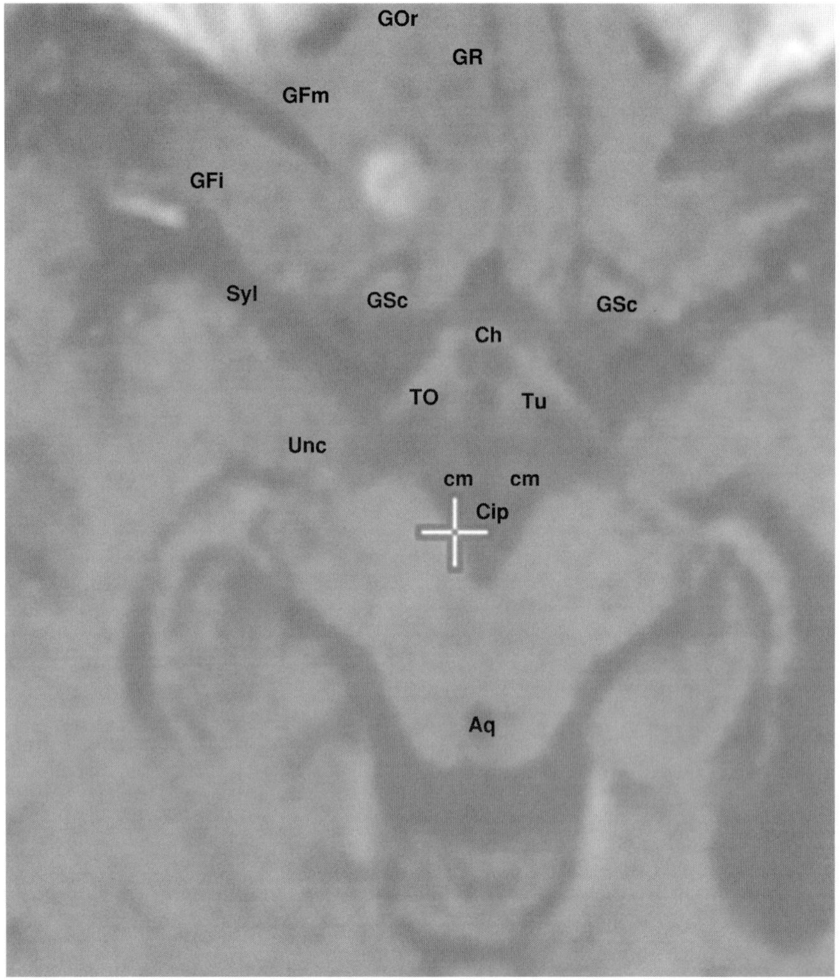

FIG. 3-1B.

FIG. 3-2. Simultaneous bilateral metastases from primary lung carcinoma to the motor-sensory cortex of the high convexity region, T_1-weighted, contrast-enhanced stereotactic axial MRIs (**A and B**) separated by 3 mm from inferior to superior, respectively. **A:** The inferior portion of the left-sided tumor and edema are shown within the precentral gyrus (GPrC). Edema widens the gyrus and displaces the precentral sulcus (SPrC) and middle frontal gyrus (GFm) anteriorly. The posterior tumor margin extends across the central sulcus (SCR), displaces it posteriorly, and exerts pressure upon the adjacent anterior edge of the postcentral gyrus (GPoC). Essentially the same anatomical relationships are seen in **B** at the superior margin of the left-sided tumor.

Edema expands the postcentral gyrus (GPoC) in the right hemisphere below the smaller tumor nodule that appears in **B**. The right-sided tumor and edema expand the postcentral gyrus slightly but exert little mass effect upon surrounding structures. The anterior tumor margin crosses the central sulcus and indents the posterior edge of the precentral gyrus.

Although the right-sided tumor is centered 3 mm superior to the left-sided one, it is situated farther from the mid-line. Thus, both tumors lie within that portion of the sensorimotor cortex that corresponds to the contralateral arm. The patient had a right hemiparesis at the time of this MRI study. Tumor progression or tissue injury around both lesions could cause bilateral sensorimotor deficits resulting in bi-brachial paralysis or quadriparesis. *(Figure continued on following pages.)*

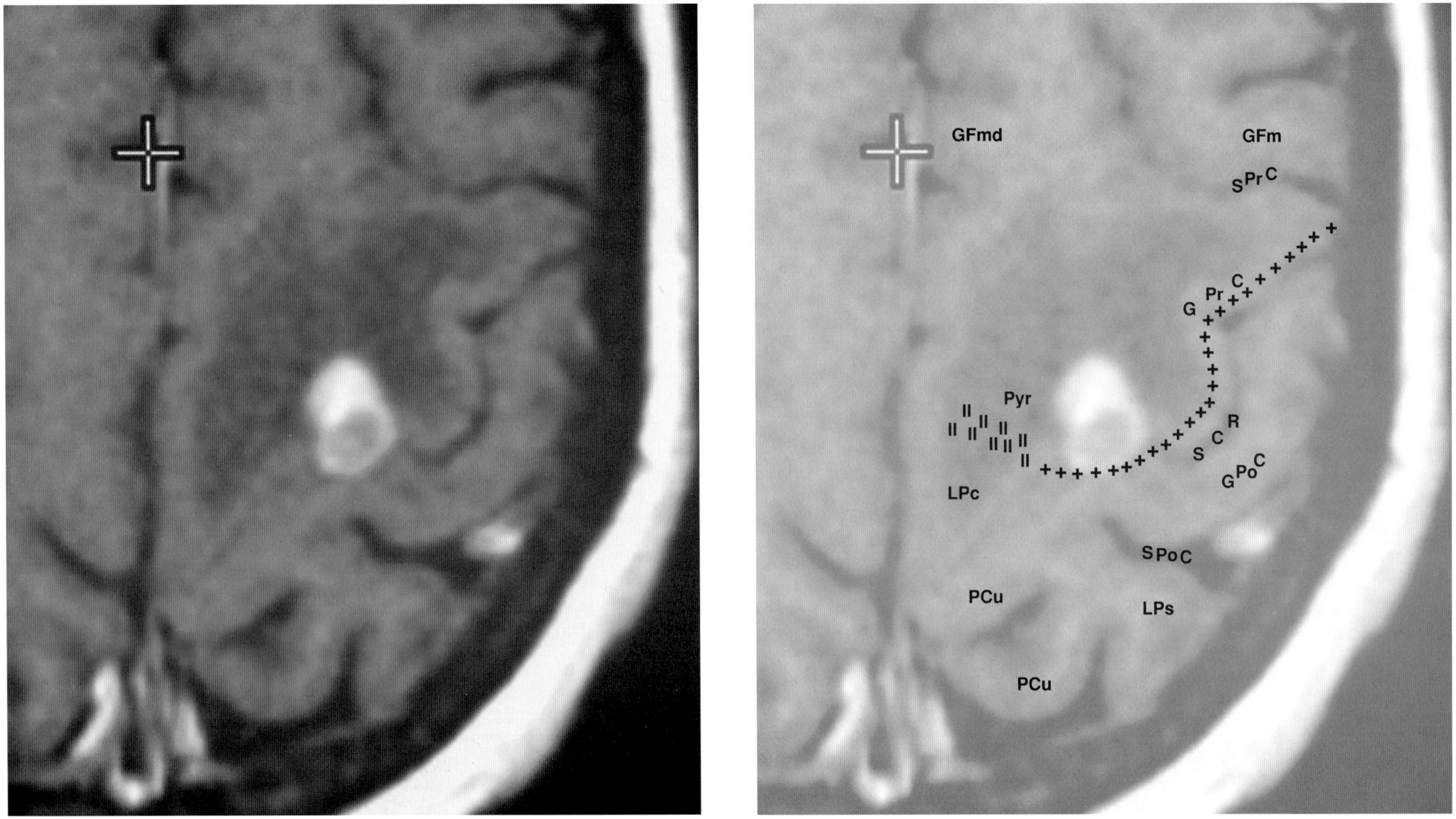

FIG. 3-2A.

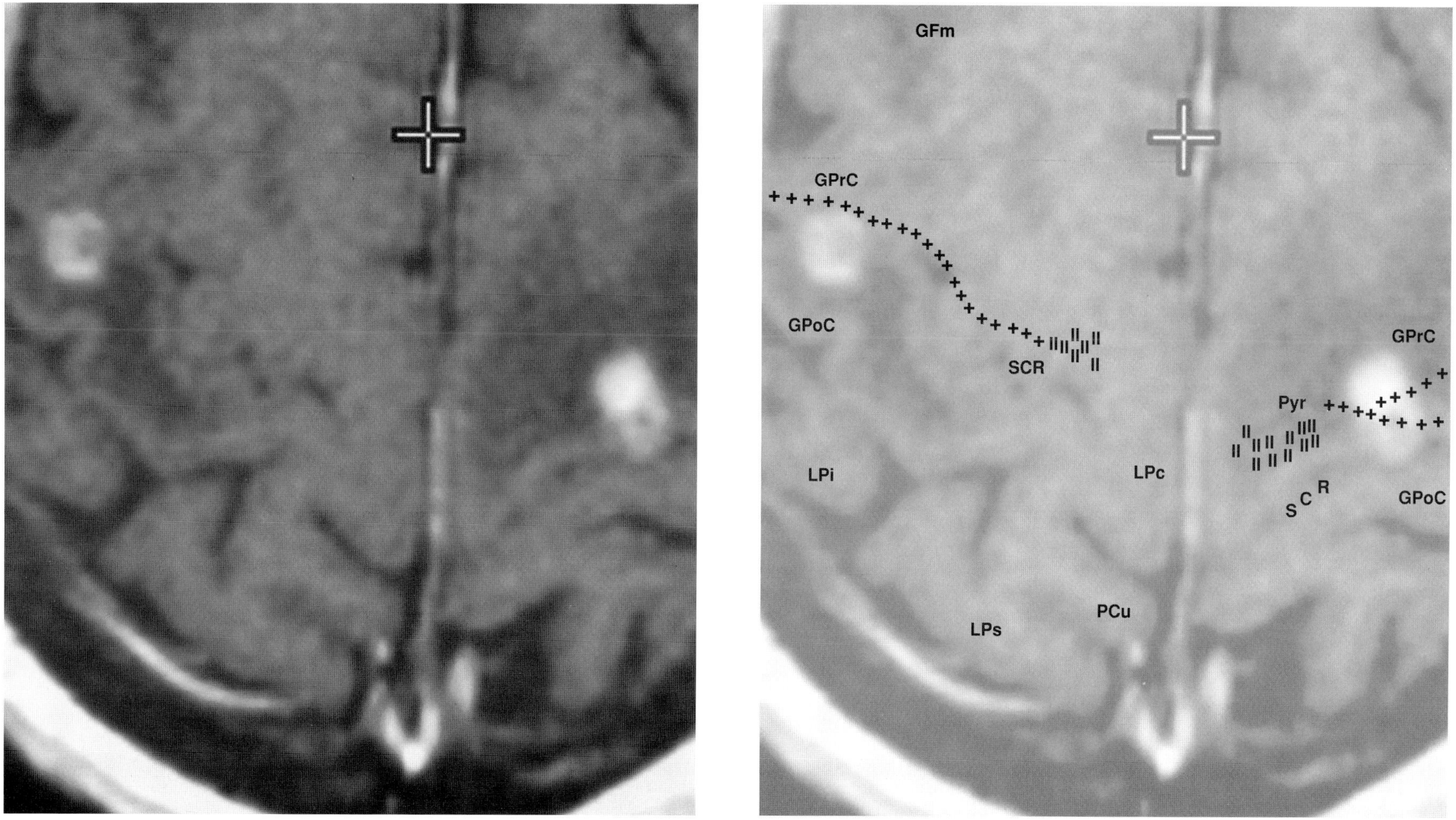

FIG. 3-2B.

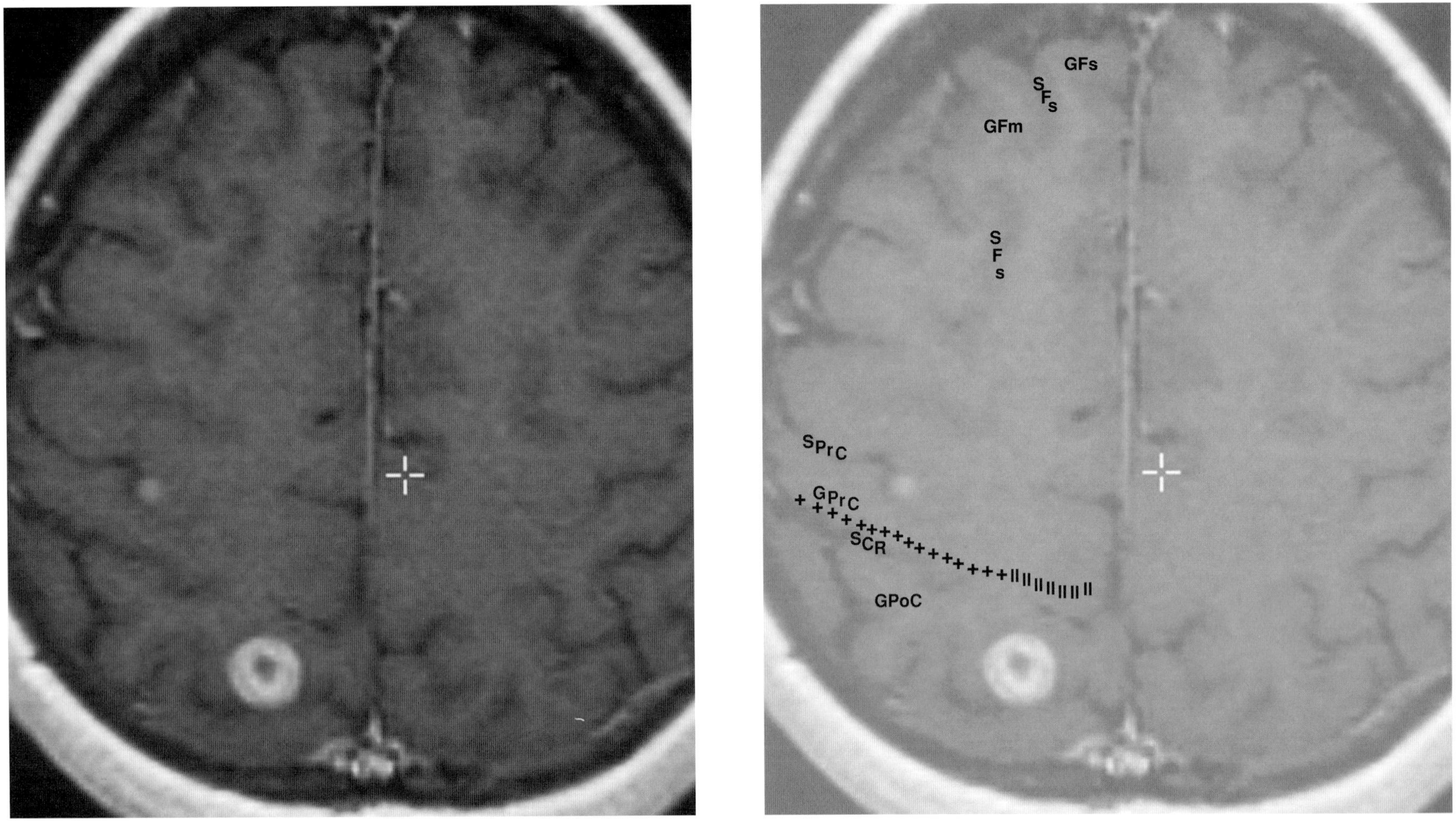

FIG. 3-3A.

FIG. 3-3. Metastatic melanomas, T_1-weighted, contrast-enhanced stereotactic axial MRIs (**A and B**) separated by 3 mm, inferior to superior, respectively. The larger, more posteriorly located tumor resides within the postcentral gyrus (GPoC) on both axial images. The center of this tumor lies approximately 2 cm from the mid-line, immediately opposite the functional regions of the precentral gyrus (GPrC, just across the central sulcus [SCR]) that control voluntary movement of the proximal lower (////) and upper (+ + +) extremities. Thus, injury to the cortex or fiber pathways in the immediate vicinity of the tumor might cause sensory loss (and less likely, weakness) in the trunk, shoulder, proximal arm, and/or proximal leg.

A second, smaller tumor (approximately 3 mm in diameter) is present in **A** just anterior to the precentral sulcus (SPrC). The functional significance of the gray matter and fiber pathways within the precentral gyrus immediately posterior to the tumor include voluntary movement of the arm and hand. *(Figure continued on following page.)*

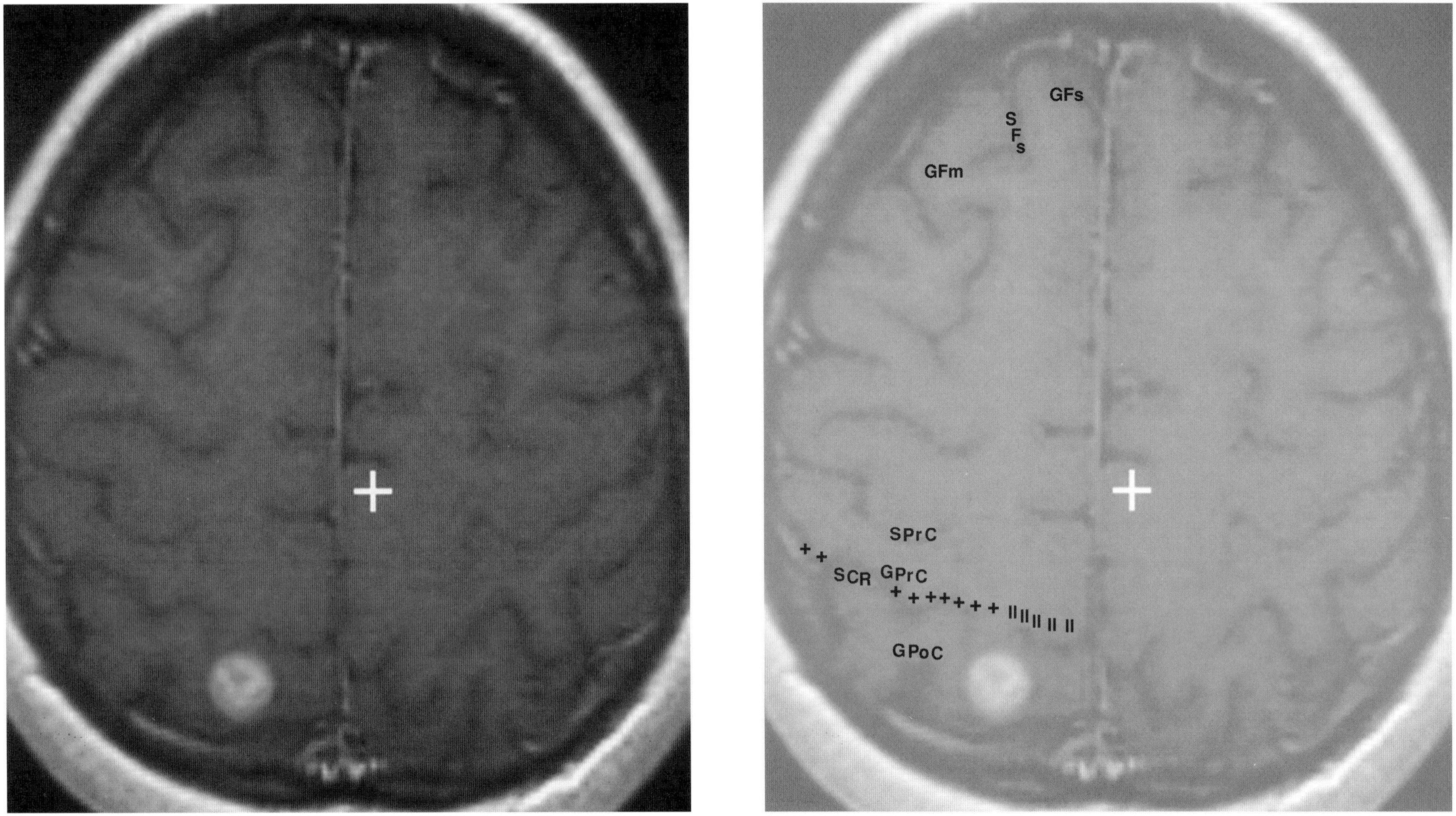

FIG. 3-3B.

FIG. 3-4. Metastatic adenocarcinoma, breast primary, to the left (**A**) and right (**B**) posterior temporal lobes, respectively. T_1-weighted, contrast-enhanced stereotactic axial MRIs separated by 9 mm from inferior to superior. The smaller left-sided tumor (**A**) is located near the confluence of the lingual (GL) and inferior occipital (GOi) gyri posteriorly, the middle occipital gyrus (GOm) anteriorly, and the fusiform gyrus (GF) medially. Although the tumor lies close to the optic radiation (RO), that pathway travels superior and lateral to the tumor (**B**). Radiosurgical treatment of this tumor would not be likely to cause a visual field defect unless tissue damage (or tumor growth) extended another 10 mm or more superiorly from the axial level of **A**.

The right-sided tumor in **B** is located within the white matter immediately lateral and inferior to the occipital horn of the lateral ventricle (not seen on this image). The choroid plexus (ChP) within the temporal horn is located approximately 14 mm anterior to the tumor margin. The middle occipital and medial occipitotemporal gyri (GOm and GOT) flank the tumor on the lateral and medial sides, respectively. The middle temporal gyrus (GTm) lies well anterior to the tumor margin. Thus, the tumor is situated within the course of the optic radiations (RO). Damage to this pathway caused by the tumor itself, surgical intervention, or as a complication of radiosurgery would be expected to cause a congruous contralateral (left-sided) visual field defect. *(Figure continued on following pages.)*

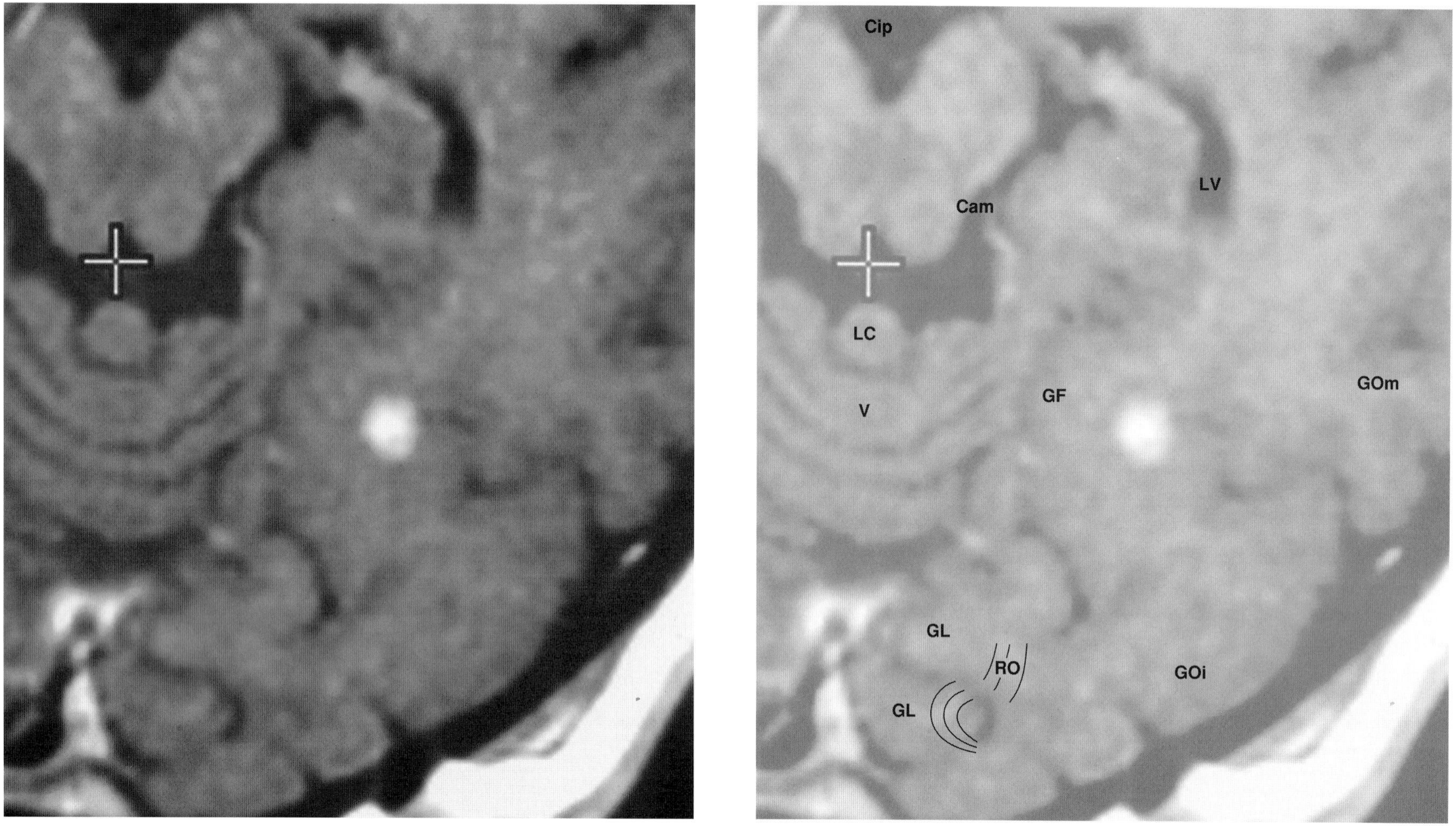

FIG. 3-4A.

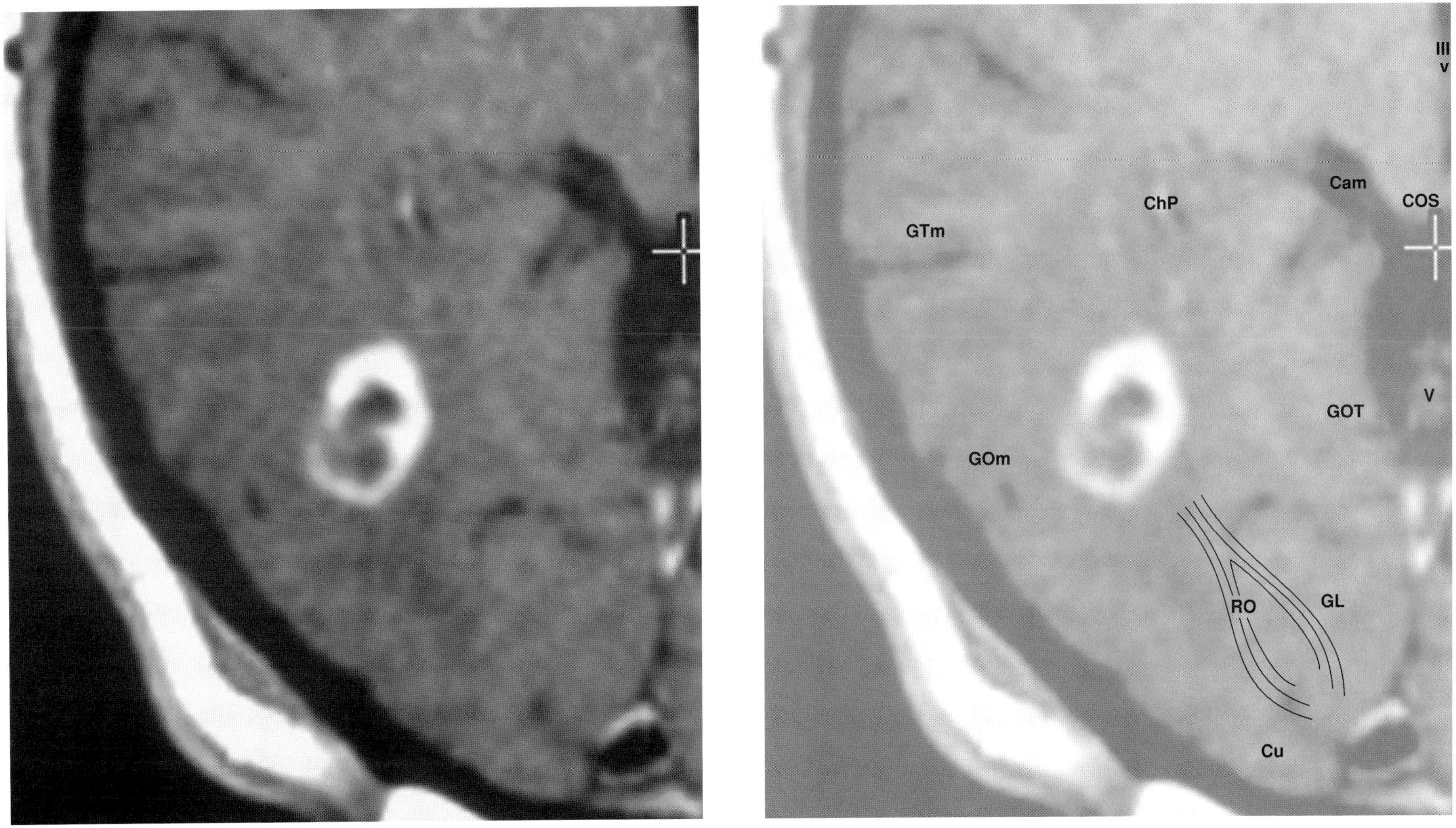

FIG. 3-4B.

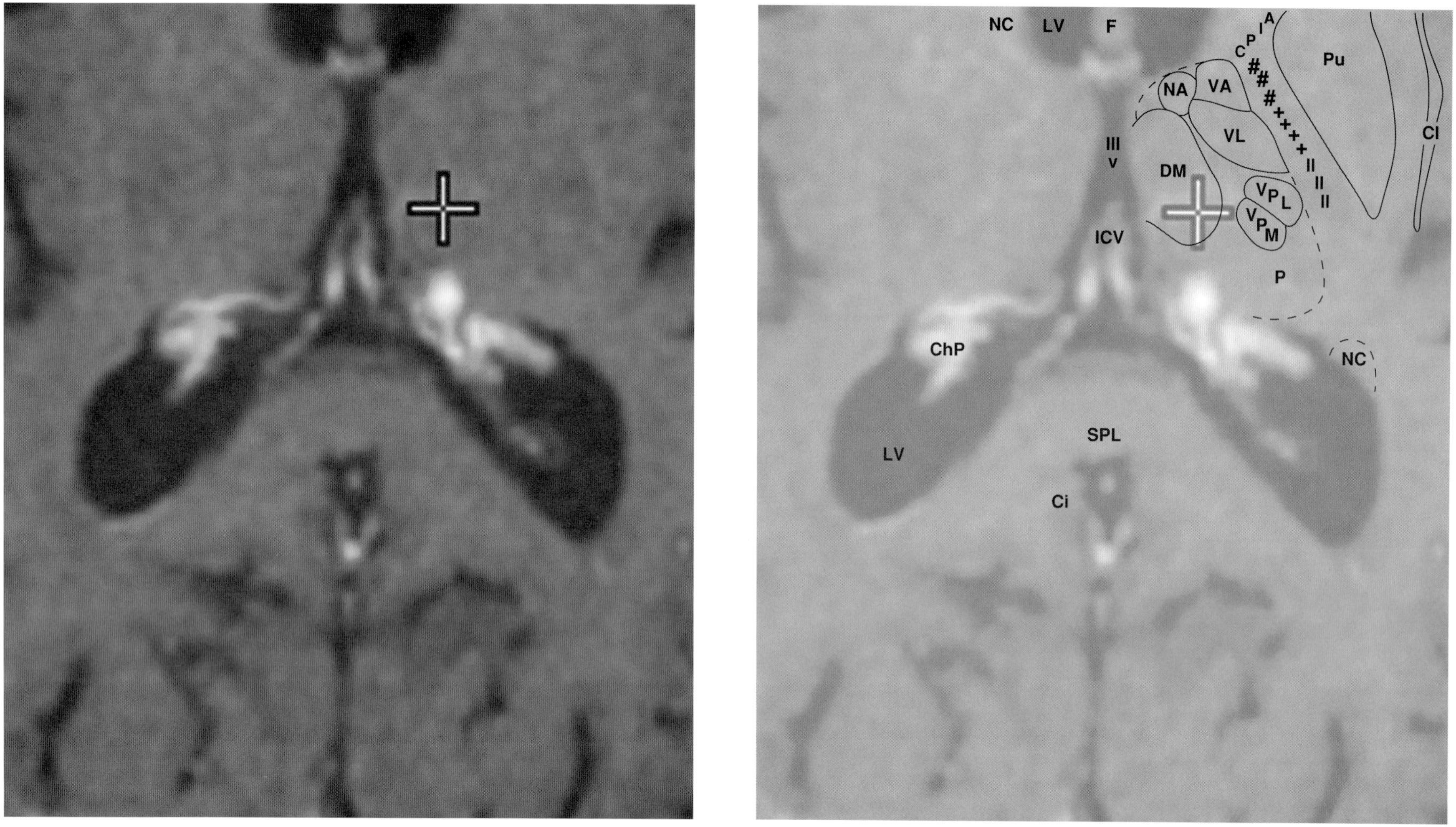

FIG. 3-5A.

FIG. 3-5. Metastatic hypernephroma (renal cell carcinoma) involving the left posterior thalamus and choroid plexus. Contrast enhanced, T_1-weighted stereotactic axial MRIs separated by 3 mm from inferior to superior. **A:** The inferior portion of the tumor appears to reside within the posterior portion of the pulvinar (P). An enhancing vascular pedicle connects the tumor to the choroid plexus (ChP) located posteriorly within the atrium of the left lateral ventricle (LV). **B:** Three millimeters more superiorly, the tumor is situated at the thalamus–cerebrospinal fluid interface, having its anterior portion within the pulvinar and its posterior half within the choroid plexus. The splenium of the corpus callosum (SPL) lies well posterior to the tumor, across the fluid-containing space of the lateral ventricle. The internal cerebral veins (ICV) lie several millimeters medial to the tumor within the posterior third ventricle (IIIv). At the level of **A** the thalamic sensory relay nuclei (VPL, VPM) are located anterior to the pulvinar, whereas more superiorly in **B** the lateral posterior nucleus (LP) is found occupying a similar position within the dorsal tier of thalamic nuclei. In both axial planes the posterior (sensory) portion of the posterior limb of the internal capsule (CPIP) lies lateral to the pulvinar and separates the thalamus from the putamen (Pu) and external capsule (CPE).

Because the pulvinar is a silent region of the thalamus, no neurologic deficit would be expected unless tumor growth, surgical injury, or radiation-induced tissue damage extended well beyond the margins of the tumor illustrated here. *(Figure continued on following page.)*

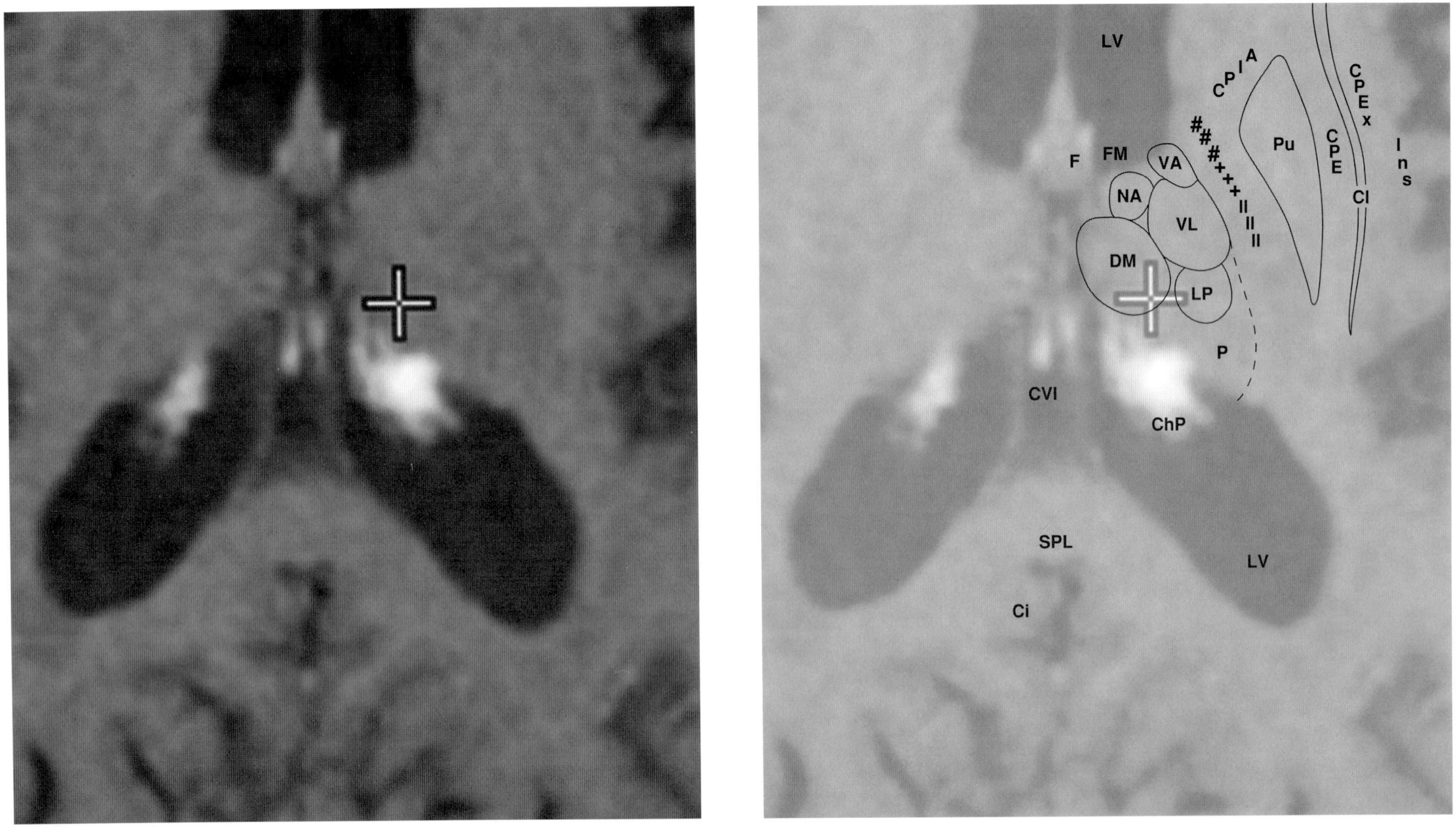

FIG. 3-5B.

FIG. 3-6. Metastatic malignant melanoma involving the margin of the body of the right lateral ventricle, T_1-weighted, contrast-enhanced stereotactic axial MRI. This 15-mm tumor actually resides within the body of the right caudate nucleus (NC), which forms the lateral ventricular margin (LV) at this level. The medial tumor margin bulges into the cerebrospinal fluid–filled cavity of the ventricle, whereas the lateral margin encroaches upon the corona radiata. Fibers of the corticospinal (pyramidal, Pyr) tract, in their superolateral-to-inferomedial course toward the internal capsule, pass along the lateral margin of the tumor. The somatotopic order of the pyramidal tract is illustrated from anterior to posterior as face (##), arm (+ + +), and leg (////), respectively.

Thus, damage to neural tissue along the lateral tumor margin caused by surgery, radiosurgery, or tumor growth would result in a contralateral hemiparesis involving the face as well as the arm and leg. *(Figure continued on following page.)*

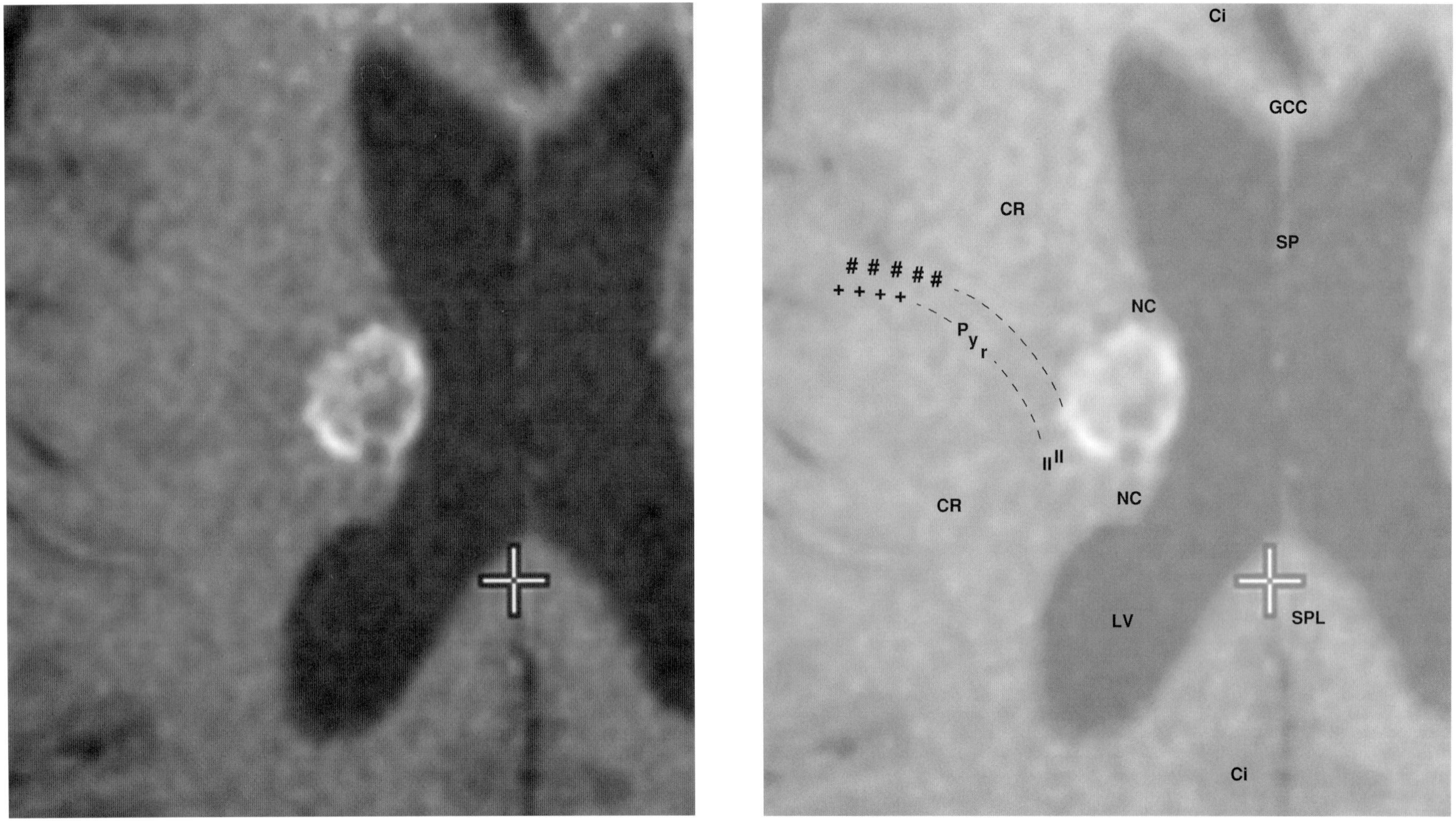

FIG. 3-6.

FIG. 3-7. Metastatic carcinoma, non–small cell lung primary, within the splenium of the corpus callosum (SPL). T_1-weighted, contrast-enhanced stereotactic axial MRI (same patient and MR series as in Fig. 3-19). This 12-mm ovoid tumor occupies the posterior two thirds of the splenium, exactly in the mid-line. Anteriorly, beyond the remaining tissue of the corpus callosum, the internal cerebral veins (ICV) lie within the velum interpositum. The posterior portion of the body of the fornix (F) lies between the splenium and the posterior thalamus on either side of the mid-line. The lateral dorsal (LD) nucleus and pulvinar (P) of the thalamus form the posterior thalamic margin at this level. The posterior tumor margin abuts the cingulate gyrus (Ci) on either side but does not appear to involve that structure. The precuneus (PCu) lies just posterior to the cingulate gyrus at this level.

Because this tumor involves only a portion of the corpus callosum, radiosurgical treatment would not be expected to cause an interhemispheric disconnection syndrome. *(Figure continued on following page.)*

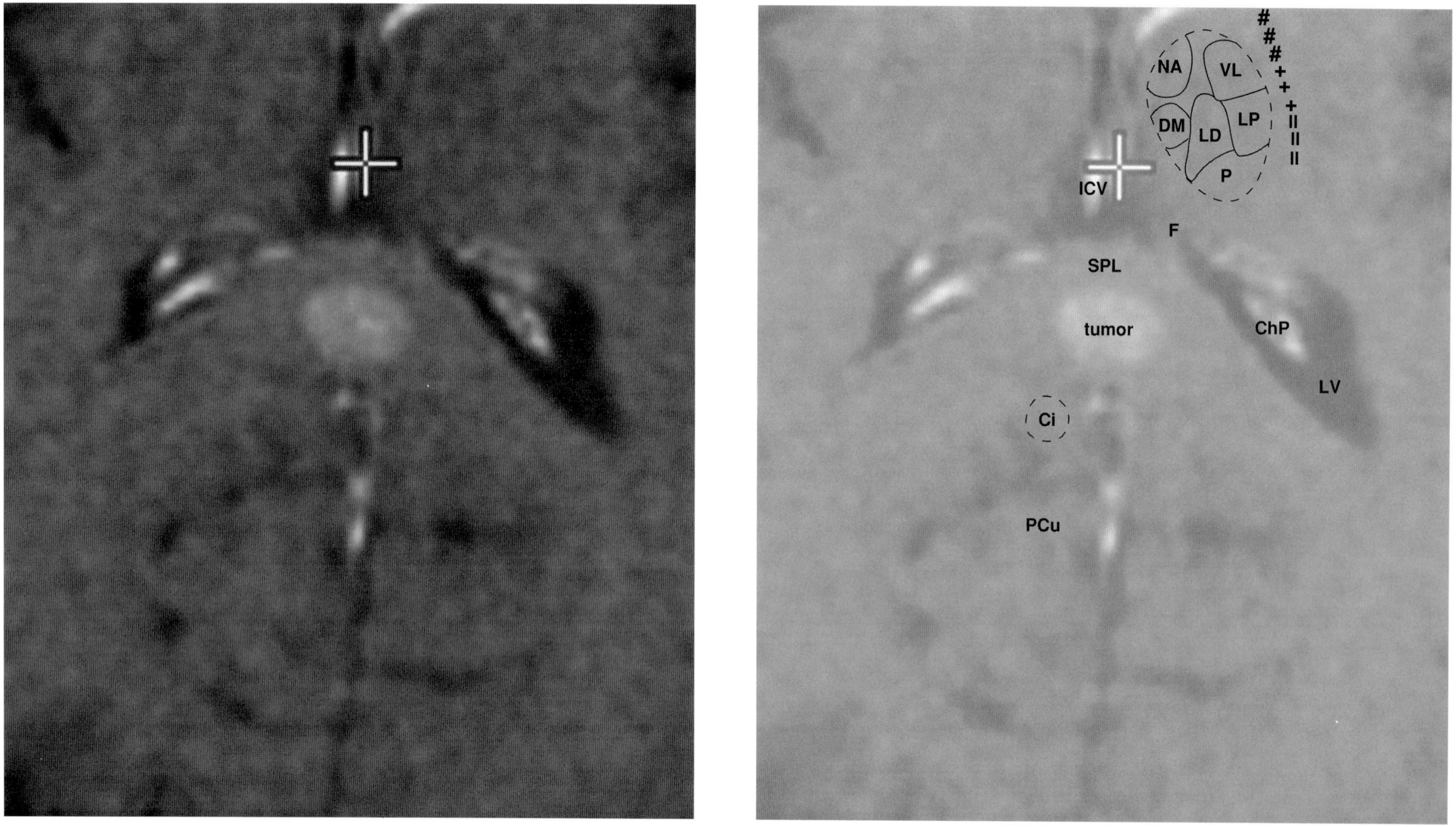

FIG. 3-7.

FIG. 3-8. Metastatic malignant melanoma deep in the left frontal lobe at the level of the head of the caudate nucleus, T_1-weighted, contrast-enhanced stereotactic axial MRIs separated by 6 mm from inferior to superior. The 11-mm diameter anterior tumor almost touches the head of the caudate nucleus (NC) at the anteromedial tumor margin. Moderate surrounding edema and mass effect displace the claustrum (Cl), extreme capsule (CPEx), and insular cortex (Ins) laterally. At this axial level, the lateral tumor margin also crosses the most superior edge of the putamen (Pu). The posterior limb of the internal capsule (CPIP) lies within 8 mm of the posterior tumor margin. The most inferior fibers of the pyramidal tract cross above the claustrum just superior to this plane of section and pass within 3 mm of the tumor margin to form the most anterior portion of the posterior limb of the internal capsule (CPIP). An open surgical approach to this tumor, a complication of radiosurgery that caused an expanding zone of necrosis, or uncontrolled tumor growth all could cause a contralateral (right-sided) hemiparesis that involved the hand (+ + +) and face (###), corresponding to the closest fibers of the corticospinal pathway.

The posterior tumor (**B**) resides within the cortex of the superior border of the insula at the level of the postcentral gyrus (GPoC) and postcentral sulcus. The pyramidal tract (Pyr) crosses deep, anterior, and medial to the tumor, whereas the most inferior edge of the inferior parietal lobule (LPi), including the supramarginal gyrus (GSm), lies posterior and lateral to the tumor. Still more posteriorly, the extreme superior edge of the superior temporal gyrus (GTs) can be seen within the posterior portion of the sylvian fissure (Syl). *(Figure continued on following pages.)*

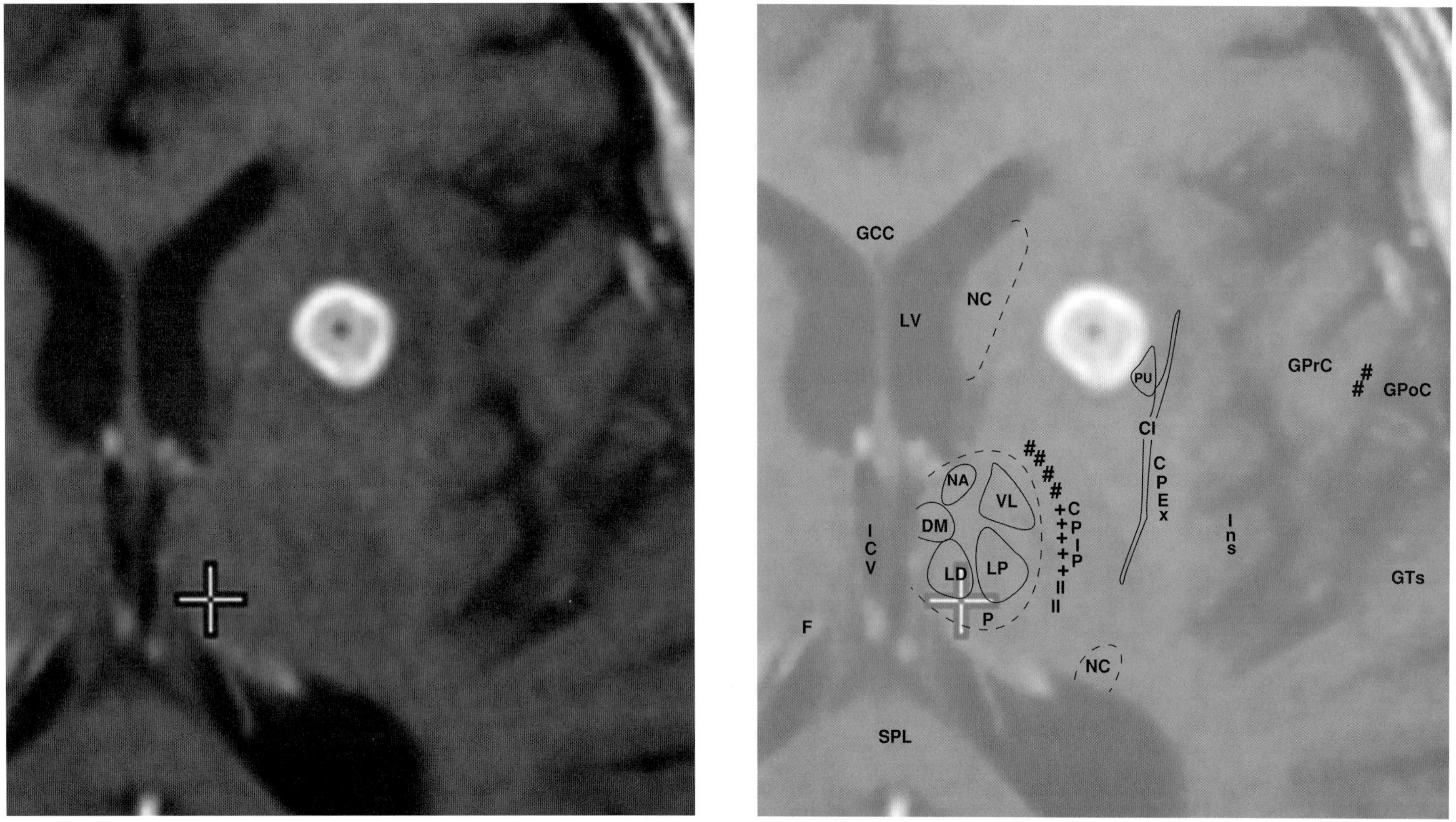
GCC
NC
LV
PU
GPrC
GPoC
CI
CPEx
NA
VL
DM
ICV
LD
LP
CPIP
P
F
Ins
GTs
NC
SPL

FIG. 3-8A.

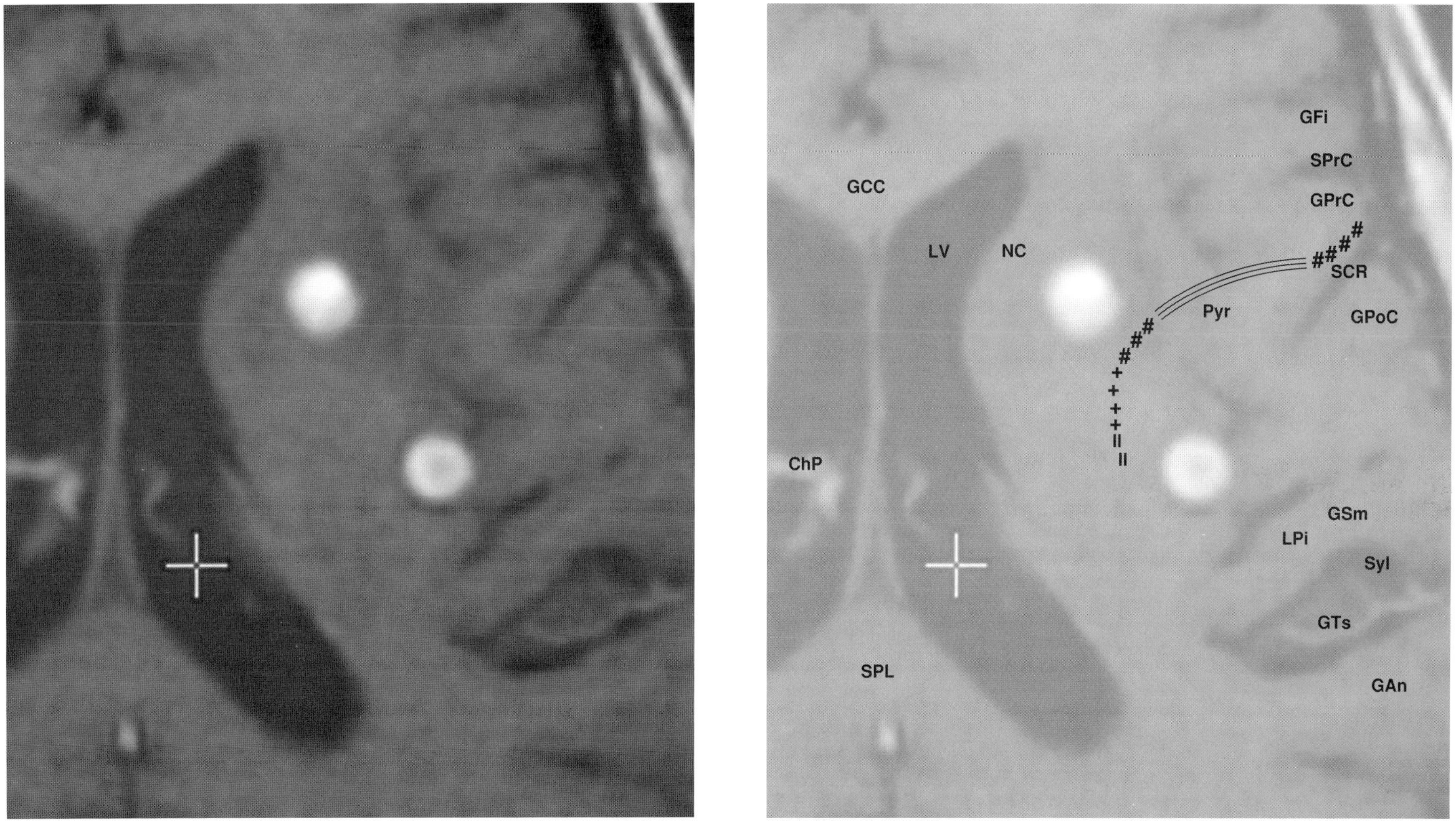

FIG. 3-8B.

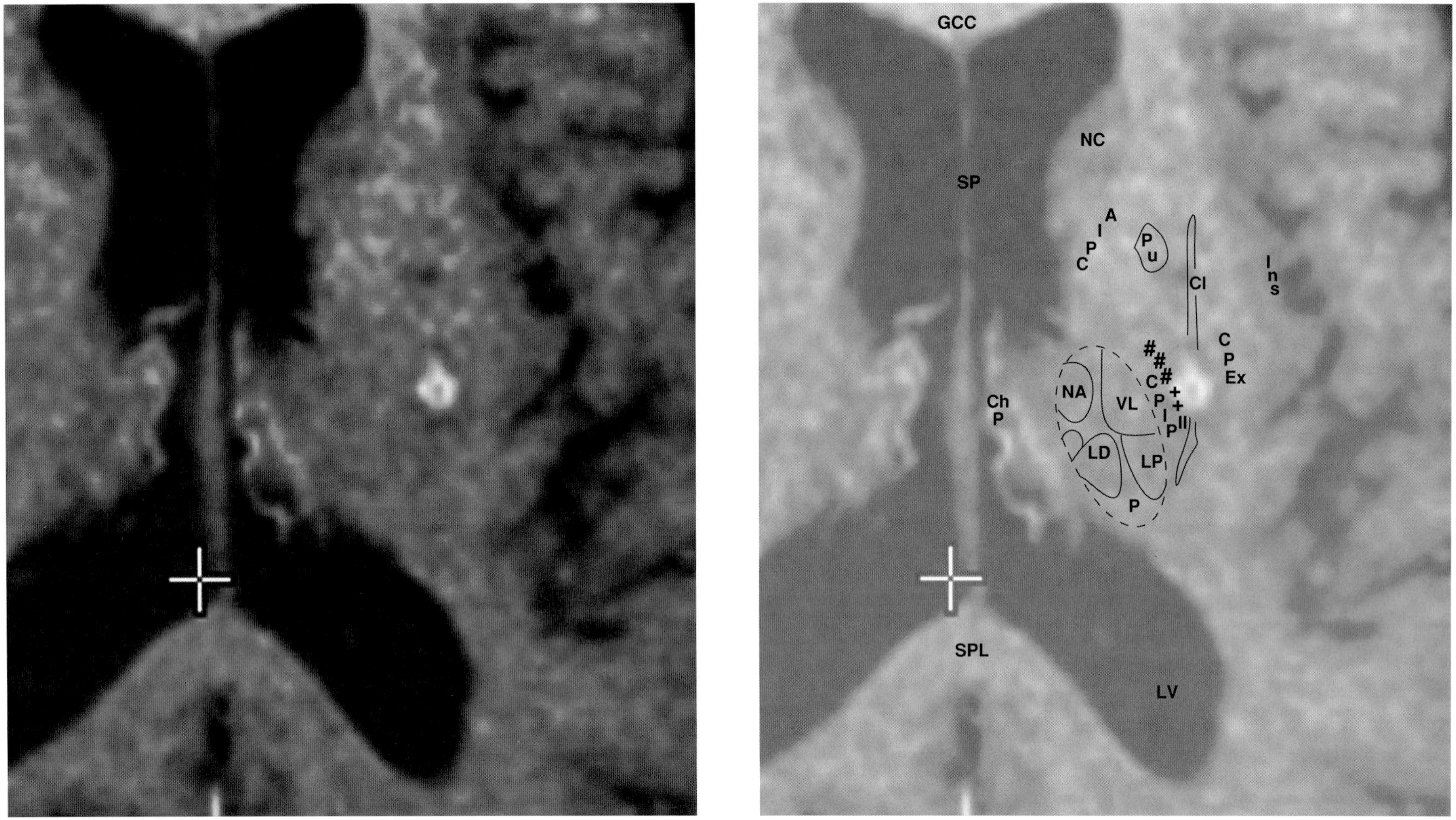

FIG. 3-9.

FIG. 3-9. Metastatic malignant melanoma to the left internal capsule, same patient and T_1-weighted, contrast-enhanced stereotactic axial MRI series as in Fig. 3-6, only 9 mm more inferior. This tumor lies at the superolateral edge of the posterior limb of the internal capsule (CPIP) on the left side. The medial tumor margin involves the corticospinal pathways that control voluntary motion of the arm (+ +) and face (##) on the right side. The lateral tumor margin crosses the external capsule and claustrum (Cl). The dorsal tier of thalamic nuclei lie well away from the tumor, medial to the internal capsule.

When this tumor and the one illustrated in Fig. 3-6 are considered together, one can appreciate that treatment-induced tissue injury or unchecked tumor growth around both lesions could lead to quadriparesis, which in reality would represent a bilateral hemiparesis.

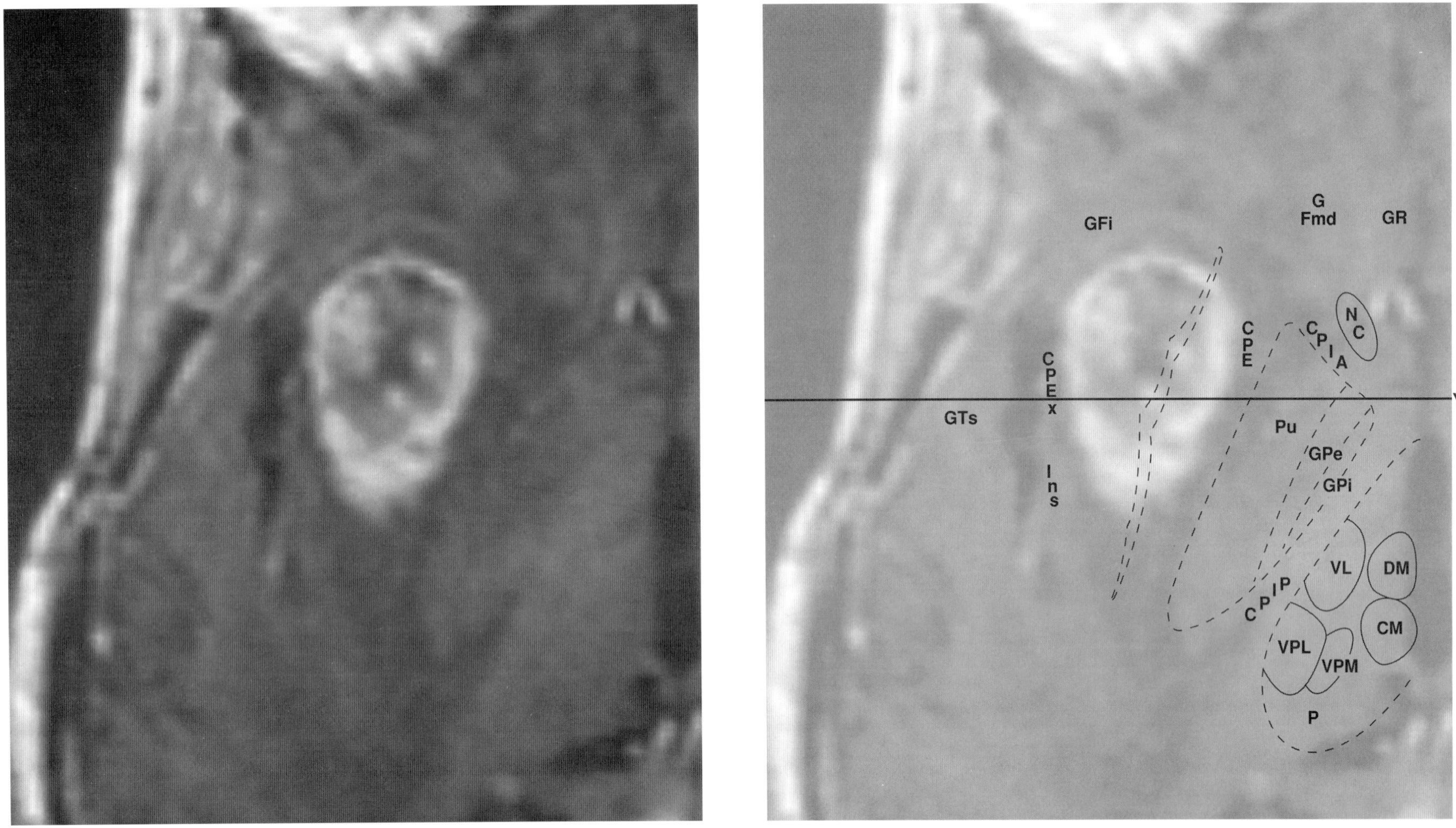
GFi
G
Fmd
GR
N
C
C
P
I
A
C
P
E
C
P
E
x
Y
GTs
Pu
GPe
GPi
I
n
s
VL
DM
C
P
I
P
CM
VPL
VPM
P

FIG. 3-10A.

FIG. 3-10. Metastatic carcinoma to the right basal ganglia and frontal operculum, non–small cell lung primary. T_1-weighted, contrast-enhanced stereotactic MRIs in the axial (**A**) and coronal (**B**) planes. Line Y on the axial image (**A**) denotes the coronal plane of **B**; line Z on the coronal image (**B**) denotes the axial plane of **A**. The patient is positioned within the stereotactic frame with the neck extended somewhat. Therefore, the plane of **B** passes through the anterior commissure (AC), infundibular recess of the third ventricle (IIIv), and optic tract (TO). In **A**, the medial tumor margin lies in the plane approximately 4 mm inferior to the anterior commissure, whereas the imaging plane of the posterior third ventricle passes through the stria medullaris thalami at a considerable distance superior to the intercommissural line.

The tumor lies lateral to the anterior half of the putamen (Pu) and appears to engulf most of the claustrum (Cl), external capsule, and extreme capsule (CPE, CPEx). The inferior frontal gyrus (GFi) and the anterior limb of the internal capsule (CPIA) are compressed and displaced anteriorly; the insula (Ins), extreme capsule, sylvian fissure (Syl), and superior temporal gyrus (GTs) are displaced laterally; and the stem of the temporal lobe, and probably the temporal horn of the lateral ventricle, are compressed inferiorly by the respective tumor margins. Significant edema and mass effect displace the external capsule, lentiform nucleus (Pu and GP), caudate nucleus (NC), and ventricular system medially, from right to left. The most inferior fibers of the pyramidal tract (Pyr) that correspond to the face area (##) of the precentral gyrus pass from lateral to medial above the tumor in **B** and leave the plane of imaging as they travel toward the posterior limb of the internal capsule (CPIP).

More posteriorly in **A**, peritumoral edema displaces the posterior limb of the internal capsule and the lateral border of the thalamus toward the mid-line. The principal danger of this tumor is its mass effect upon the basal ganglia, internal capsule, and ventricular system rather than direct neoplastic involvement of those structures. *(Figure continued on following page.)*

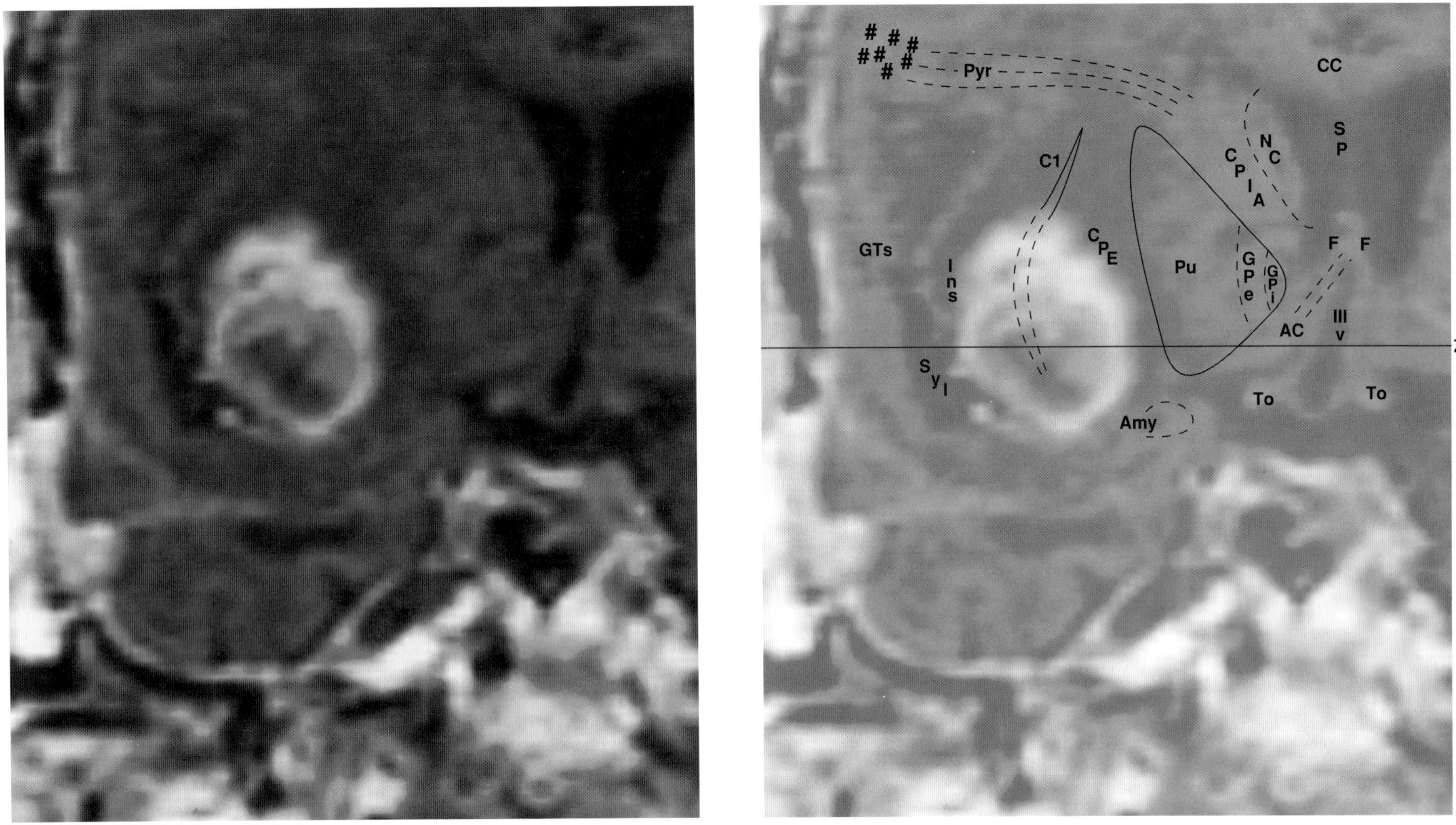
Pyr
CC
SP
NC
CPIA
C1
CPE
GTs
Ins
Pu
GPe
GPi
F
F
AC
III v
Z
Syl
To
To
Amy

FIG. 3-10B.

FIG. 3-11. Metastatic carcinoma, breast primary, to the right basal ganglia and upper brain stem. T_1-weighted, contrast enhanced stereotactic MRIs in the axial plane separated by 3 mm from inferior to superior (**A and B**) and in the coronal plane through the center of the tumor (**C**). On the axial images the anterior tumor margin appears to invade and/or displace the posterior margin of the putamen (Pu) and globus pallidus (GPe, GPi). A portion of the posterior limb of the internal capsule (CPIP) also appears to be engulfed by the anterior and medial edges of the tumor. The medial tumor margin just reaches the subthalamic nucleus (CL) anteriorly and approaches the edge of the substantia nigra (SN) more posteriorly. The lateral geniculate body (CGl) is surrounded by the posteromedial tumor margin, whereas the optic radiation (RO) is interrupted by the posterior and posterolateral tumor margins.

Similar anatomical relationships are illustrated in the coronal plane (**C**). Here the superolateral tumor margin occupies the caudal portion of the putamen and globus pallidus, whereas the medial tumor margin invades and displaces the posterior limb of the internal capsule (CPIP). A thin sliver of internal capsule remains between the tumor and the thalamus (VL and VPL nuclei). Again, the inferomedial tumor margin encroaches upon the subthalamic nucleus and substantia nigra. More laterally, the inferior edge of the tumor crosses the choroidal fissure and temporal horn of the lateral ventricle (LV) to indent the superior edge of the hippocampal formation (H).

Neurologic deficits likely to arise from this tumor would include a left hemiparesis (internal capsule) and left homonymous hemaniopsia (optic radiations, lateral geniculate body), both of which were present in this patient. *(Figure continued on following pages.)*

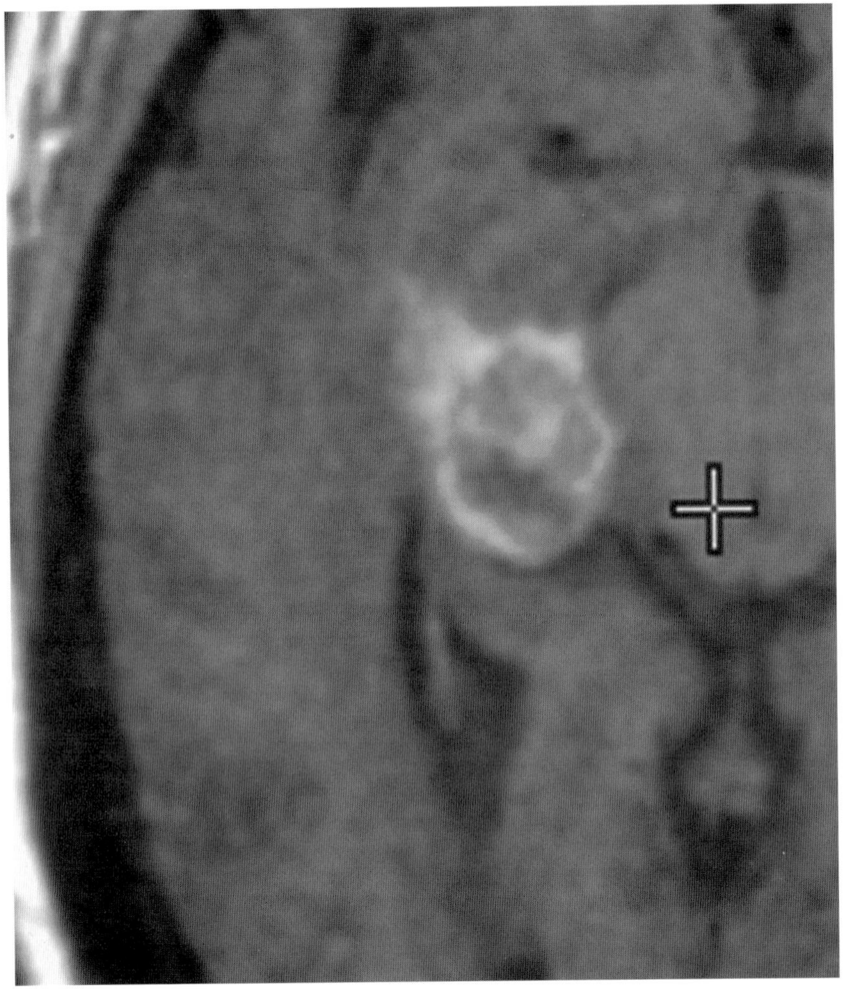

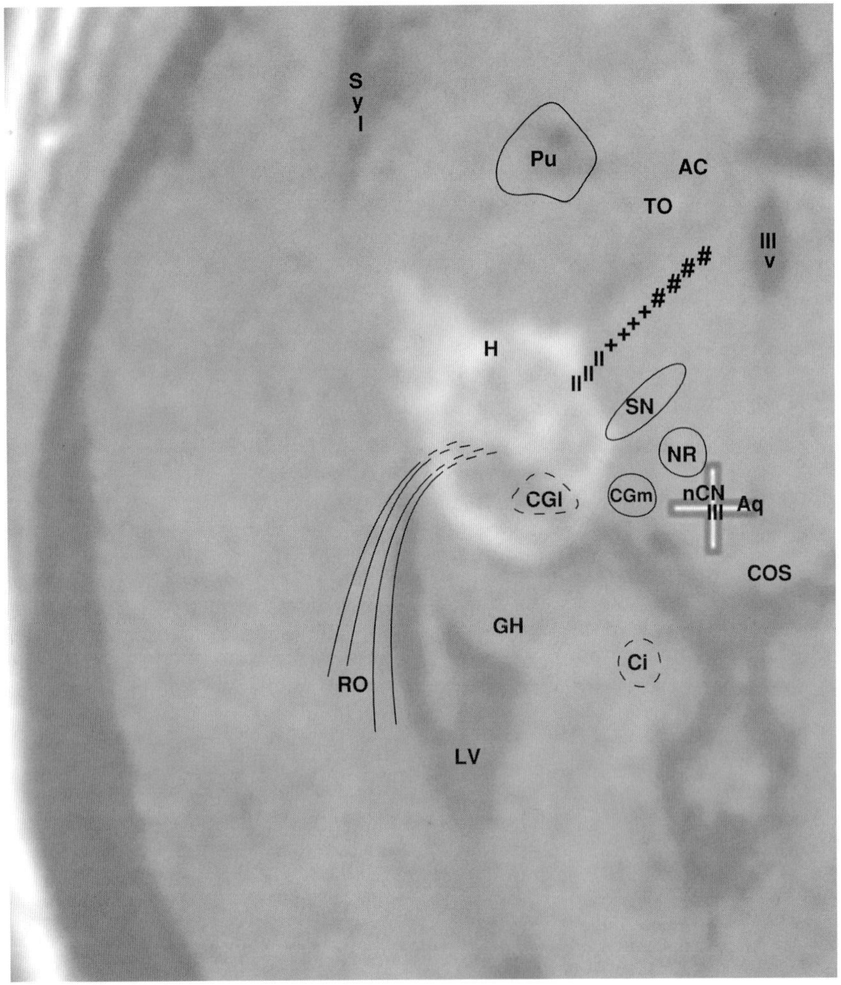

FIG. 3-11A.

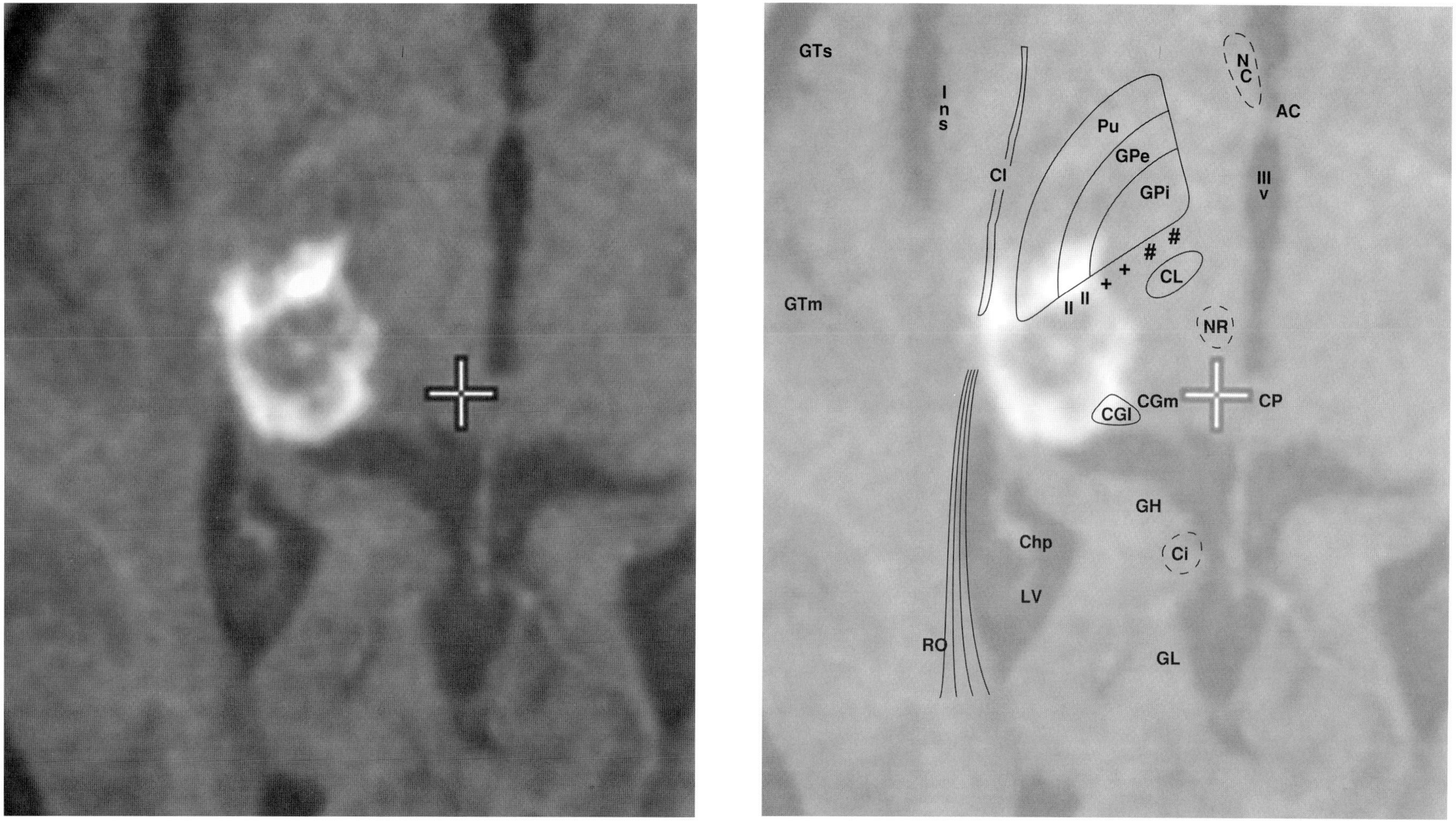
GTs
Ins
Cl
Pu
GPe
GPi
NC
AC
III v
GTm
CL
NR
CGl
CGm
CP
GH
Chp
Ci
LV
RO
GL

FIG. 3-11B.

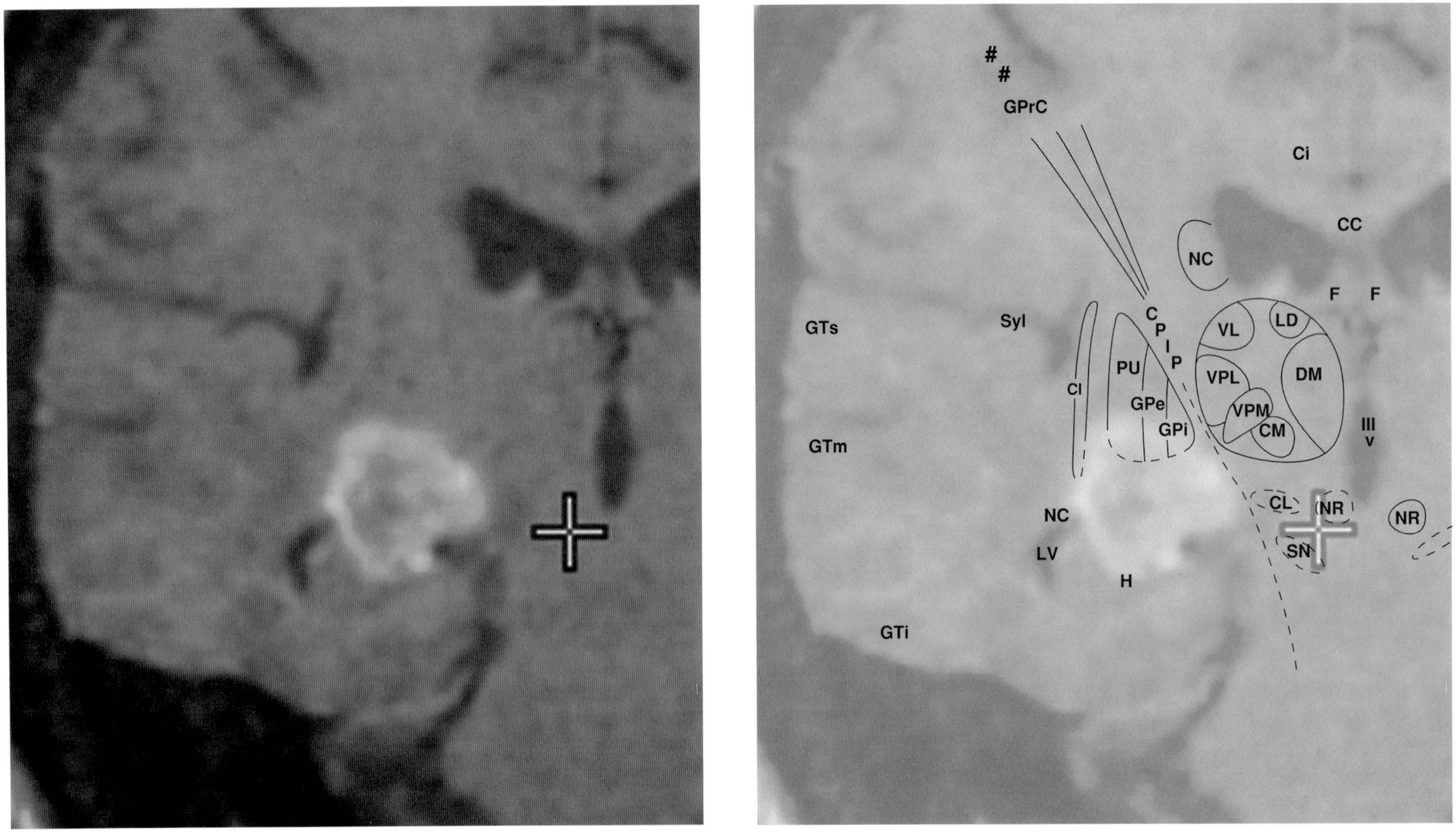
#
#
GPrC
Ci
CC
NC
F
F
GTs
Syl
C
P
I
P
LD
VL
PU
DM
VPL
Cl
GPe
VPM
GPi
CM
III
v
GTm
CL
NR
NR
NC
SN
LV
H
GTi

FIG. 3-11C.

FIG. 3-12. Metastatic carcinoma, lung primary, within the left thalamus, hypothalamus, and third ventricle. T_1-weighted, contrast-enhanced stereotactic axial MRIs separated by 6 mm from inferior to superior. The axial plane of **A** passes through the anterior commissure (AC) and through the habenular commissure (CmHb). **B** passes through the foramen of Monro (FoM) parallel to **A**. The tumor occupies and/or displaces a substantial portion of the left thalamus (NA, VA, VL, DM, and CM nuclei), fills the central portion of the third ventricle (IIIv), completely occludes the left foramen of Monro, and causes asymmetric obstructive hydrocephalus (more severe on the left side). The tumor appears to cross the third ventricle (alternatively, it may traverse and enlarge the masa intermedia of the thalamus) to exert mass effect upon the anterior portion of the right thalamus.

The anterior tumor margin displaces the fornix (F) anteriorly in both imaging planes and tilts the left side of the anterior commissure forward in **A**. The anterolateral tumor margin nearly obliterates the genu and anterior half of the posterior limb of the internal capsule (CPIP) and pushes the medial corner of the globus pallidus (GPi) laterally. The corticospinal fibers within the internal capsule that correspond to the face (###) and upper extremity (+ + +) are affected most. *(Figure continued on following pages.)*

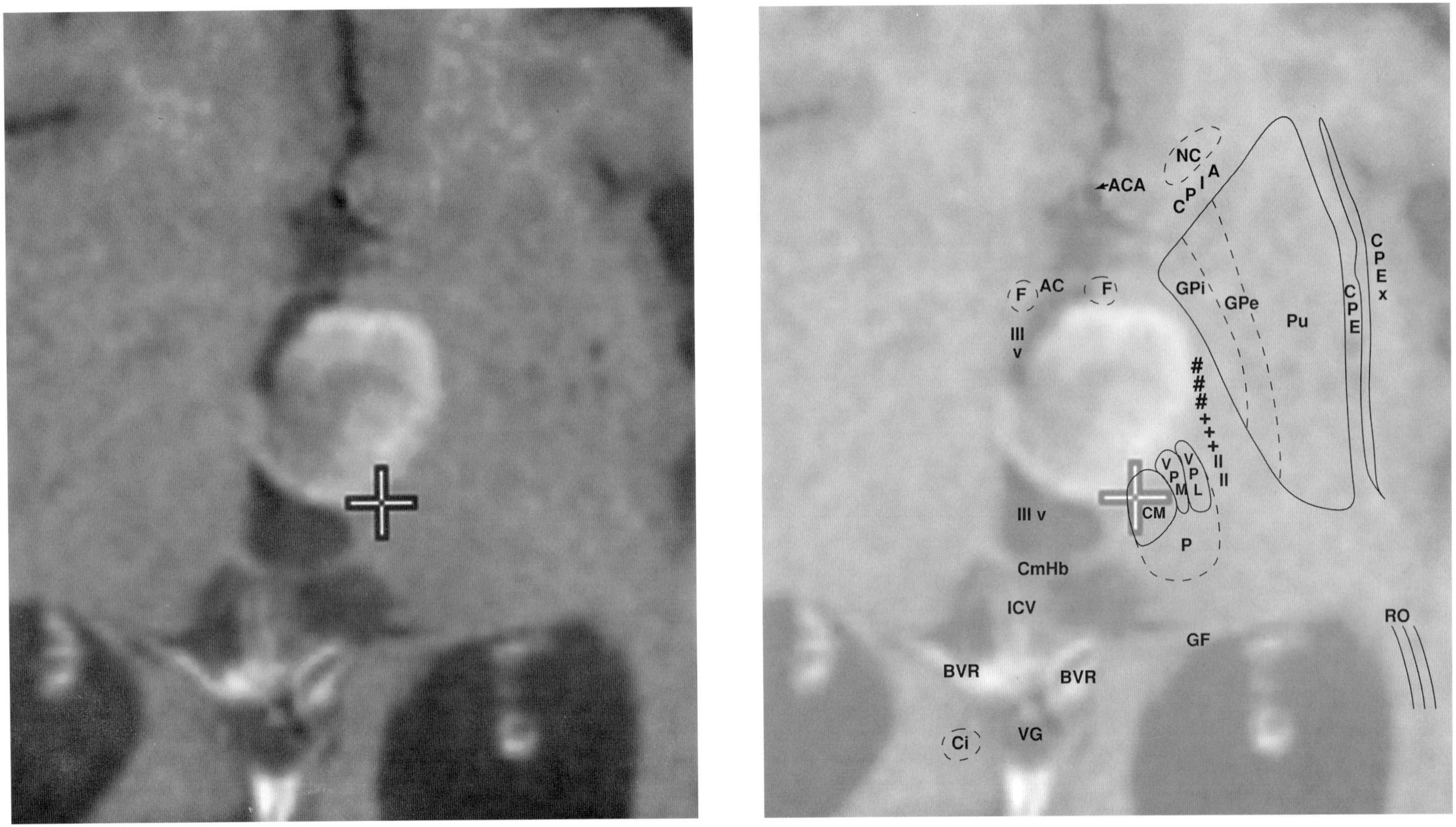

NC
ACA
C P I A
C P E x
F
AC
F
GPi
GPe
Pu
C P E
III v
# # #
+ + +
II II
V P M
V P L
CM
III v
P
CmHb
ICV
RO
GF
BVR
BVR
Ci
VG

FIG. 3-12A.

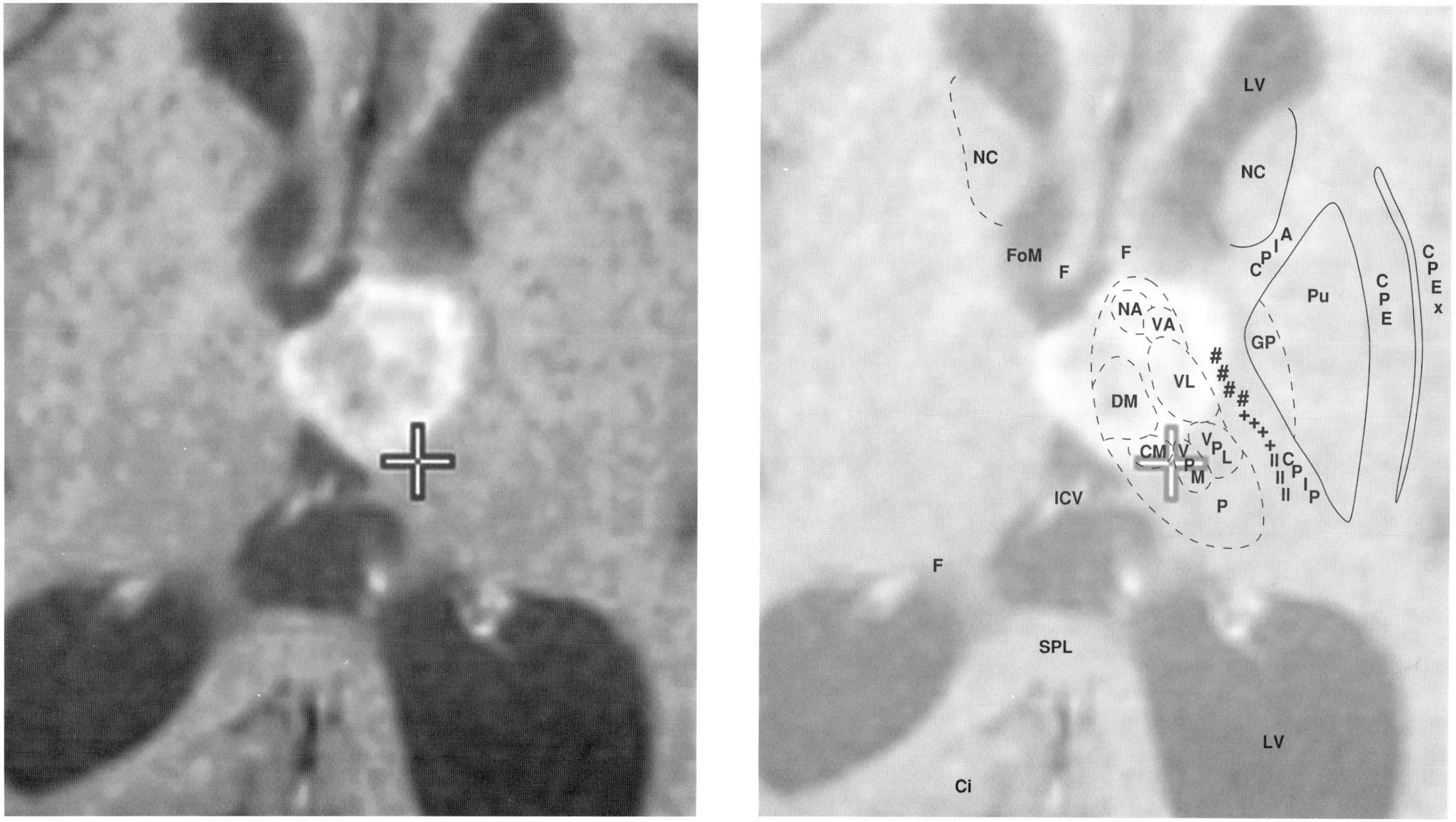
LV
NC
NC
FoM
F
F
CPIA
Pu
GP
CPE
CPEx
NA
VA
VL
DM
CM
VPL
VPM
P
CPIP
ICV
F
SPL
LV
Ci

FIG. 3-12B.

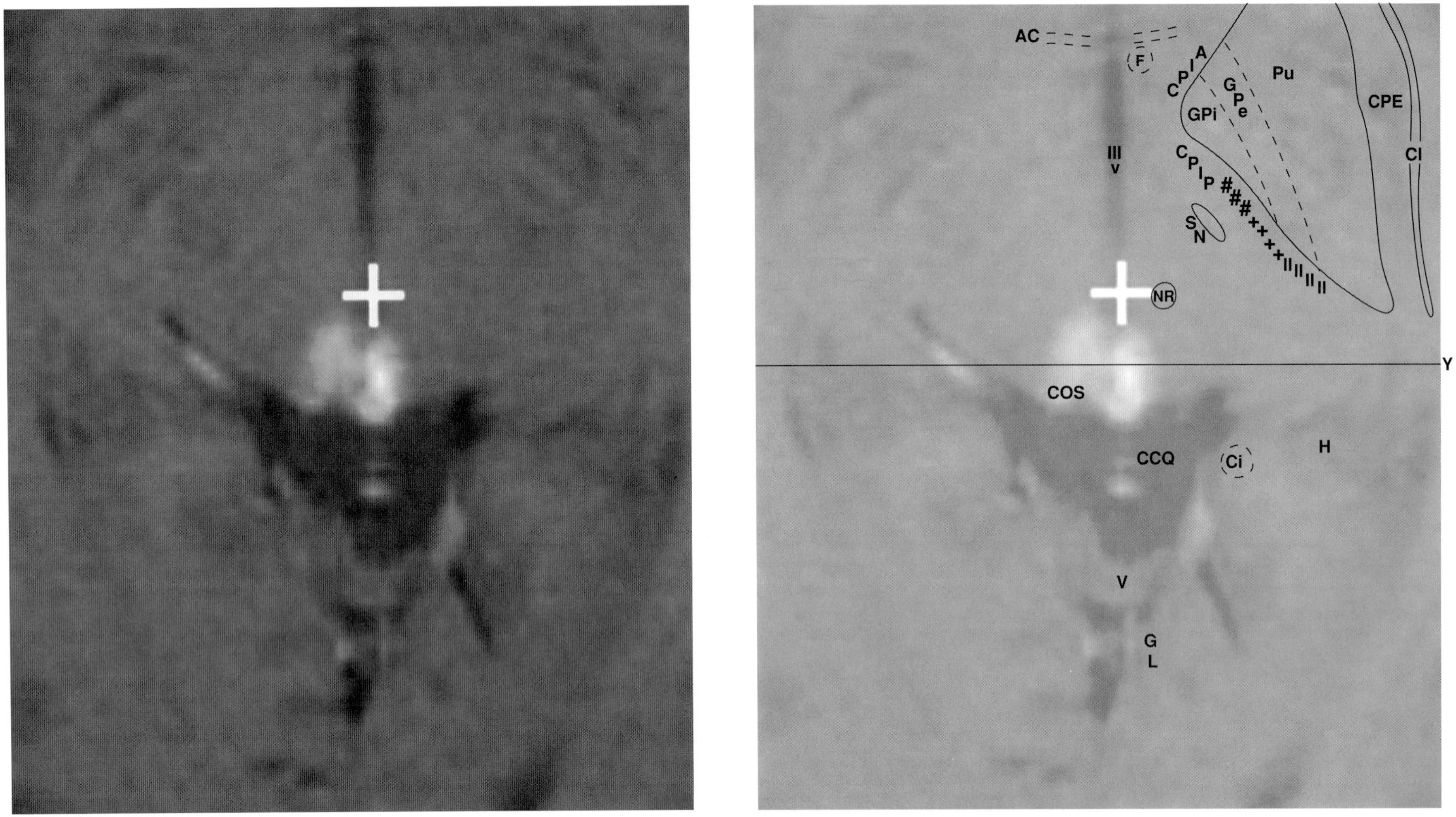

FIG. 3-13A.

FIG. 3-13. Glioblastoma multiforme of the pineal region. T_1-weighted, contrast-enhanced stereotactic MRIs separated by 6 mm from inferior to superior in the axial plane (**A and B**) and through the center of the tumor in the coronal plane (**C**). The axial levels of **A** and **B** are shown in **C** as lines Z_1 and Z_2, respectively. Likewise, line Y on the axial images indicates the plane of **C**.

The anterior inferior tumor margin invades the dorsal mid-brain and posterior third ventricle (IIIv) through the level of the posterior commissure (which is engulfed by the tumor), whereas the posterior tumor margin protrudes into the quadrigeminal plate cistern (CCQ). The superior edge of the red nuclei on either side (NR) lie 2 mm anterior to the tumor. The superior edge of the substantia nigra (SN) and corticospinal fibers of the internal capsule (CPIP) lie much farther anterolateral to the tumor in **A**. The central and superior portion of the tumor invades the posterior thalamus almost symmetrically on both sides. At the level of **B**, the internal cerebral veins (ICV) and basal vein of Rosenthal (BVR) join the vein of Galen immediately behind the posterior tumor margin. Because the pineal gland itself cannot be identified distinct from the tumor on any imaging plane, the tumor is presumed to arise from that structure.

The most likely clinically detectable effects of tissue damage immediately surrounding this tumor would be a Parinaud's syndrome as a consequence of injury to the posterior commissure region at the inferior tumor margin. Hydrocephalus also could arise secondary to posterior third ventricular or aqueductal obstruction. *(Figure continued on following pages.)*

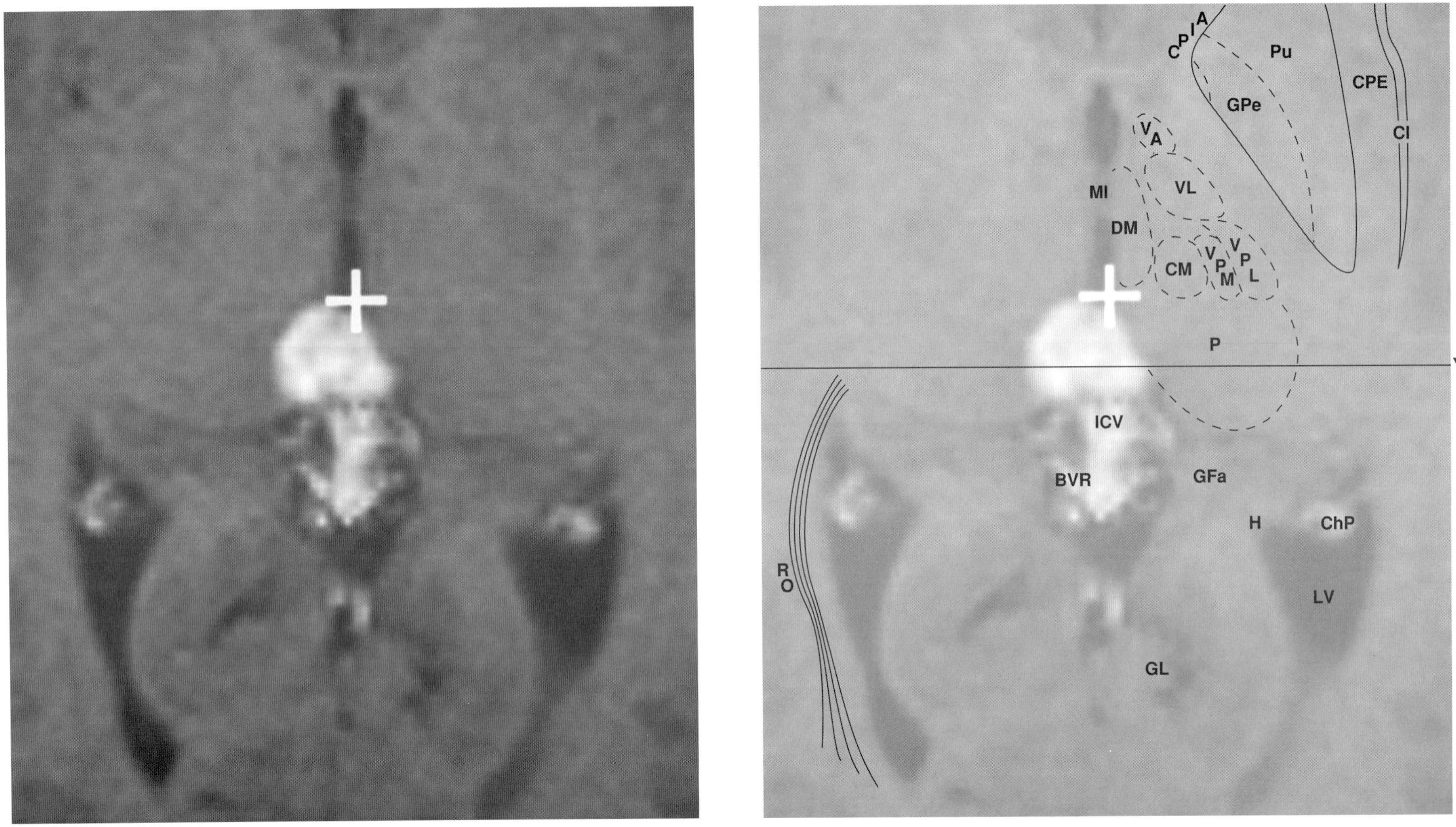
CPIA
Pu
CPE
GPe
CI
VA
MI
VL
DM
CM
VPM
VPL
P
Y
ICV
BVR
GFa
H
ChP
RO
LV
GL

FIG. 3-13B.

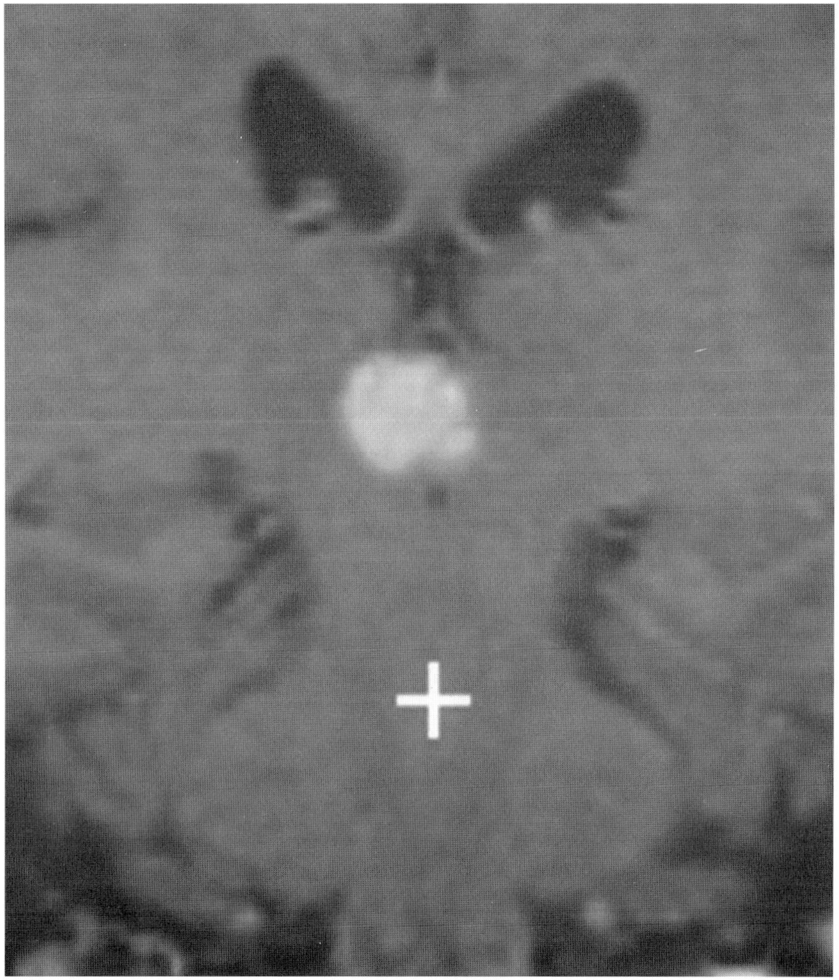

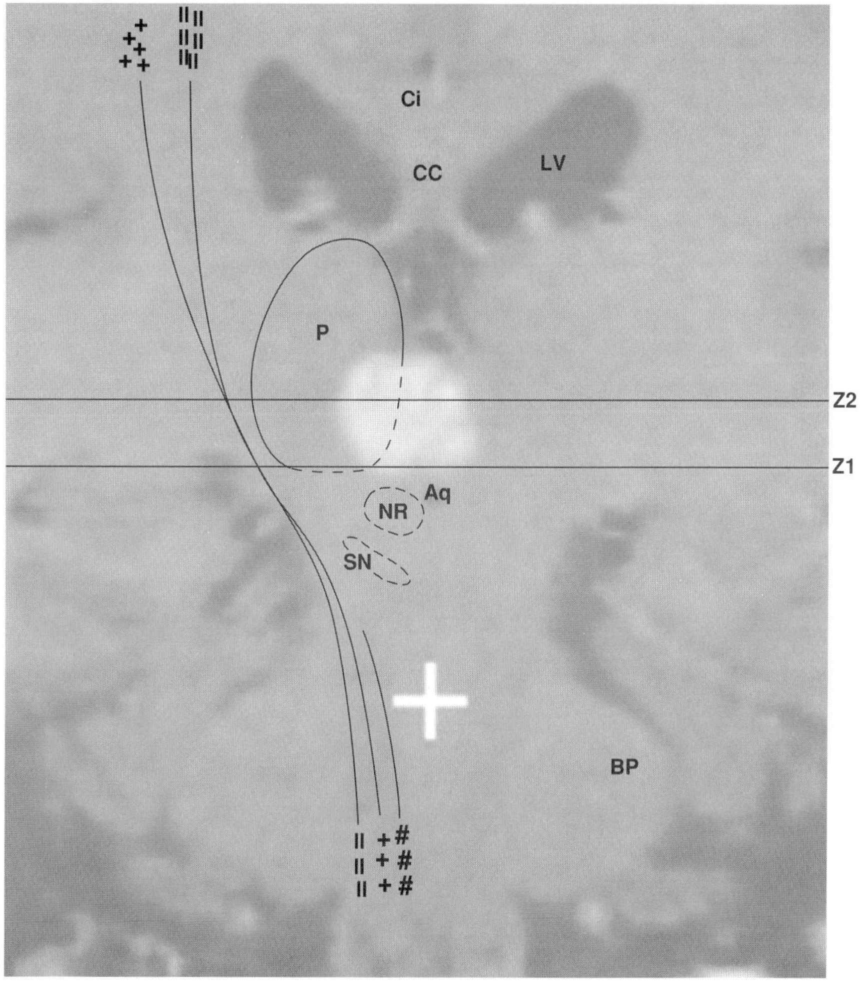

FIG. 3-13C.

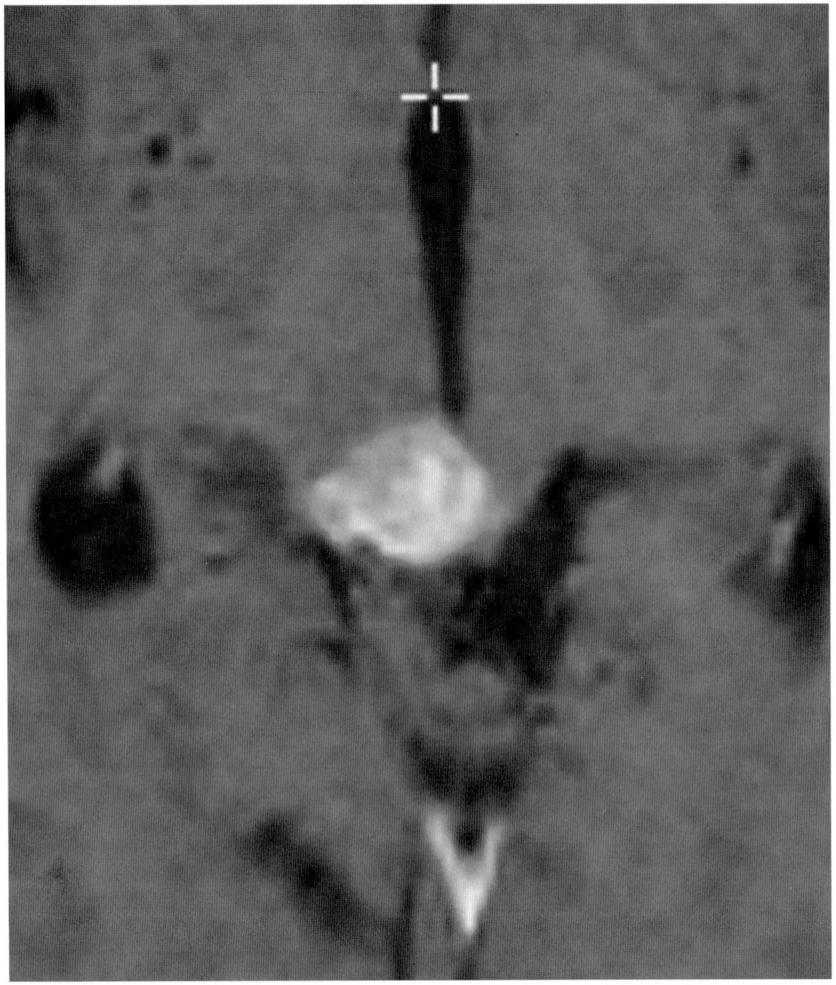

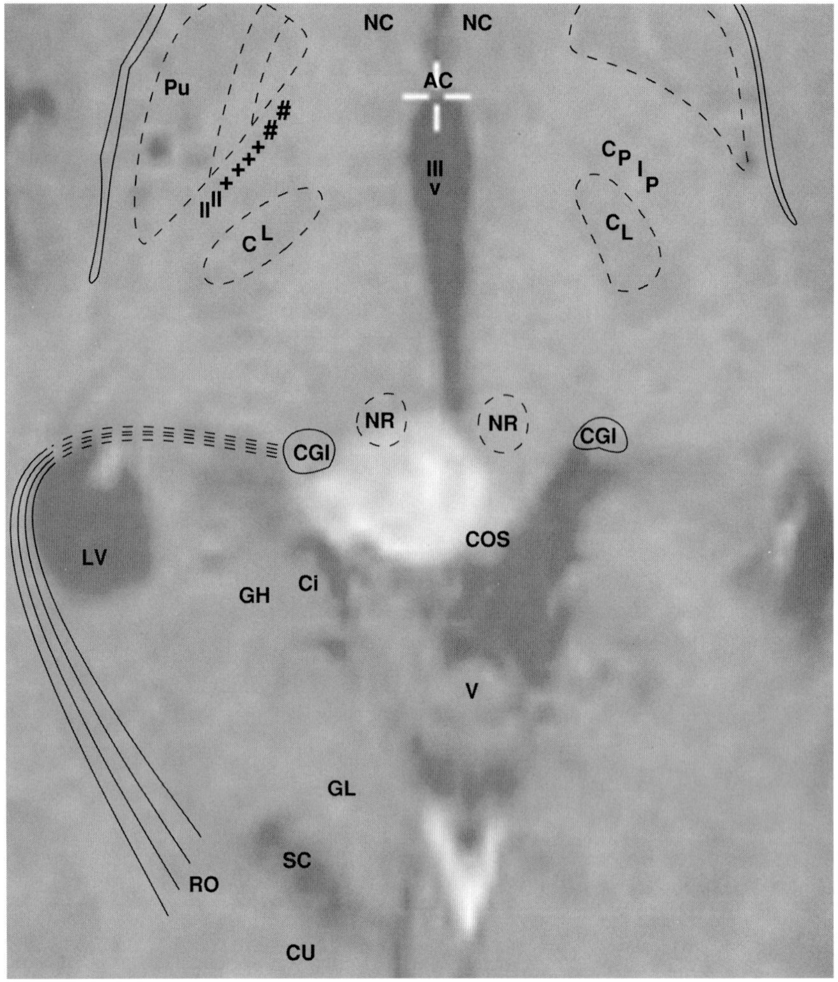

FIG. 3-14A.

FIG. 3-14. Giant cell glioblastoma multiforme involving the right posterior thalamus and thalamus–mid-brain junction. Stereotactic T_1-weighted, contrast-enhanced axial MRIs (**A and B**) separated by 6 mm inferior to superior, respectively. The enlarged atrium of the right lateral ventricle (LV) is postoperative in nature, the patient having undergone removal of a large intraventricular component of the tumor several months before this MRI study.

A: The inferior tumor margin lies approximately in the intercommissural plane. The anterior commissure (AC) is seen just anterior to the crosshair cursor. The posterior commissure is obscured by the medial tumor margin, which extends across the mid-line toward the superior edge of the left superior colliculus (COS). At this level, the anterior margin of the tumor appears to engulf or displace the superior portion of the red nucleus (NR). Six millimeters more superiorly in **B**, the anterior edge of the tumor invades and/or displaces the pulvinar (P, labeled on left), centromedian (CM), and dorsomedian (DM) thalamic nuclei. The lateral tumor margin extends to the pial surface from the caudal edge of the retropulvinaric cistern up into the porencephalic surgical defect within the medial wall of the ventricular atrium. **B:** The medial tumor margin abuts the third ventricle (IIIv) anteriorly and obliterates the posterior and habenular commissures to fill the cistern of the velum interpositum around the internal cerebral veins (ICV) and to reach the left pulvinar posteriorly. At both levels, the cingulate bundle (Ci) travels posterolateral to the tumor at the anteromedial edge of the hippocampal gyrus (GH). The posterior limb of the internal capsule (CPIP) is separated from the anterolateral tumor margin by the remaining ventral thalamus and rostral mid-brain tegmentum.

Despite the invasive appearance of this tumor and extensive previous surgery, the patient was neurologically normal. Potential neurologic deficits that could result from further neural injury might include a left-sided visual field defect (optic radiations [RO], inferolateral to tumor), right-sided rubral tremor (ipsilateral red nucleus), left hemisensory loss (VPM, VPL nuclei), and left hemiparesis (internal capsule). *(Figure continued on following page.)*

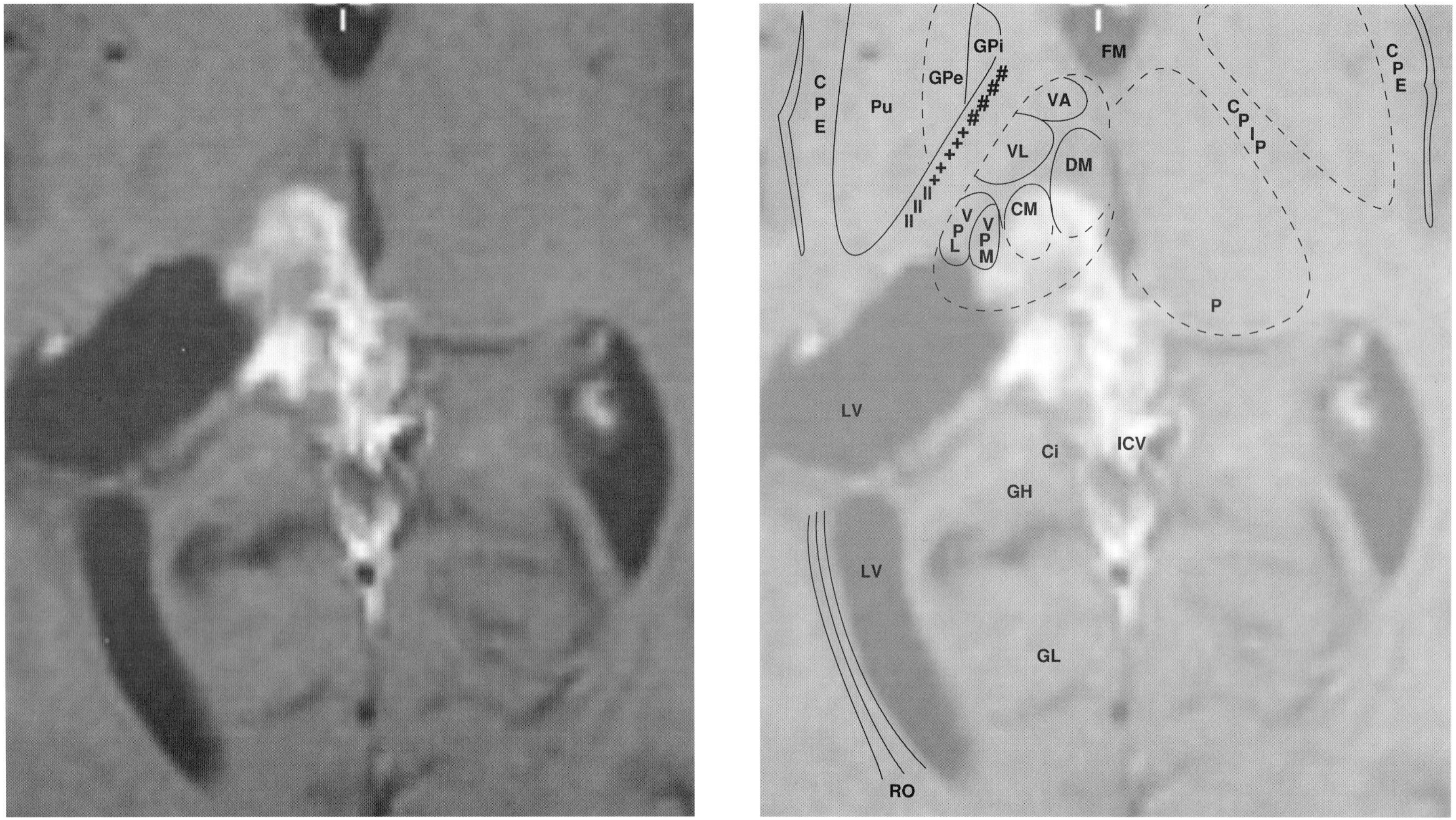
C
P
E
Pu
GPe
GPi
FM
VA
VL
DM
CM
V
P
L
V
P
M
C
P
I
P
C
P
E
P
LV
Ci
ICV
GH
LV
GL
RO

FIG. 3-14B.

FIG. 3-15. Metastatic malignant melanoma within the left superior colliculus (COS). T_1-weighted, contrast-enhanced axial (**A**) and coronal (**B**) MRIs through the center of the tumor in each imaging plane. This 5-mm diameter tumor lies within 3 mm of the rostral end of the aqueduct of Sylvius (Aq). The superior and dorsal tumor margins (seen on the coronal and axial images, respectively) reach the pial surface to barely enter the quadrigeminal plate cistern (CCQ). The medial tumor margin just touches the periaqueductal gray matter (PAG), whereas the lateral margin (**A**) displaces the brachium of the superior colliculus (BCS) laterally. The commissure of the superior colliculi lies between the tumor and the unaffected superior colliculus on the right. The pineal gland sits 3 mm superomedial to the tumor margin in **B**. The crossed dorsal trigeminal tract (DTT) forms the anterior tumor margin and separates it from the superior edge of the red nucleus (NR). *(Figure continued on following page.)*

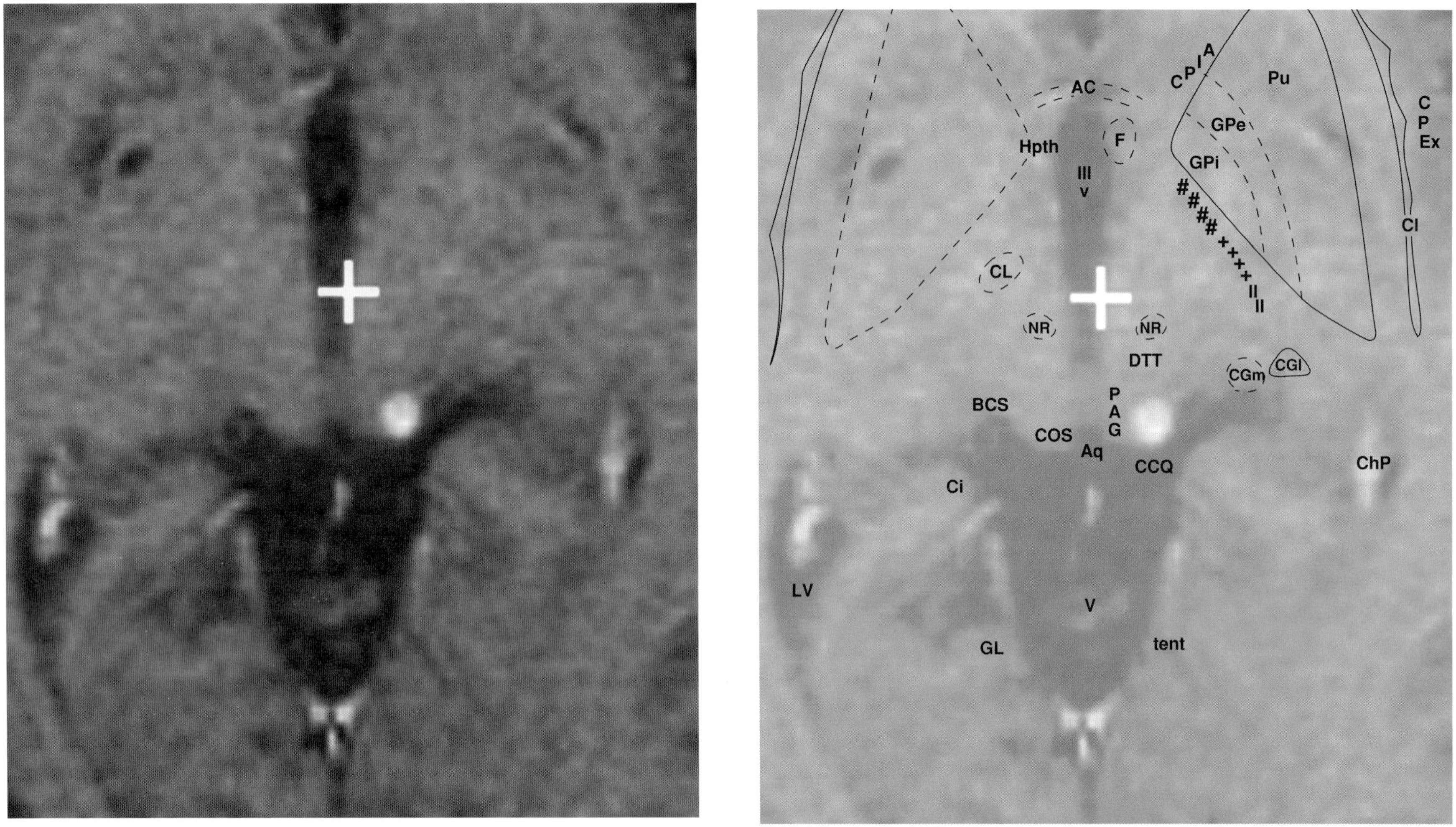
AC
CPIA
Pu
CPEx
Hpth
F
III V
GPe
GPi
Cl
CL
NR
NR
DTT
CGm
CGl
BCS
PAG
COS
Aq
CCQ
ChP
Ci
LV
V
GL
tent

FIG. 3-15A.

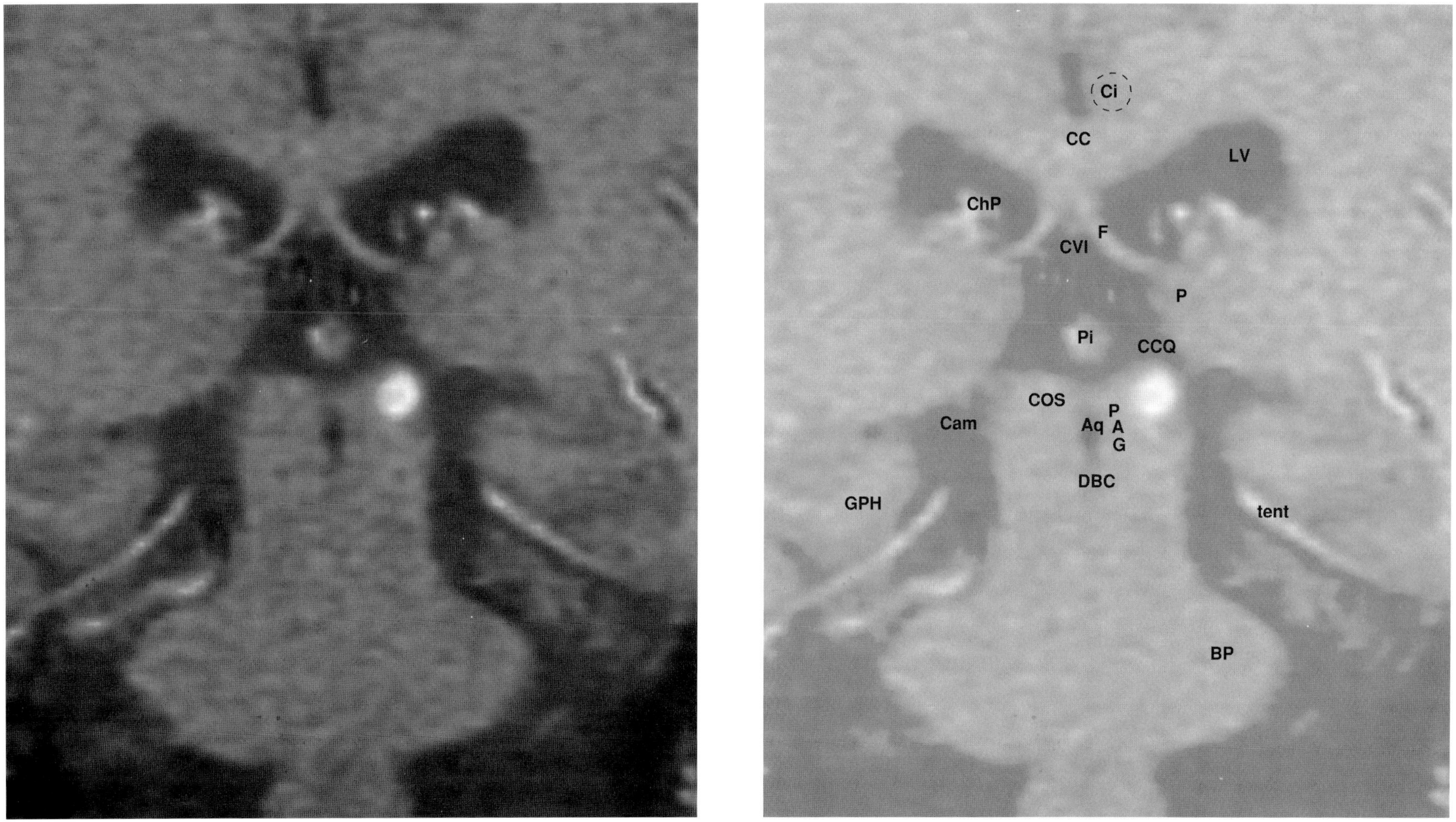

FIG. 3-15B.

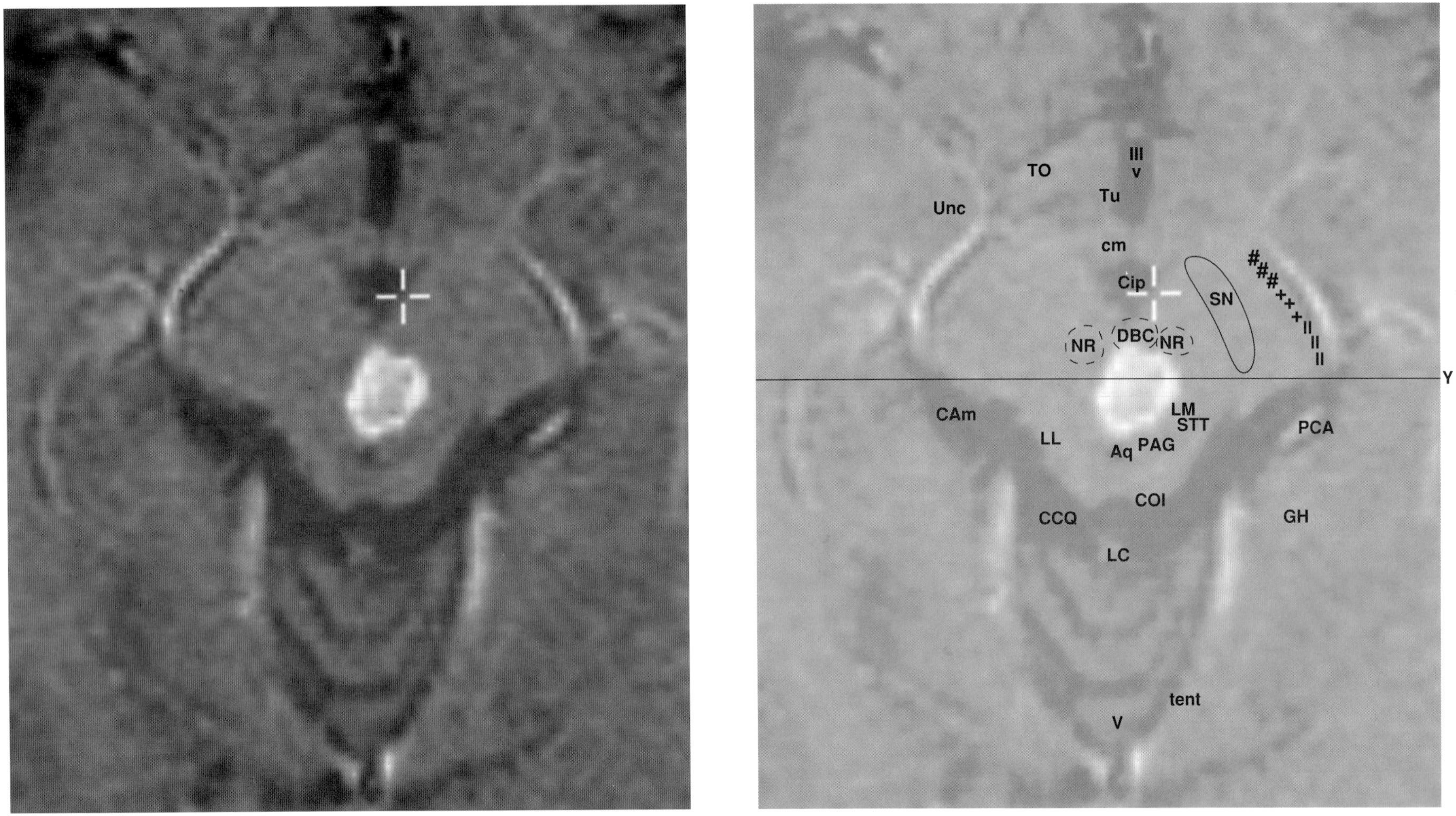
III
V
TO
Tu
Unc
cm
Cip
SN
NR
DBC
NR
Y
CAm
LM
STT
PCA
LL
Aq
PAG
COI
CCQ
GH
LC
tent
V

FIG. 3-16A.

FIG. 3-16. Metastatic neuroendocrine carcinoma, lung primary, within the central mid-brain tegmentum, somewhat eccentric to the left side. Contrast-enhanced, T_1-weighted stereotactic axial MRI (**A**) at the level of the inferior colliculi (COI), optic tracts (TO), and mammillary bodies (cm, corpora mammillare), and stereotactic coronal image (**B**) orthogonal to the plane of **A** and through the center of the tumor as indicated by line Y. Line Z in **B** indicates the axial plane of **A**.

The 10-mm diameter tumor lies entirely within the mid-brain, ventral to the aqueduct of Sylvius (Aq), centered slightly to the left of the mid-line. It displaces the decussation of the superior cerebellar peduncles (DBC) ventrally toward the interpeduncular cistern (Cip). The left red nucleus (NR) is displaced and/or distorted in the ventrolateral direction by the tumor margin. The substantia nigra (SN), located just ventral and lateral to the red nucleus, also may be deviated slightly in the same direction. The pyramidal (corticospinal) tract (Pyr), which in turn is located ventral and lateral to the substantia nigra, does not appear to be affected by the tumor.

The medial lemniscus (LM) on the left side appears to be displaced laterally and dorsally by the tumor. Just lateral and dorsal to the medial lemniscus, the spinothalamic tract (STT) and lateral lemniscus (LL) occupy the remaining sliver of tissue just beneath the lateral edge of the mid-brain that abuts the cisterna ambiens (CAm). The dorsal tumor margin encroaches slightly upon the aqueduct some 3.5 to 4.0 mm ventral to the center of the inferior colliculi (COI).

Although this patient's only findings were asymmetric oculomotor nerve paresis, tumor progression or injury to surrounding tissue might cause any combination of the following symptoms: ataxia, tremor, bradykinesia, or other movement disorder (red nucleus, decussation of the superior cerebellar peduncle, substantia nigra), loss of sensation in the right hemibody (medial lemniscus and spinothalamic tract on the left side). Obstruction of the aqueduct also could cause hydrocephalus. *(Figure continued on following page.)*

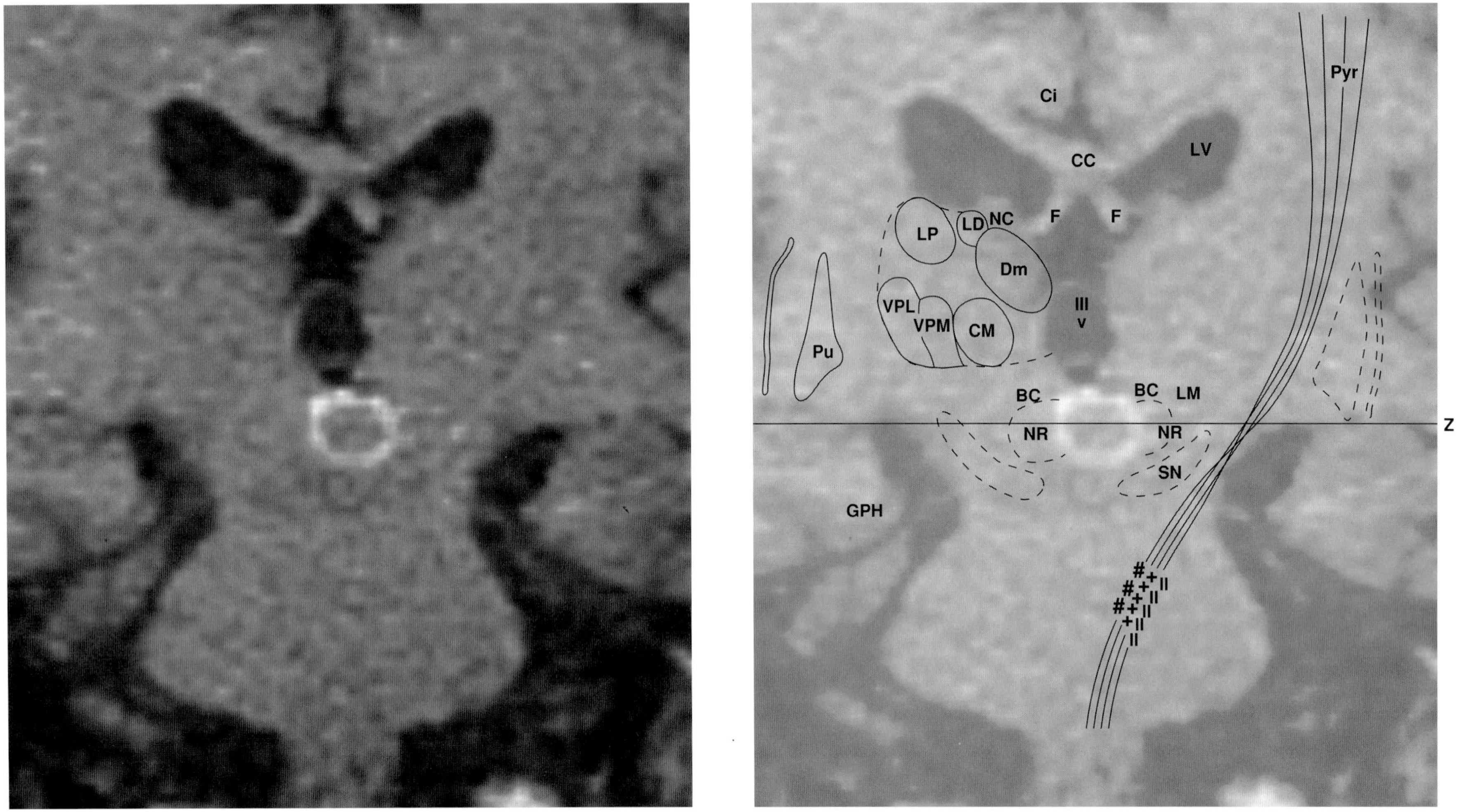

FIG. 3-16B.

FIG. 3-17. Metastatic carcinoma, non–small cell lung primary, within the tegmentum of the right side of the pons. T_1-weighted, contrast-enhanced stereotactic axial MRI at the level of the superior edge of the cisternal segment of the trigeminal nerve (V), seen within the ambient cistern (Cam) on the left side. The 8-mm diameter tumor lies entirely within the substance of pons, 2 mm deep to the right lateral surface near the entry zone of the root of the trigeminal nerve. The superior cerebellar peduncle (brachium conjunctivum, BC) abuts the dorsal margin of the tumor. Just medial to the superior cerebellar peduncle, the intramedullary fibers of the mesencephalic root of the trigeminal nerve traverse the dorsomedial tumor margin. The tumor probably displaces the central tegmental tract (Ttc) in a medial direction, the medial lemniscus (LM) in a ventral direction, and the lateral lemniscus (LL) and spinothalamic tract (STT) in a ventrolateral direction. The locus coeruleus (Coe) lies close to or against the dorsal tumor margin, between the fibers of the trigeminal mesencephalic root medially and the caudal end of the mesencephalic nucleus of the trigeminal nerve (Vme) laterally.

Still closer to the mid-line of the pons, the medial longitudinal fasciculus (MLF) and tectospinal tract (Ttsp) probably are not distorted or displaced by the tumor mass. The corticospinal (pyramidal, Pyr) tract and frontopontine fibers (Tfp) lie 6 to 10 mm ventral to the tumor margin and also do not appear to be affected.

Neurologic symptoms and signs that could arise from tumor progression or damage to surrounding structures include ipsilateral limb ataxia (superior cerebellar peduncle), trigeminal sensory or motor-proprioceptive loss (trigeminal nucleus and fibers), loss of contralateral hemibody lemniscal, pain or temperature sensations (medial lemniscus, spinothalamic tract), and loss of auditory integration or reflex function (lateral lemniscus). *(Figure continued on following page.)*

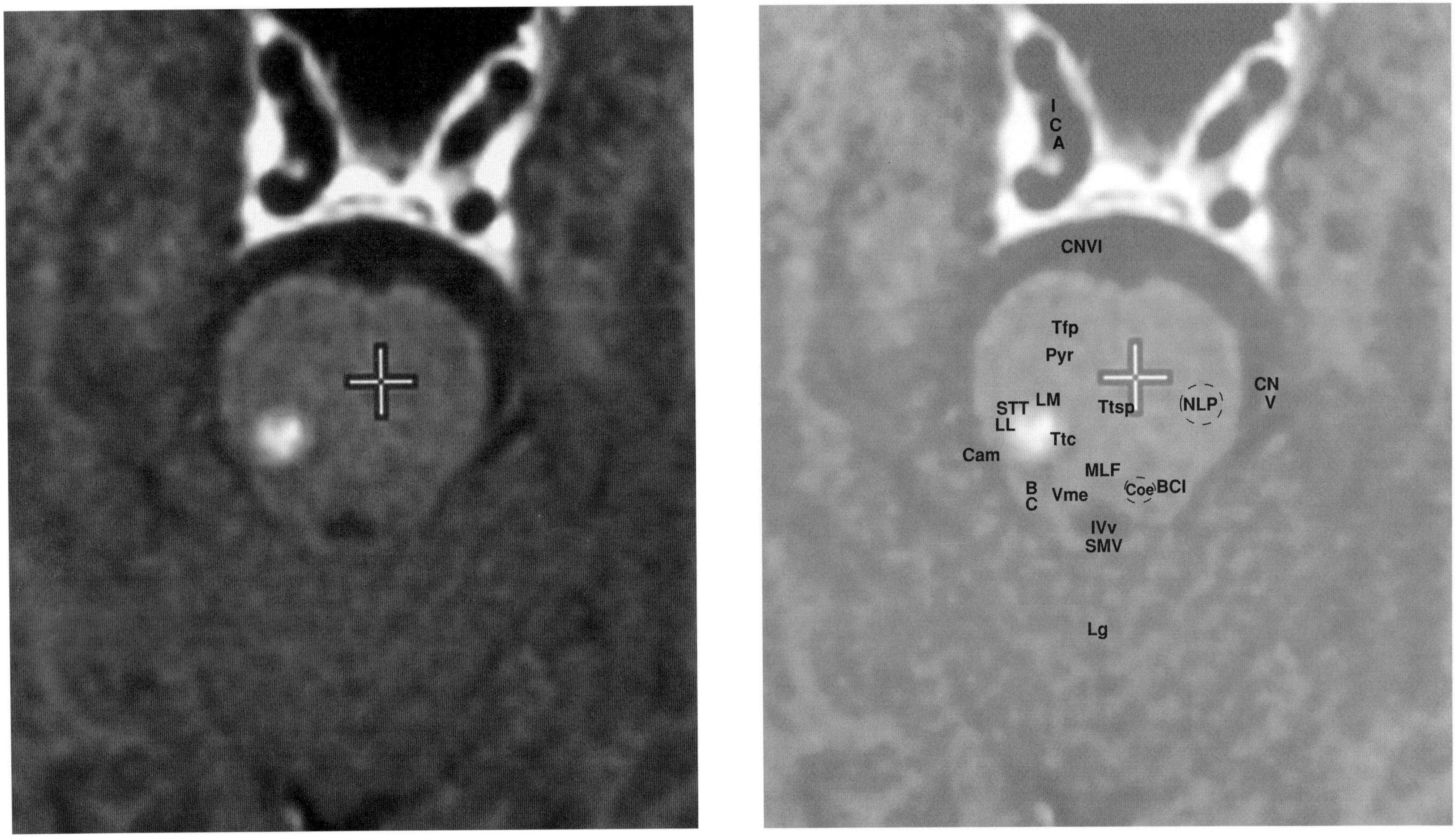

I
C
A
CNVI
Tfp
Pyr
CN
V
STT
LM
LL
Ttsp
NLP
Ttc
Cam
MLF
Coe
BCI
B
C
Vme
IVv
SMV
Lg

FIG. 3-17.

FIG. 3-18. Metastatic renal cell carcinoma to the medulla oblongota near the caudal end of the fourth ventricle, T_1-weighted, contrast-enhanced stereotactic axial MRI. The tumor is situated entirely within the substance of the brain stem, centrally in the dorsoventral plane and slightly eccentric to the right side. The tumor probably displaces the medial lemniscus (LM) in the ventral (anterior) direction and the tectospinal tract (Ttsp) in the dorsolateral direction. The spinothalamic tract (STT) lies just lateral to the center of the tumor on the right side, whereas the right solitary tract (Ts) lies dorsolateral to the tumor. The descending spinal trigeminal tract (Vst) is located just lateral to the solitary tract, and the inferior cerebellar peduncle (ICP) passes just lateral to the spinal trigeminal tract. All three structures (ICP, Vst, Ts) are displaced dorsolaterally by the tumor mass. The hypoglossal nucleus (XII) resides in the mid-line dorsal to the center of the tumor, whereas the vagal nucleus (X) lies just dorsolateral to the hypoglossal nucleus. The dorsal and ventral spinocerebellar tracts are located more superficially along the dorsolateral surface of the medulla and are affected much less, if at all, by the tumor.

The pyramid and olive (Pyr, Oli) abut the ventral and ventrolateral tumor margins, respectively, and also appear to be displaced by the tumor mass. Although this patient was neurologically normal, multiple cranial nerve deficits (trigeminal, glossopharyngeal, vagal, hypoglossal) and long tract signs (spinocerebellar, spinothalamic, corticospinal) could be caused by tumor progression or by damage to structures immediately surrounding the lesion. *(Figure continued on following page.)*

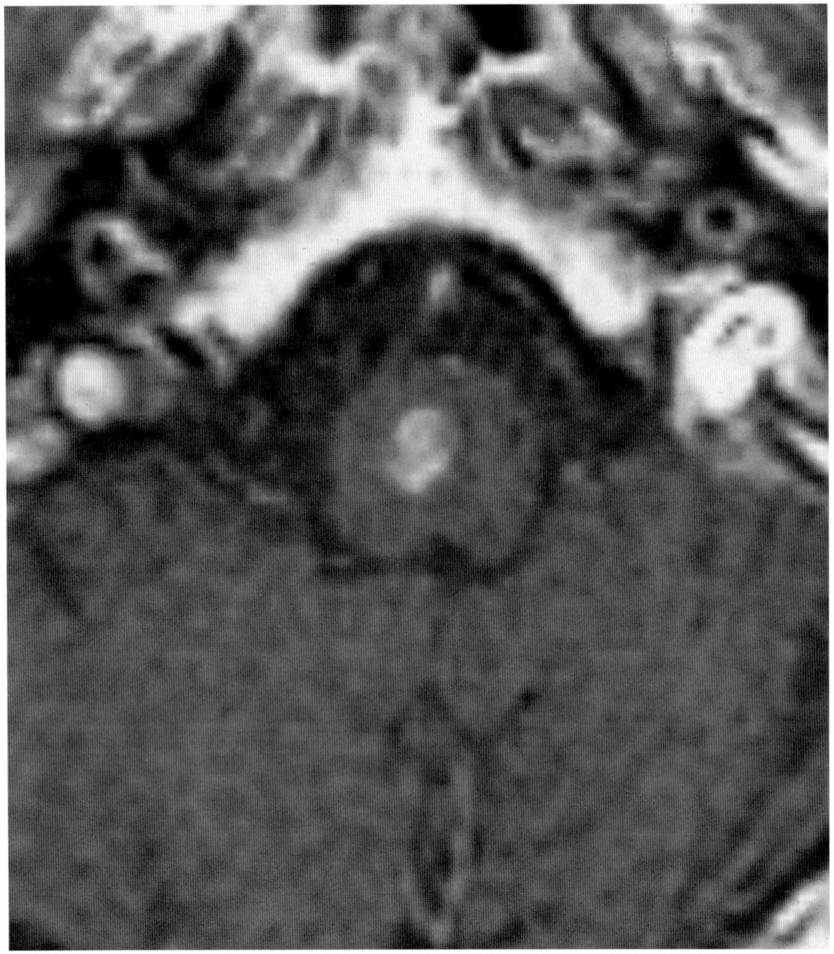

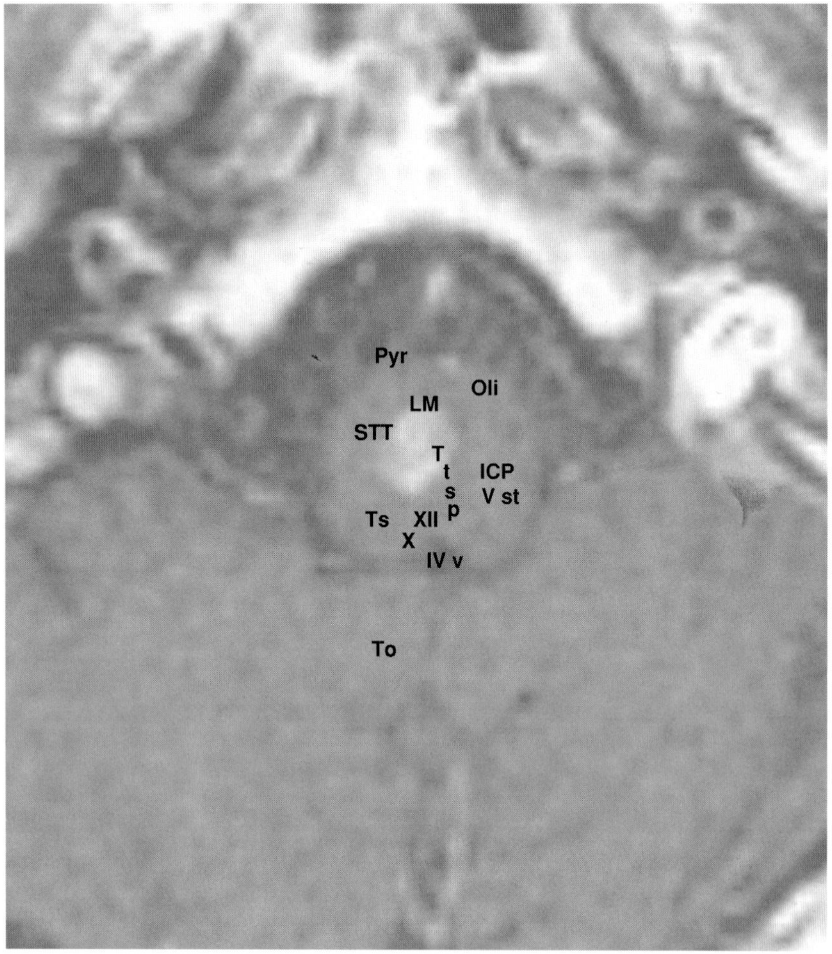

FIG. 3-18.

FIG. 3-19. Metastatic carcinoma, non–small cell lung primary, within the nodulus of the cerebellum. T_1-weighted, contrast-enhanced stereotactic axial MRI (same patient and MRI series as in Fig. 3-7). The tumor appears to have replaced the nodulus entirely, leaving that segment of the cerebellar vermis unrecognizable. The uvula (Uv) and pyramis (Pr) are displaced posteriorly by the tumor. Anteriorly, the tumor mass fills the fastigium of the fourth ventricle (IVv) and blunts the superolateral recesses on either side. The lateral tumor margin abuts and probably displaces the globose nuclei (Gl) on both sides. The remainder of the more laterally situated cerebellar roof nuclei (emboliform, Eb; fusiform, Fu; and dentate, Dt) are affected to a lesser degree. Anterolateral to the tumor, the superior cerebellar peduncles (brachium conjunctivum, BC) may be slightly displaced anterolaterally. The remainder of the pontine nuclei and tracts lie sufficiently distant from the tumor that they remain in their normal locations.

The patient's only neurologic symptom was nausea. Additional damage to the cerebellar vermis or deep cerebellar nuclei (due to tumor growth or treatment-induced side effects) could cause truncal or gait ataxia and/or dysmetria of the extremities on either side. *(Figure continued on following page.)*

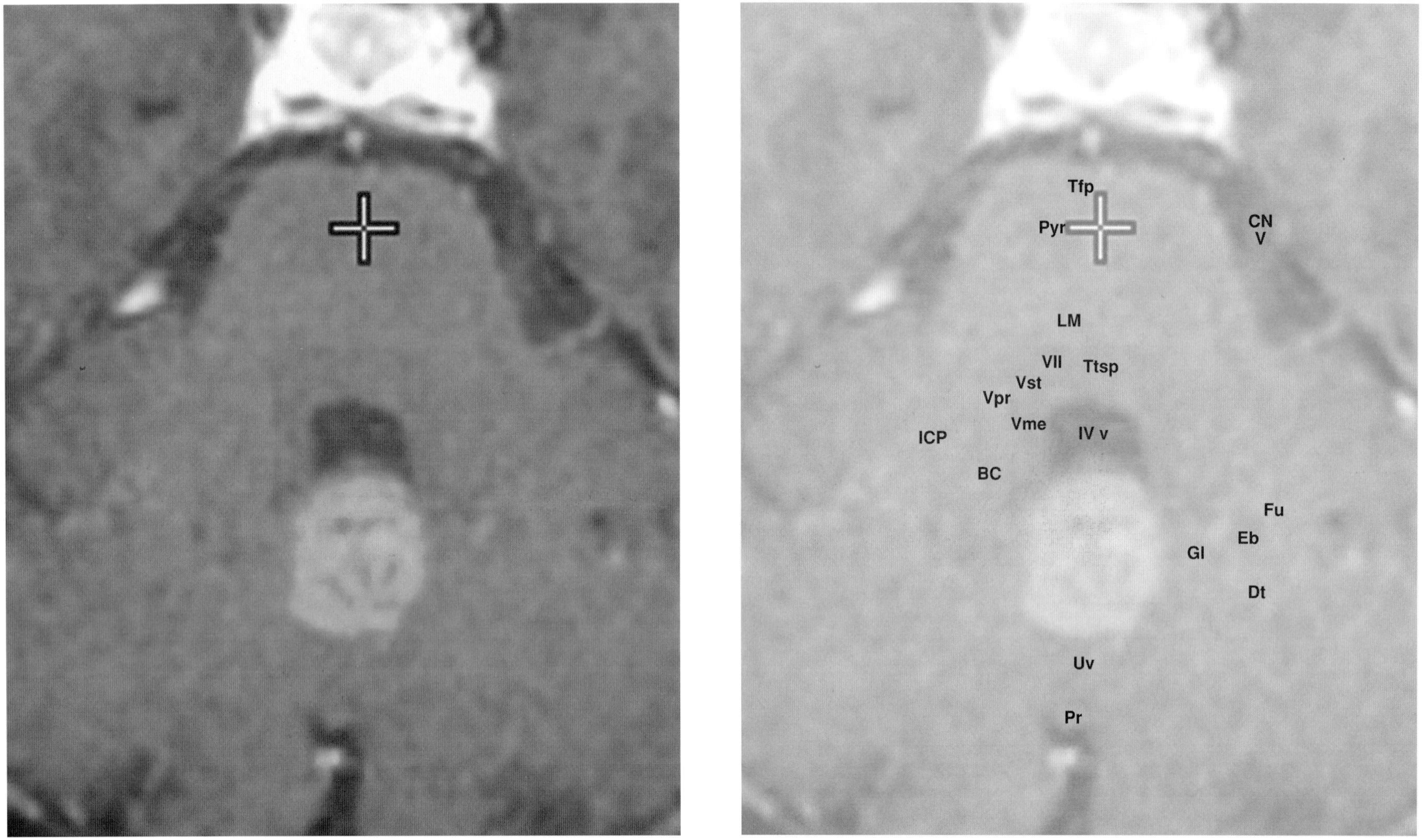

FIG. 3-19.

FIG. 3-20. Metastases from non–small cell lung carcinoma to the right cerebellar tonsil and left cerebellar hemisphere in the region of the dentate nucleus. T_1-weighted, contrast-enhanced stereotactic axial MRI through the medulla, fourth ventricle, and cerebellum at the level of the inferior olive (Oli), ventral cochlear nucleus (VIIcv), and uvula (Uv). The 16-mm diameter irregular tumor on the right side occupies most of the cross-sectional area of the tonsil (To) in this plane; only the most medial portion of the tonsil can be seen. Although the right cerebellar hemisphere appears mildly swollen, little displacement of tissue has occurred. The ventrolateral tumor margin enters the medial edge of the flocculus (Fl), which also appears slightly enlarged. Contrast enhancement extends from the ventromedial tumor margin to involve the floor of the fourth ventricle including the dorsal spinocerebellar tract (Tspcd) and vestibular nucleus (VIIIv). Immediately anterior to the tumor the inferior cerebellar peduncle (ICP) is flanked by the ventral cochlear nucleus (VIIIcv) and ventral spinocerebellar tract (Tspcv). The fibers of the vagal nerve (X) and descending spinal trigeminal tract (Vsp) lie medial to the inferior cerebellar peduncle. Neurologic risks associated with progression or treatment of this tumor predominantly involve the vestibular-spinal-cerebellar interconnections that maintain postural stability.

The smaller (10 mm) tumor in the left cerebellar hemisphere occupies the caudal portion of the dentate nucleus. Damage to that structure could cause ipsilateral limb ataxia, resting tremor, and/or intention tremor. *(Figure continued on following page.)*

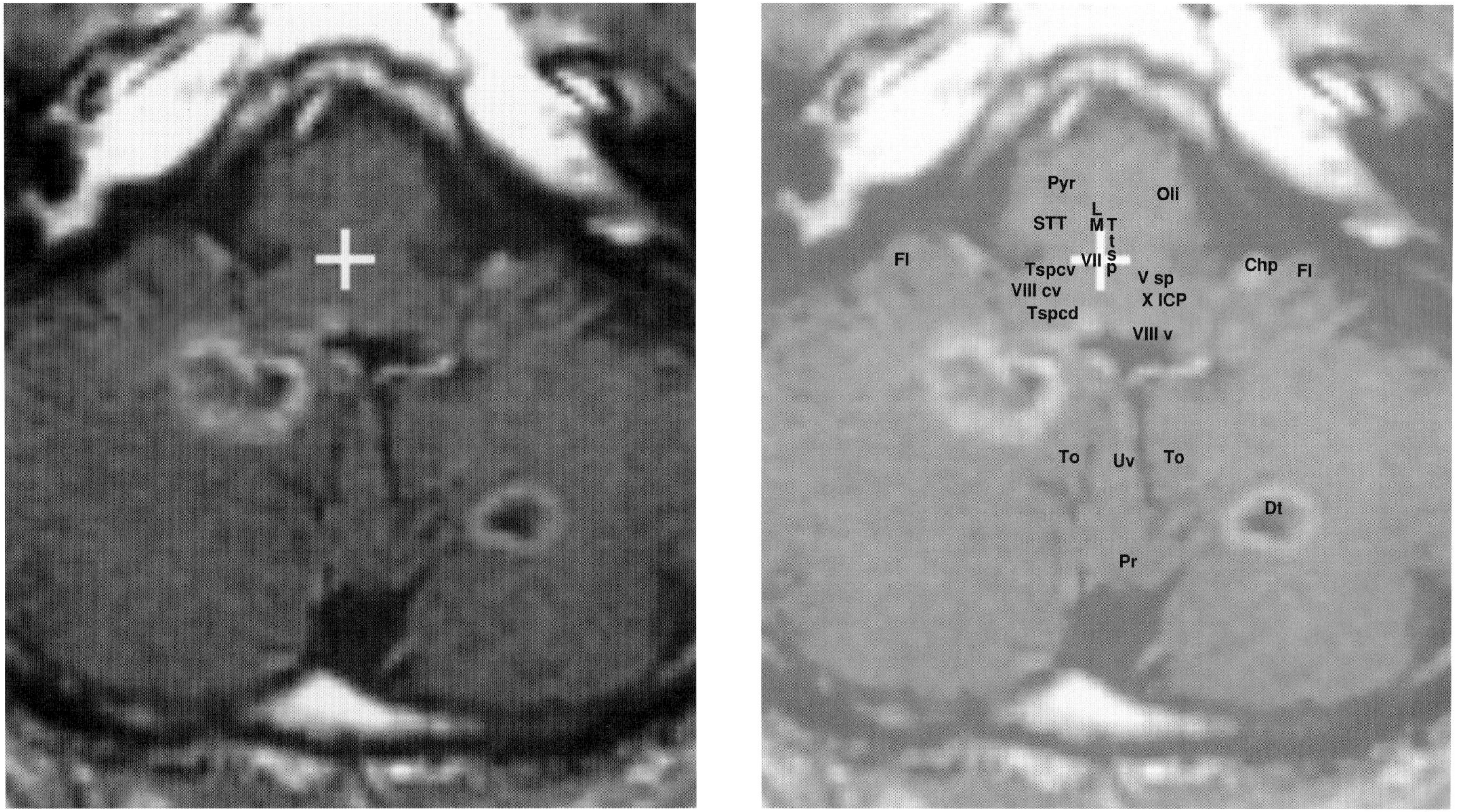
Pyr
Oli
L
STT
M
T
t
s
p
VII
Fl
Tspcv
Chp
Fl
V sp
VIII cv
X ICP
Tspcd
VIII v
To
Uv
To
Dt
Pr

FIG. 3-20.

Chapter 4

Arteriovenous Malformations

The order in which the arteriovenous malformations are presented in this chapter follows the same general sequence as that established for tumors in the foregoing sections: from anterior to posterior within the cranial cavity, and from superficial to deep within the cerebral substance. Every case includes a PA and/or lateral stereotactic angiographic image and at least one MRI (most often using stereotactic technique as well) through the center of the AVM nidus. Whenever applicable, the PA angiogram is presented first, followed by the coronal MRIs, lateral angiogram, sagittal MRI, and axial MRIs. This arrangement facilitates comparison between the angiographic projection images and the corresponding MR cross-sectional images (PA versus coronal, and lateral versus sagittal). The millimeter scale that appears near the margin of each stereotactic angiogram is corrected for magnification at the center of each AVM nidus. Because most of the angiographic images are life size, readers can appreciate the dimensions, depth, and orientation of the AVM and surrounding structures fairly accurately. In contrast, the fainter shadows caused by coordinate indicators on the stereotactic headframe vary in size considerably according to the target-to-film distance.

As in previous chapters, the AVM cases selected for inclusion here are anatomical or location-specific prototypes. Although not exhaustive, the catalogue that follows should give the reader an overview of the functional significance of the cerebral structures within and around commonly encountered cerebral AVMs.

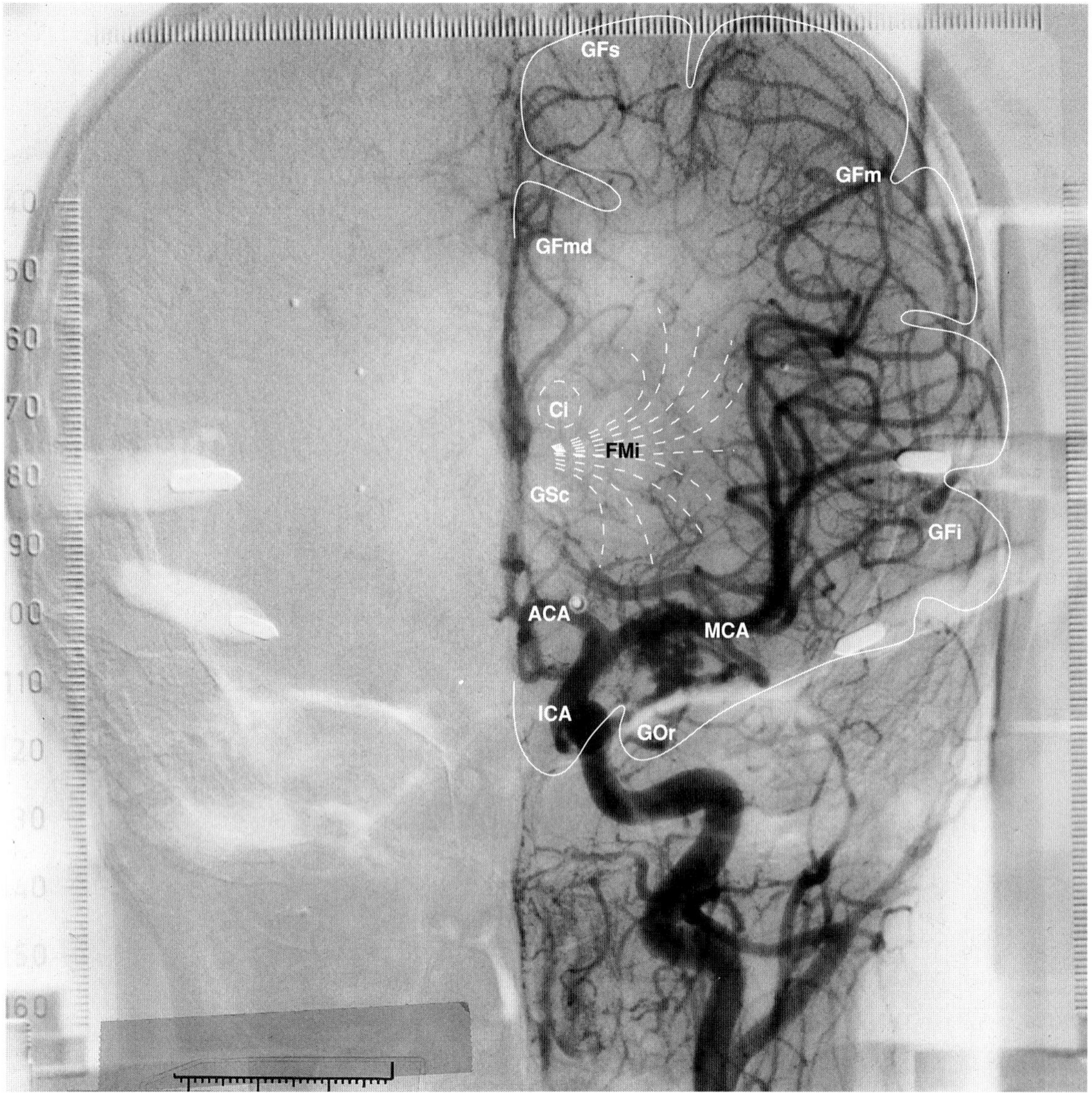

FIG. 4-1A.

FIG. 4-1. Small arteriovenous malformation of the left orbitofrontal cortex in a 10-year-old child, PA and lateral stereotactic left carotid angiogram films (**A and B**), and proton density-weighted MRI (**C**). The feeding artery appears to be a middle cerebral artery (MCA) branch that runs along the orbital surface of the frontal lobe between the medial and lateral orbital gyri (GOr). The draining vein (vv) runs anteriorly along the floor of the anterior cranial fossa before turning medially to enter the superior sagittal sinus. Although this AVM projects beneath the M_1 segment of the MCA on the PA view (**A**), the nidus is located far anteriorly, within the white matter superior to the orbital gyri and deep to the middle and inferior frontal gyri (GFm and GFi).

Because this small AVM is surrounded by relatively silent regions of the brain, either surgical or radiosurgical treatment should be associated with minimal neurologic risk. *(Figure continued on following pages.)*

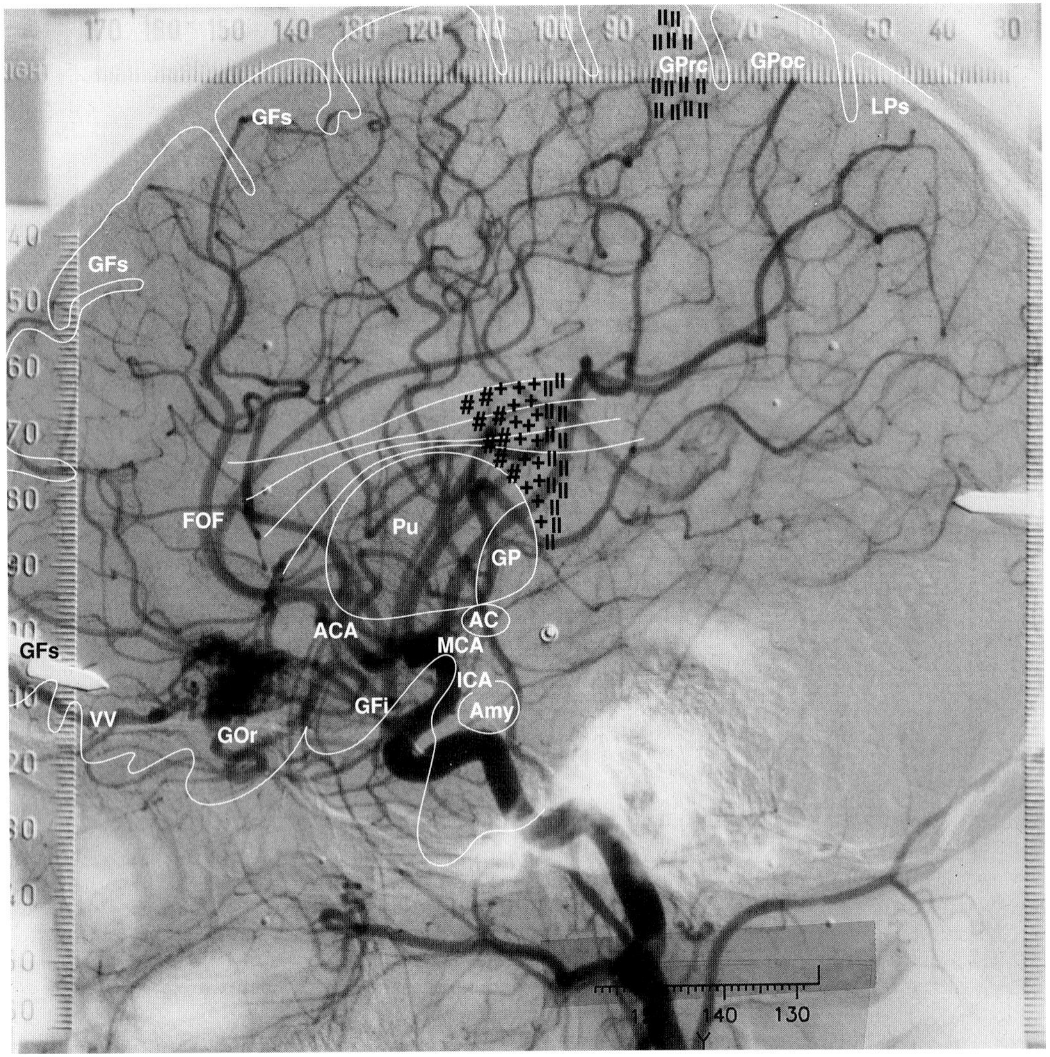

FIG. 4-1B.

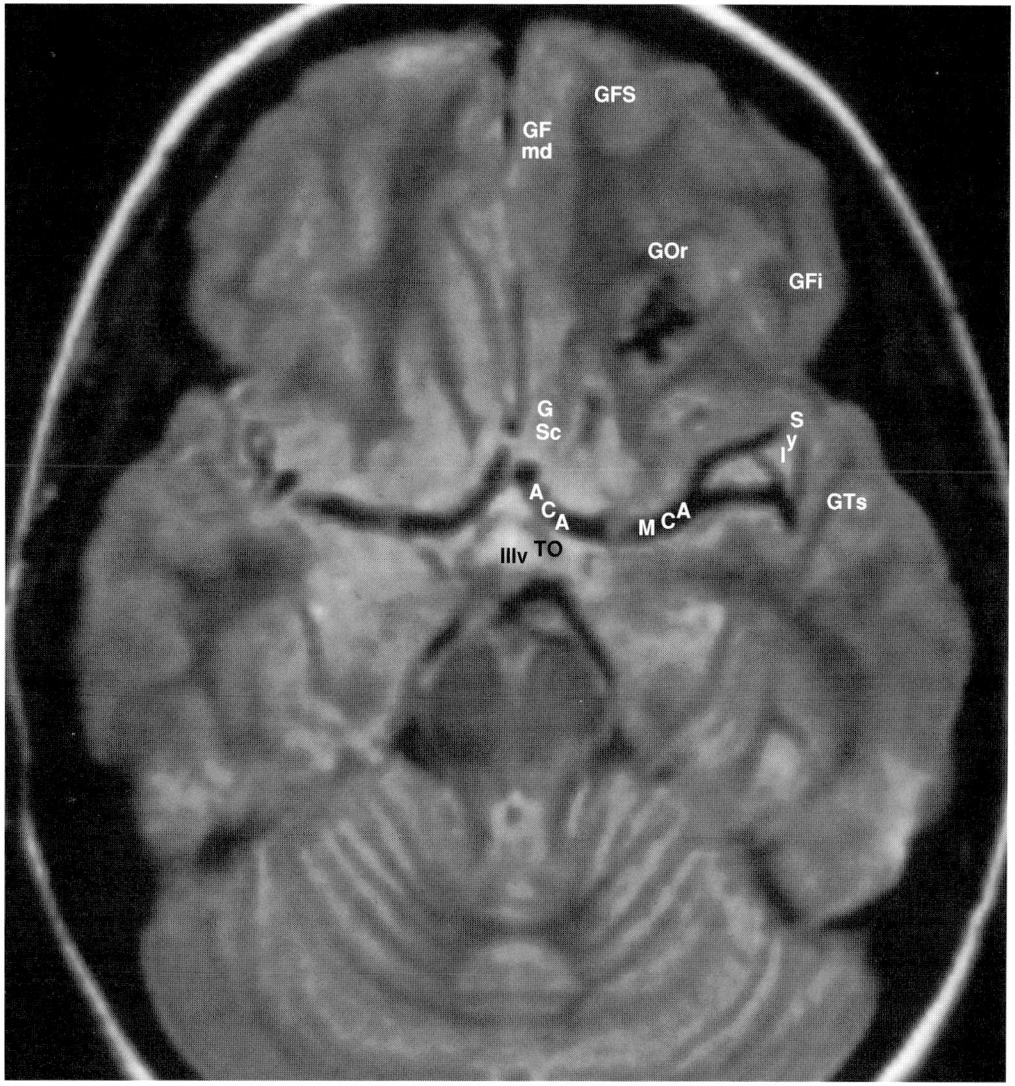

FIG. 4-1C.

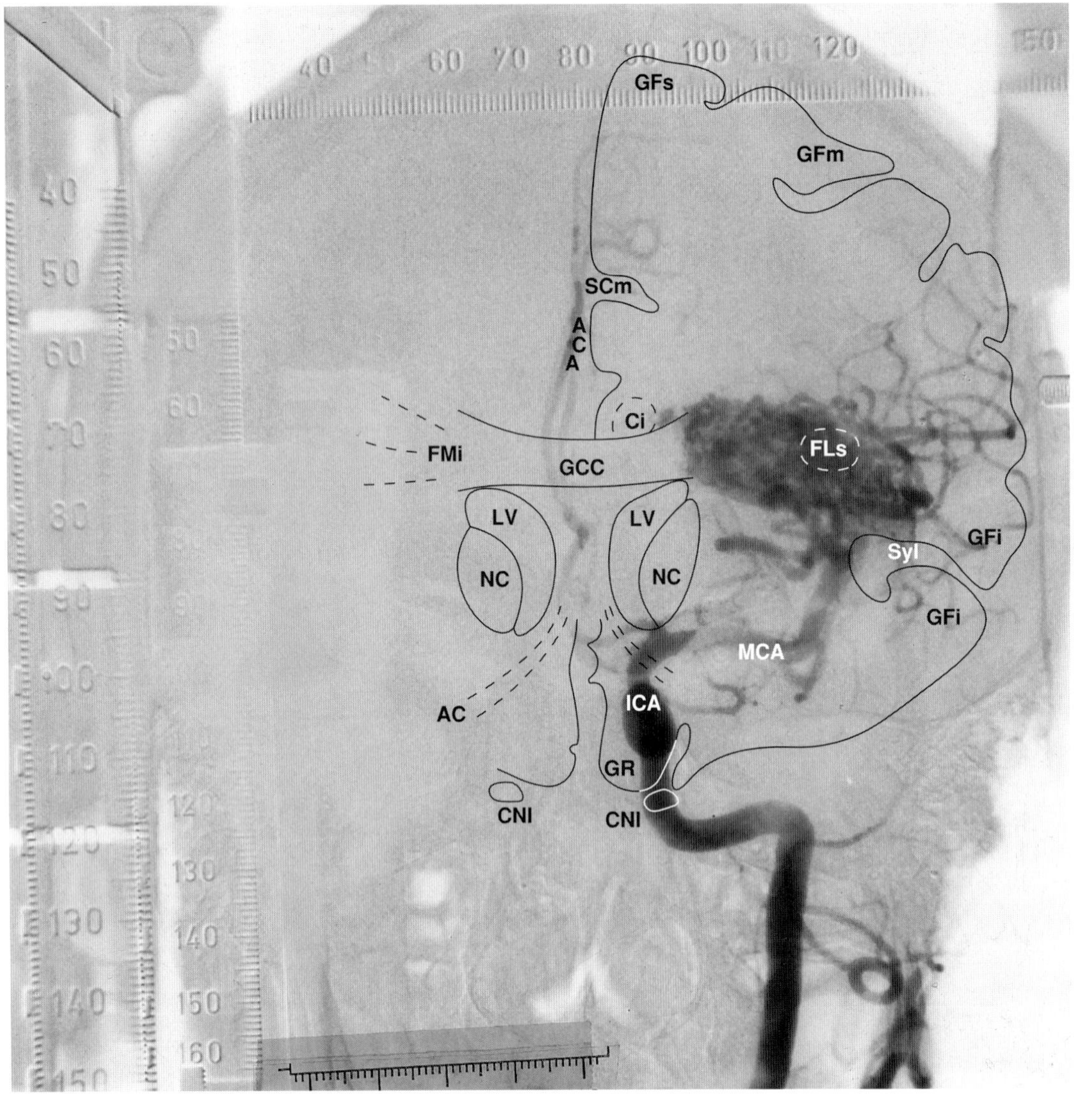
GFs
GFm
SCm
A
C
A
Ci
FMi
GCC
FLs
LV
LV
NC
NC
Syl
GFi
GFi
MCA
ICA
AC
GR
CNI
CNI

FIG. 4-2A.

FIG. 4-2. Arteriovenous malformation of the deep left frontal lobe and opercular region, PA and lateral stereotactic left carotid angiogram films (**A and B**), and non-stereotactic T_1-weighted parasagittal MRI (**C**). Feeding vessels include left middle cerebral artery (MCA) branches exclusively, despite the deep medial extension of the AVM nidus. The major draining vein (vv, illustrated only in the lateral view, **B**) courses anteriorly, then superficially around the nidus to enter the superior sagittal sinus at the level of the middle frontal gyrus (GFm).

The nidus has an ovoid shape with its long axis in the medial-lateral direction. The most superficial portion of the nidus resides within the frontal operculum, just above the superior bank of the sylvian fissure (Syl). Medially, the deepest edge of the nidus reaches the superior edge of the genu of the corpus callosum (GCC), just above the frontal horn of the lateral ventricle (LV) and head of the caudate nucleus (NC). The cingulate bundle (Ci) passes deep to the medial edge of the nidus, and the superior longitudinal fasciculus (FLs) courses just above the top edge of the AVM. Motor fibers of the pyramidal tract (Pyr) pass more than 3 cm behind the posterior margin of the AVM.

Neurologic risks associated with treatment of this malformation could include a language disorder and/or buccofacial dyspraxia from involvement of Broca's area and the adjacent subcortical white matter, and frontal gaze palsy from involvement of the FLs and deep superior frontal white matter. *(Figure continued on following pages.)*

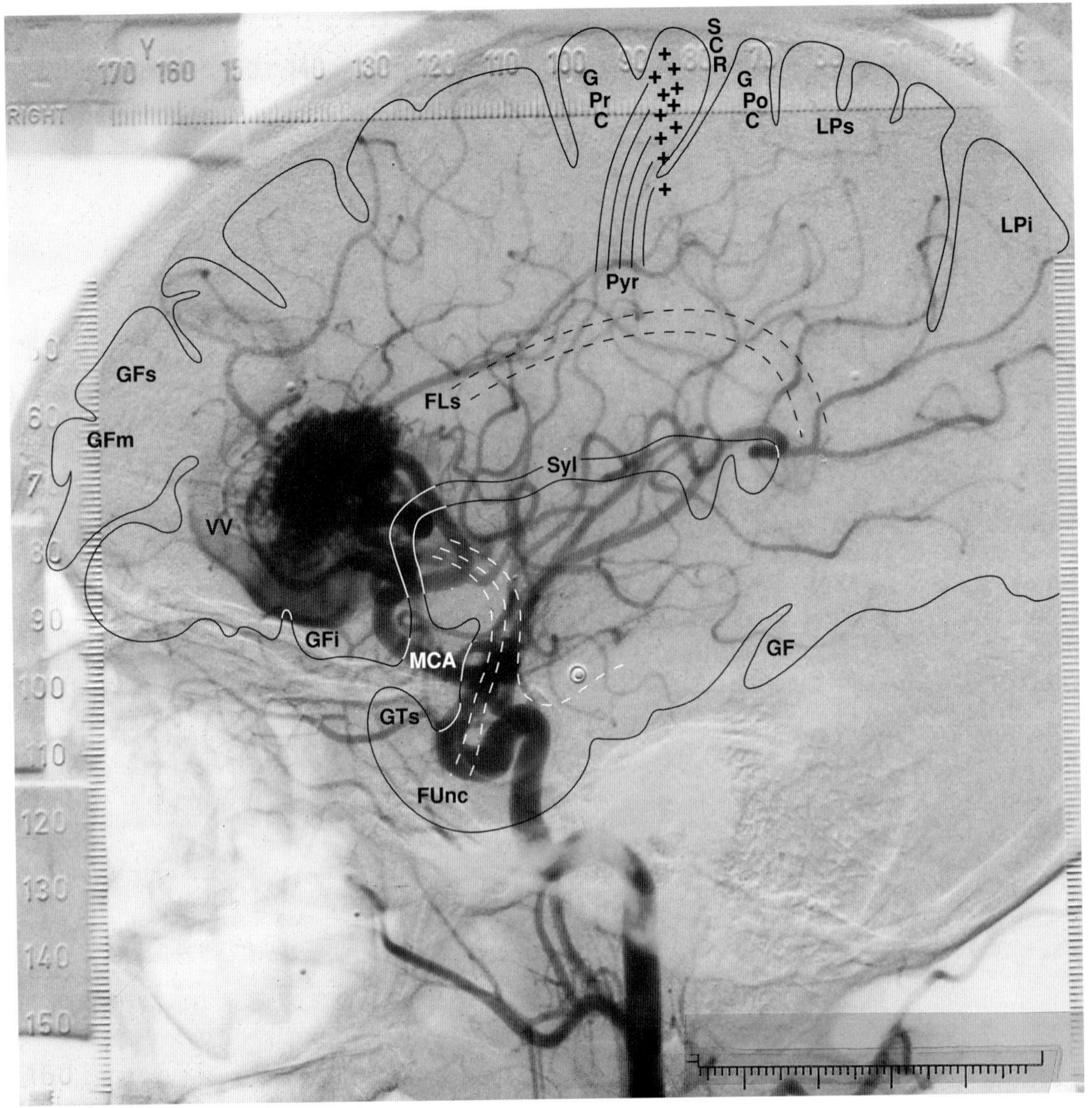

FIG. 4-2B.

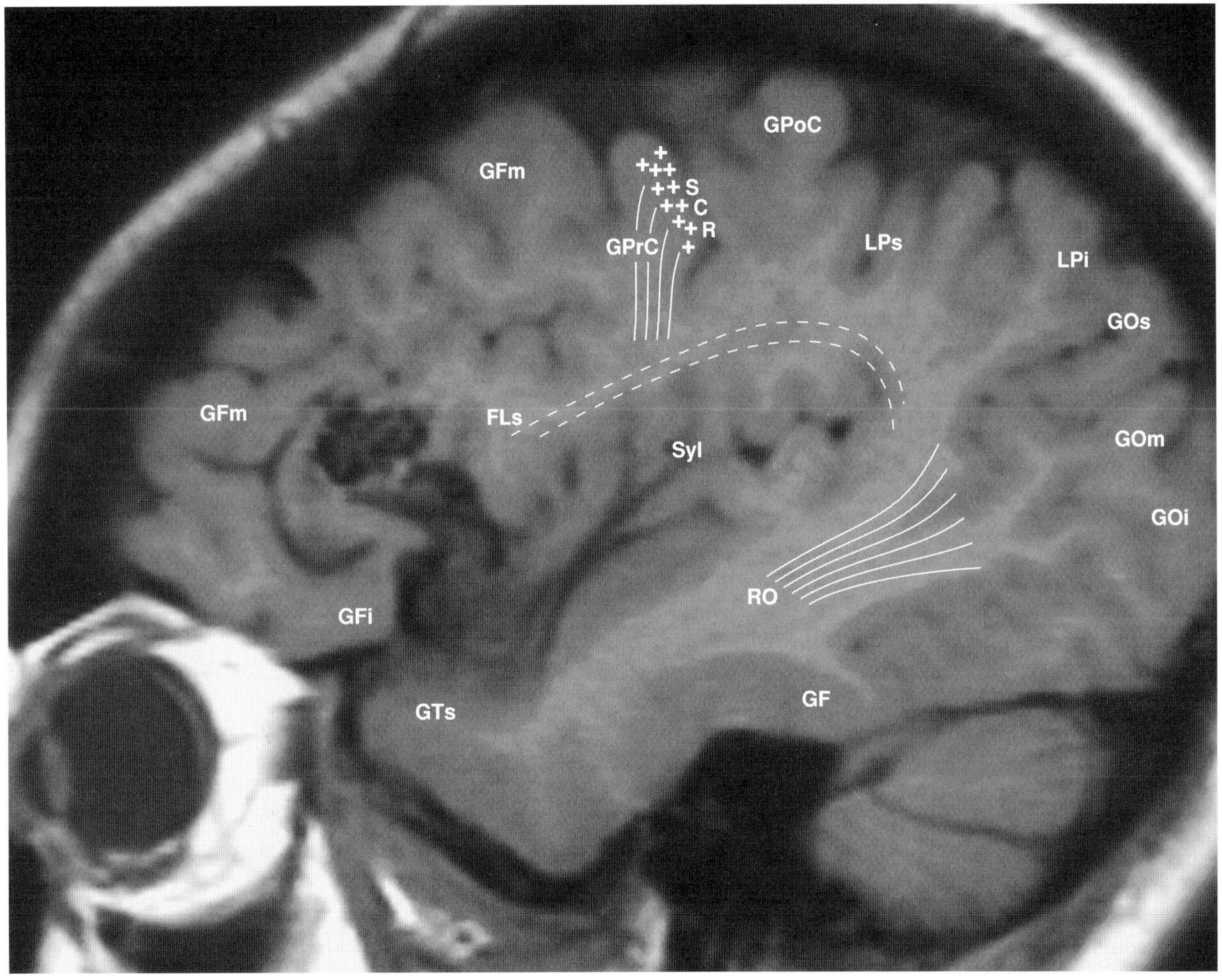

FIG. 4-2C.

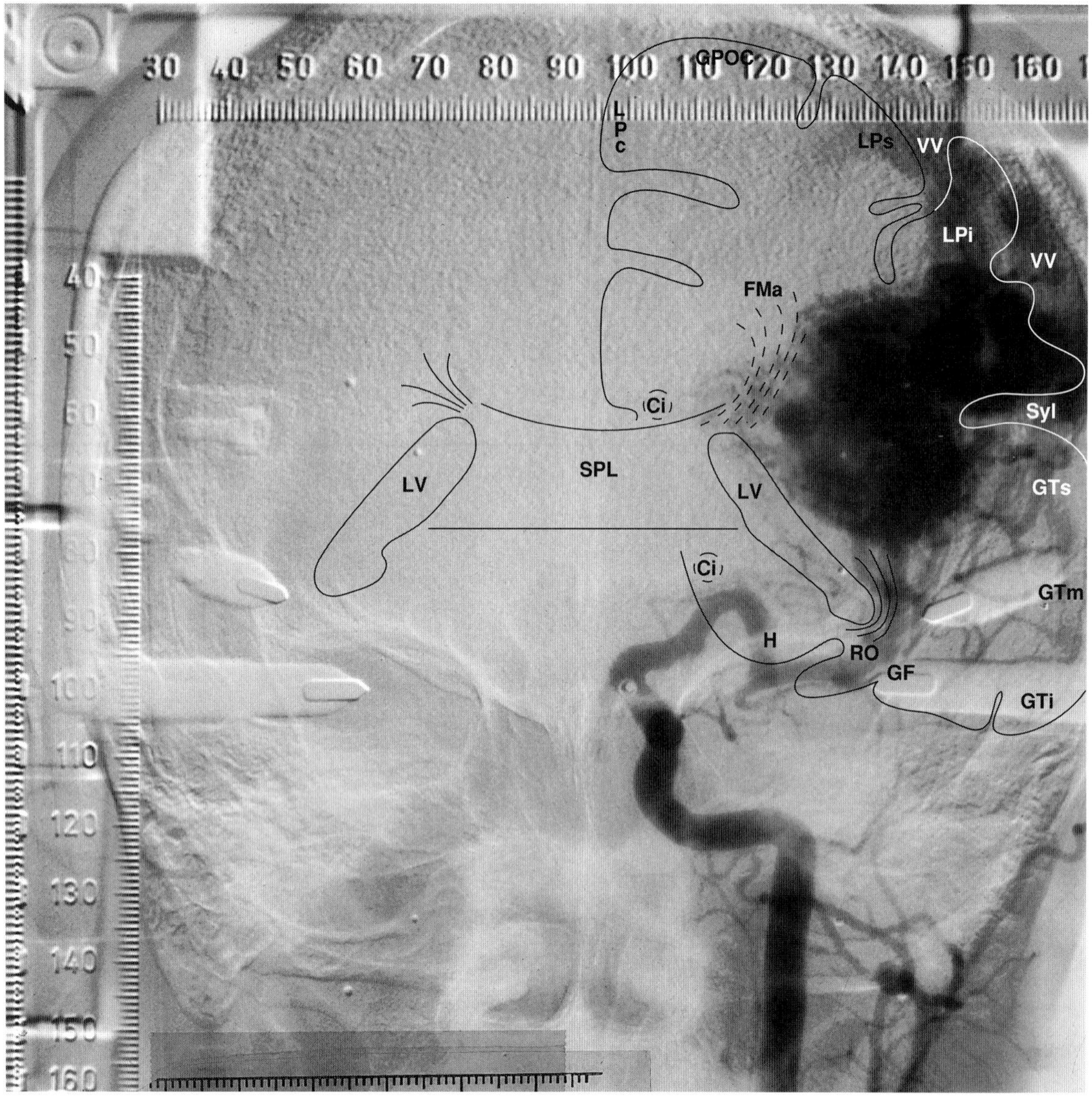

FIG. 4-3A.

FIG. 4-3. Arteriovenous malformation within the subcortical and deep left temporoparietal region. PA and lateral stereotactic left carotid angiogram films (**A and B**) and stereotactic T_1-weighted axial MRIs separated by 9 mm from inferior to superior (**C and D**). This AVM is fed by angular and parietal branches of the middle cerebral artery (MCA) and has two major superficial draining veins (vv) that arise from the anterior and superior margins of the nidus to enter the superior sagittal sinus at the level of the paracentral lobule and superior parietal lobule (LPs). Less prominent deep venous drainage is present along the anterior wall of the atrium of the lateral ventricle (LV). The superficial portion of the nidus straddles the posterior quarter of the sylvian fissure (Syl) within the subcortical white matter of the parietal operculum (inferior parietal lobule, LPi) and superior temporal gyrus (GTs). The deep margin of the nidus abuts the atrium and posterior body of the lateral ventricle, whereas the splenium of the corpus callosum (SPL) and forceps major sharply delimit the posteromedial edge of the AVM.

Fibers of the corticospinal tract (Pyr) descend within the corona radiata approximately 5 mm anterior to the leading edge of the anterior draining vein (deep and inferior to the postcentral gyrus, GPoC). Most of the nidus itself resides within the inferior parietal lobule; the inferior edge of the nidus extends into the superior temporal gyrus. Fibers of the optic radiation (RO) pass beneath the inferior edge of the nidus, whereas the superior longitudinal fasciculus (FLs) appears to pass into the AVM (or to be displaced around the superior margin).

Risks associated with treatment of this AVM might include a language disorder from injury to Wernicke's area (GTs) or the subjacent white matter, or a complete or partial Gerstmann's syndrome from injury to the dominant inferior parietal lobule. Other potential neurologic risks include cortical sensory and/or motor deficits from injury to the pyramidal tract or thalamocortical connections to the postcentral gyrus, and a visual field defect from injury to the optic radiation. *(Figure continued on following pages.)*

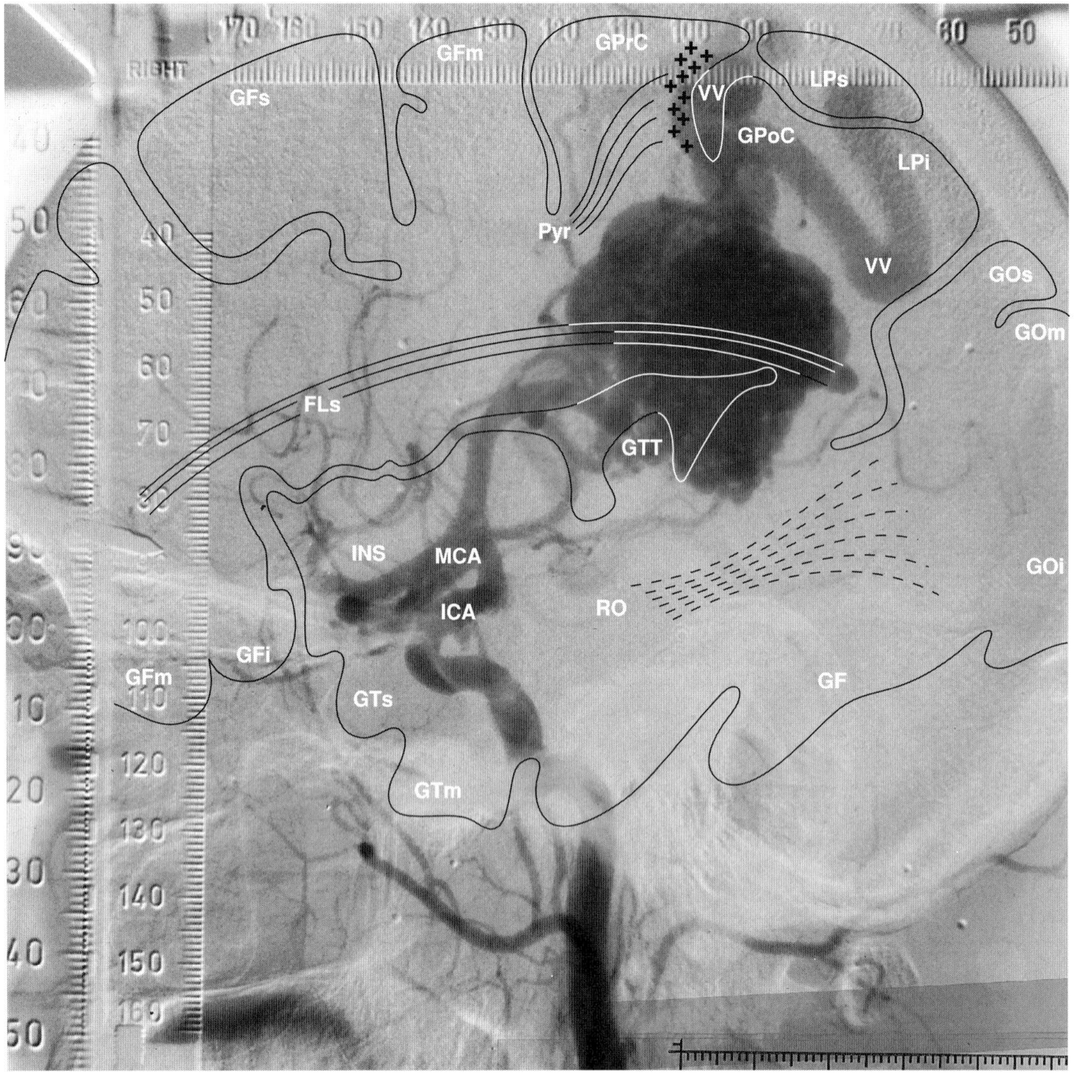
GFm
GPrC
VV
LPs
GFs
GPoC
LPi
Pyr
VV
GOs
GOm
FLs
GTT
INS
MCA
ICA
RO
GOi
GFi
GFm
GTs
GF
GTm
RIGHT

FIG. 4-3B.

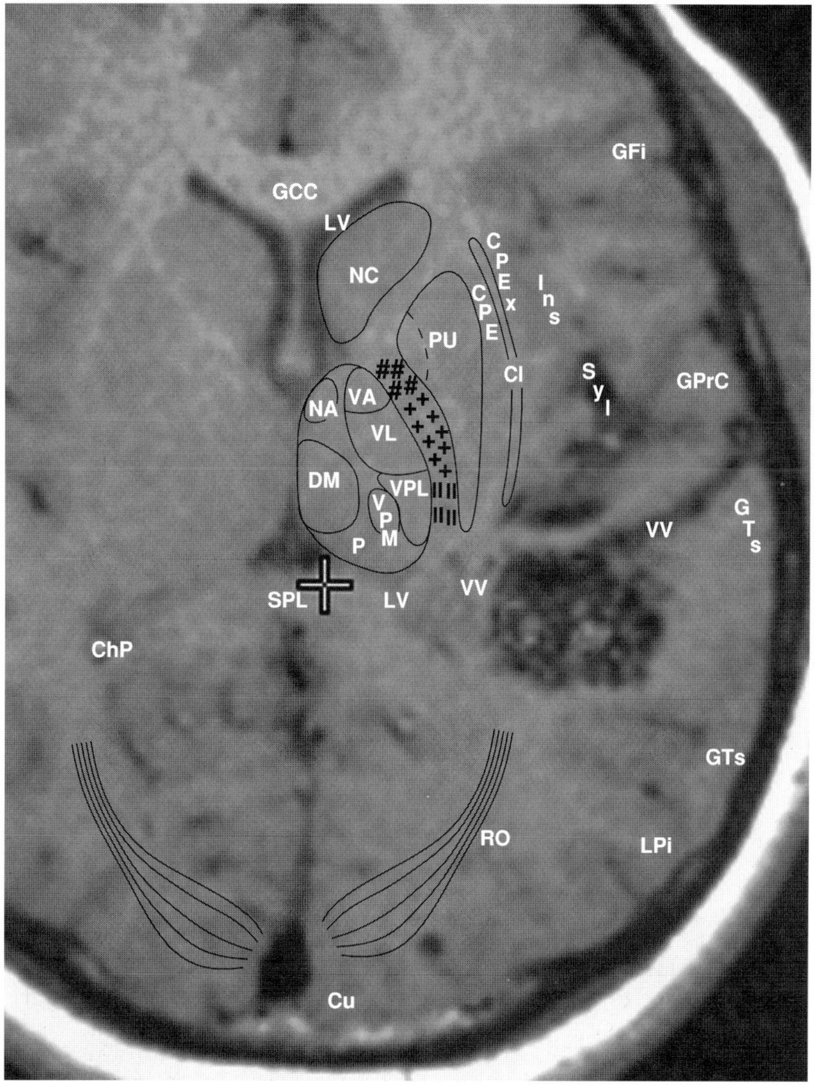
GFi
GCC
LV
NC
C
P
E
x
I
n
s
C
P
E
PU
Cl
S
y
l
GPrC
NA
VA
VL
DM
VPL
V
P
M
P
G
T
s
VV
SPL
LV
VV
ChP
GTs
RO
LPi
Cu

FIG. 4-3C.

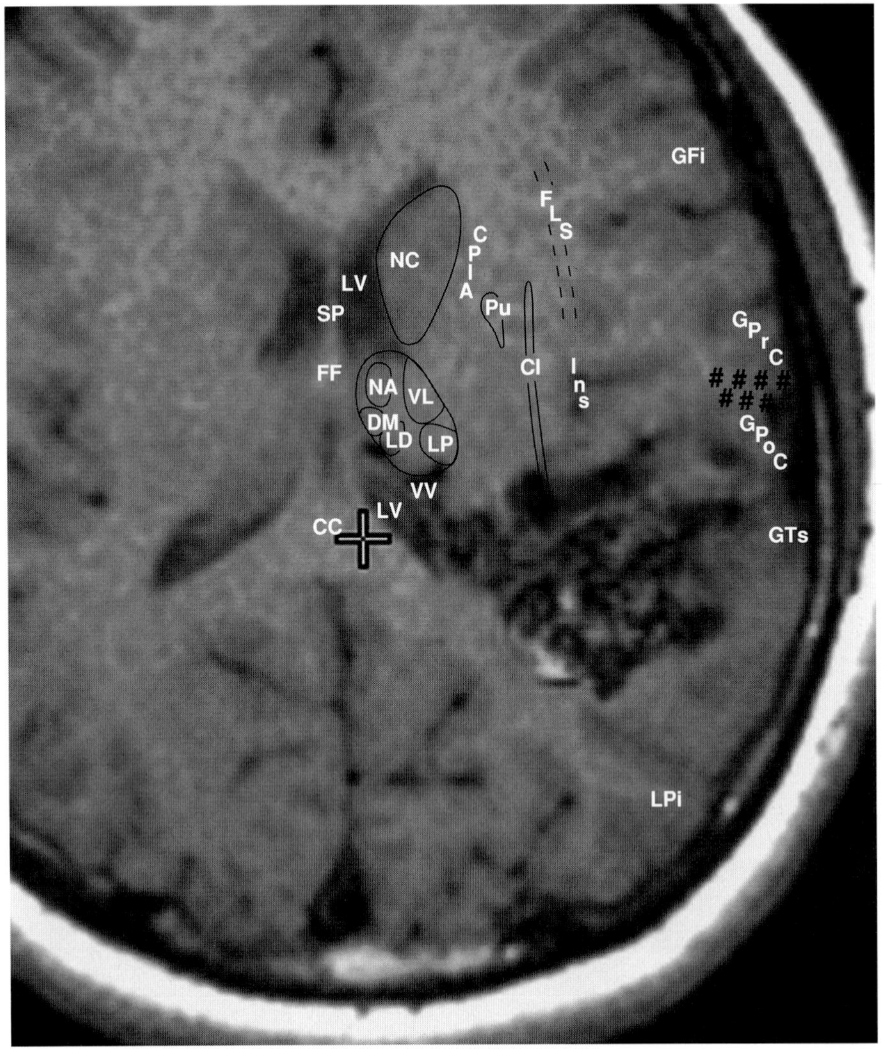
GFi
FLS
C
P
I
A
NC
LV
SP
Pu
FF
CI
Ins
GPrC
NA
VL
DM
LD
LP
GPoC
VV
LV
CC
GTs
LPi

FIG. 4-3D.

FIG. 4-4. Small arteriovenous malformation located within the posterior ramus of the left sylvian fissure, PA and lateral stereotactic left carotid angiogram films (**A and C**), and nonstereotactic T_1-weighted coronal MRI (**B** through plane Y in **C**). The principal feeding artery is the angular branch of the left middle cerebral artery (MCA), which appears to be a vessel of passage, sending small branches to the AVM as the artery continues out of the sylvian fissure (Syl) toward the angular gyrus of the inferior parietal lobule (LPi). The single inferior parietal draining vein (vv) joins the vein of Labbé, after exiting the nidus (and sylvian fissure) laterally to course inferiorly over the cortical surface toward the transverse sinus. The nidus itself is tucked into the inferior parietal lobule (LPi) approximately 1 cm deep to the cortical surface.

Either microsurgical removal or radiosurgical treatment of this malformation would be relatively straightforward. The neurologic risks associated with either treatment modality also would be similar and could involve deficits of dominant hemisphere higher cortical functions as a consequence of direct neural tissue injury or of vascular compromise. These could include Wernicke's aphasia, transcortical sensory aphasia (superior temporal gyrus or subcortical white matter, respectively), conduction aphasia (arcuate fasciculus), and/or a complete or partial Gerstmann's syndrome (angular gyrus, inferior parietal lobule). *(Figure continued on following pages.)*

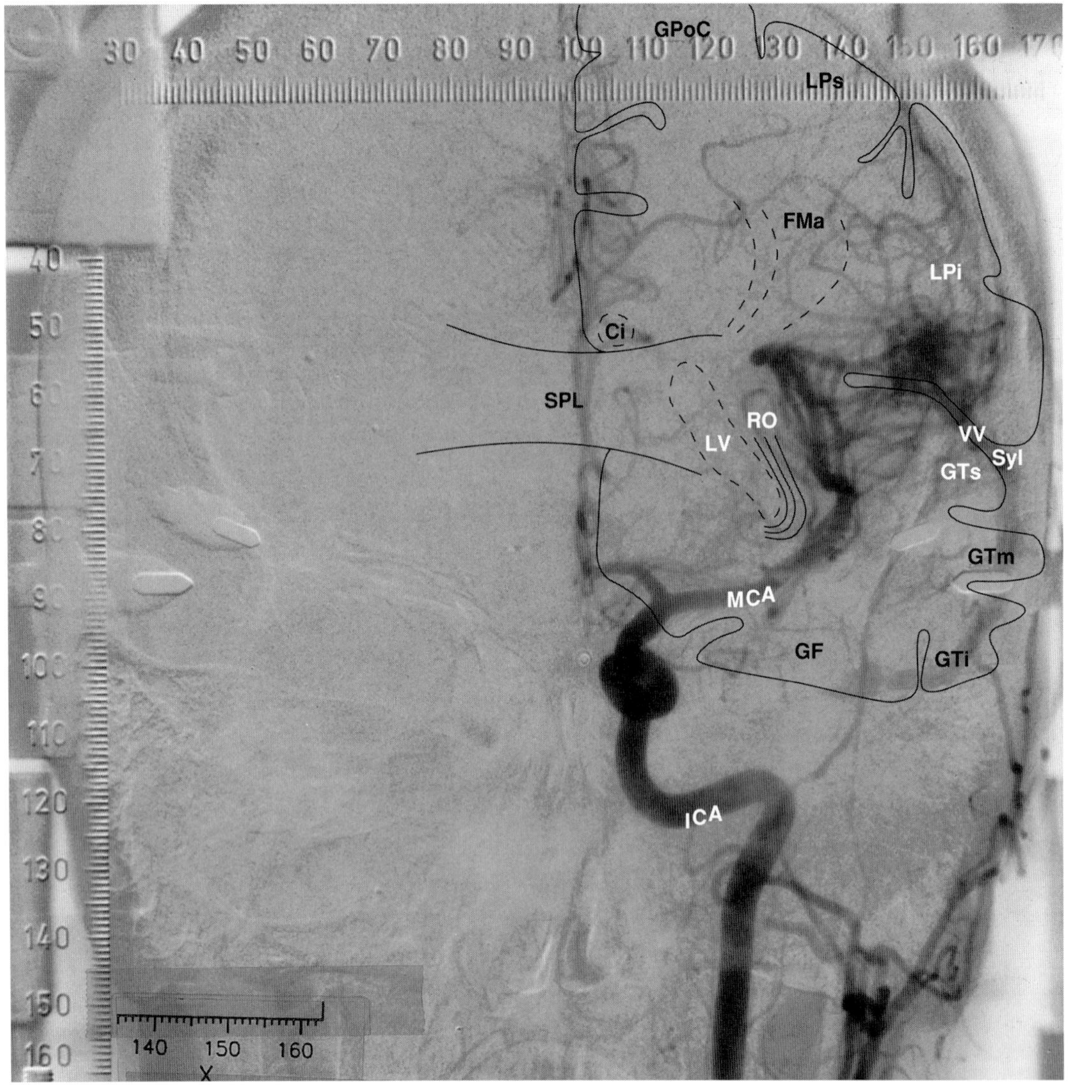

FIG. 4-4A.

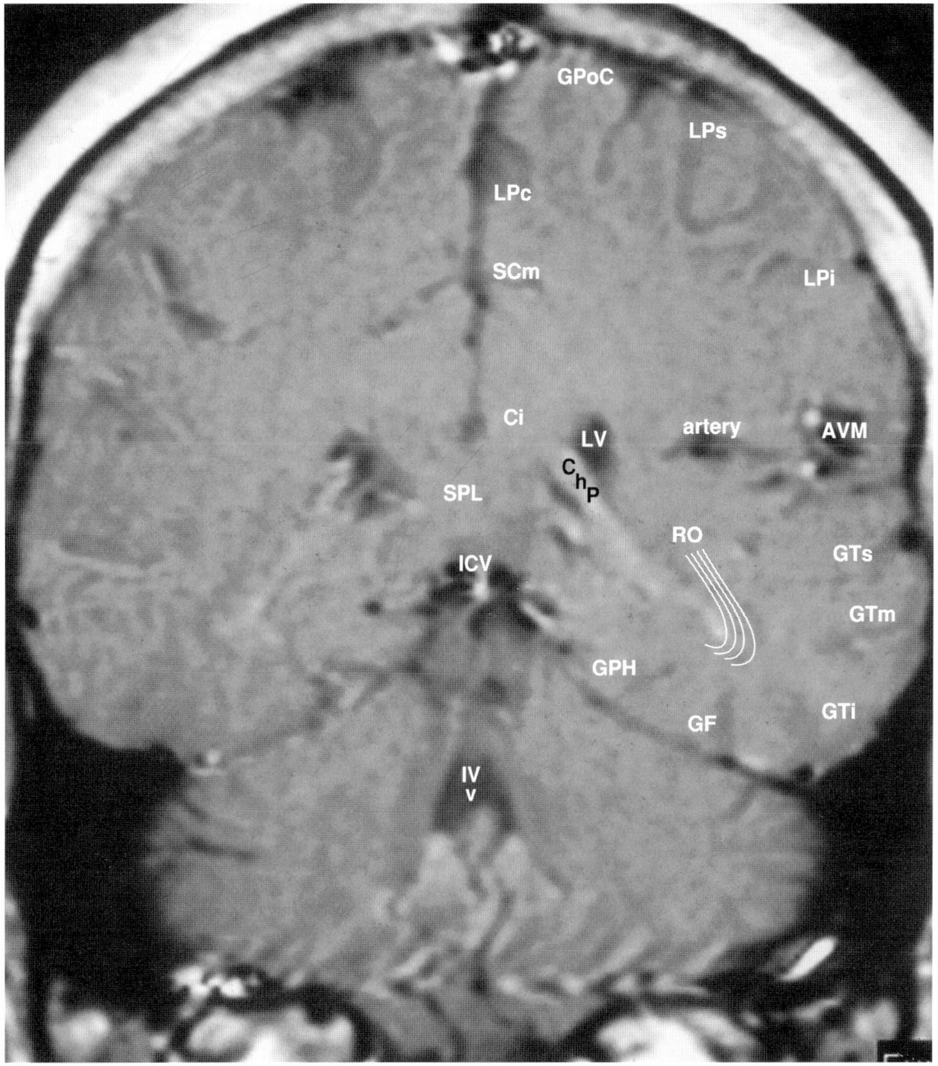
GPoC
LPs
LPc
SCm
LPi
Ci
LV
artery
AVM
ChP
SPL
RO
GTs
ICV
GTm
GPH
GF
GTi
IV
v

FIG. 4-4B.

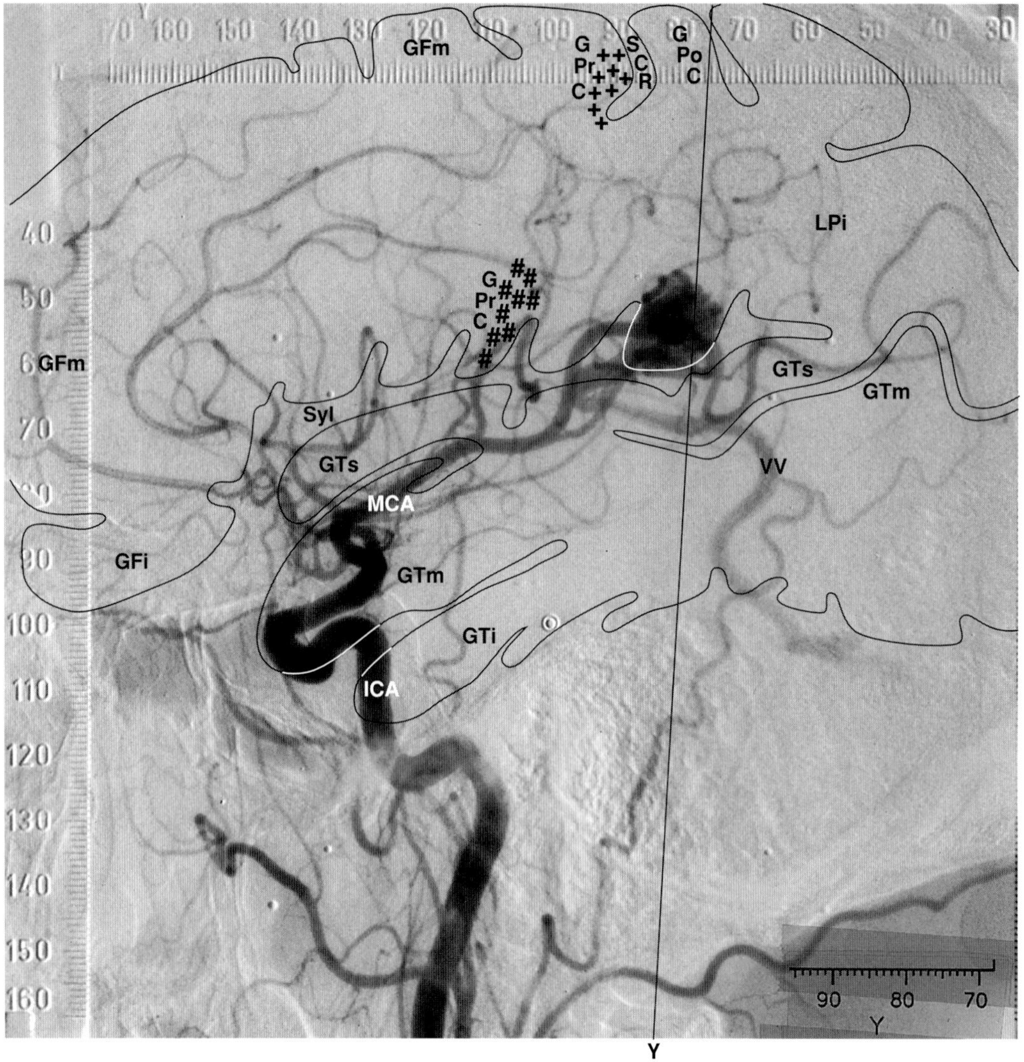
GFm
G
Pr
C
S
C
R
G
Po
C
LPi
G
Pr
C
GFm
GTs
GTm
Syl
GTs
VV
MCA
GFi
GTm
GTi
ICA
Y

FIG. 4-4C.

FIG. 4-5. Arteriovenous malformation of the left parietal lobe, PA and lateral stereotactic left carotid angiogram films (**A and C**) and nonstereotactic T_2-weighted MRIs in the coronal (**B**) and axial planes (**D** and **E** are axial images separated by 7.5 mm from inferior to superior). Line Y in **D** and **E** indicates the plane of **B**. The feeding vessels are hypertrophied angular and posterior parietal branches of the middle cerebral artery (MCA). The single visualized draining vein (vv) emerges from the posterosuperior margin of the AVM nidus to enter the superior sagittal sinus at the level of the postcentral gyrus (GPoC) and superior parietal lobule (LPs).

The nidus is located almost entirely within the inferior parietal lobule. The anterior margin of the nidus reaches the posterior bank of the postcentral sulcus (SPoC); the inferior margin of the nidus is entirely above the sylvian fissure. Somatosensory cortex of the postcentral gyrus lies across the postcentral sulcus from the AVM, whereas the arm, hand, and face areas of the motor strip (GPrC) (from superior to inferior) lie almost 2 cm anterior to the front edge of the AVM. Fibers of the corticospinal tract (Pyr) remain well anterior to the AVM as they descend through the corona radiata toward the posterior limb of the internal capsule (outside of the imaging planes illustrated here). The optic radiation (RO) passes through the temporo-occipital white matter well inferior to the margin of the AVM.

The principal neurologic risk associated with treatment of this lesion would be a complete or partial Gerstmann's syndrome due to injury of the inferior parietal lobule or its blood supply. Another risk might include cortical sensory loss due to injury of the postcentral gyrus or its afferent pathways from the thalamus. *(Figure continued on following pages.)*

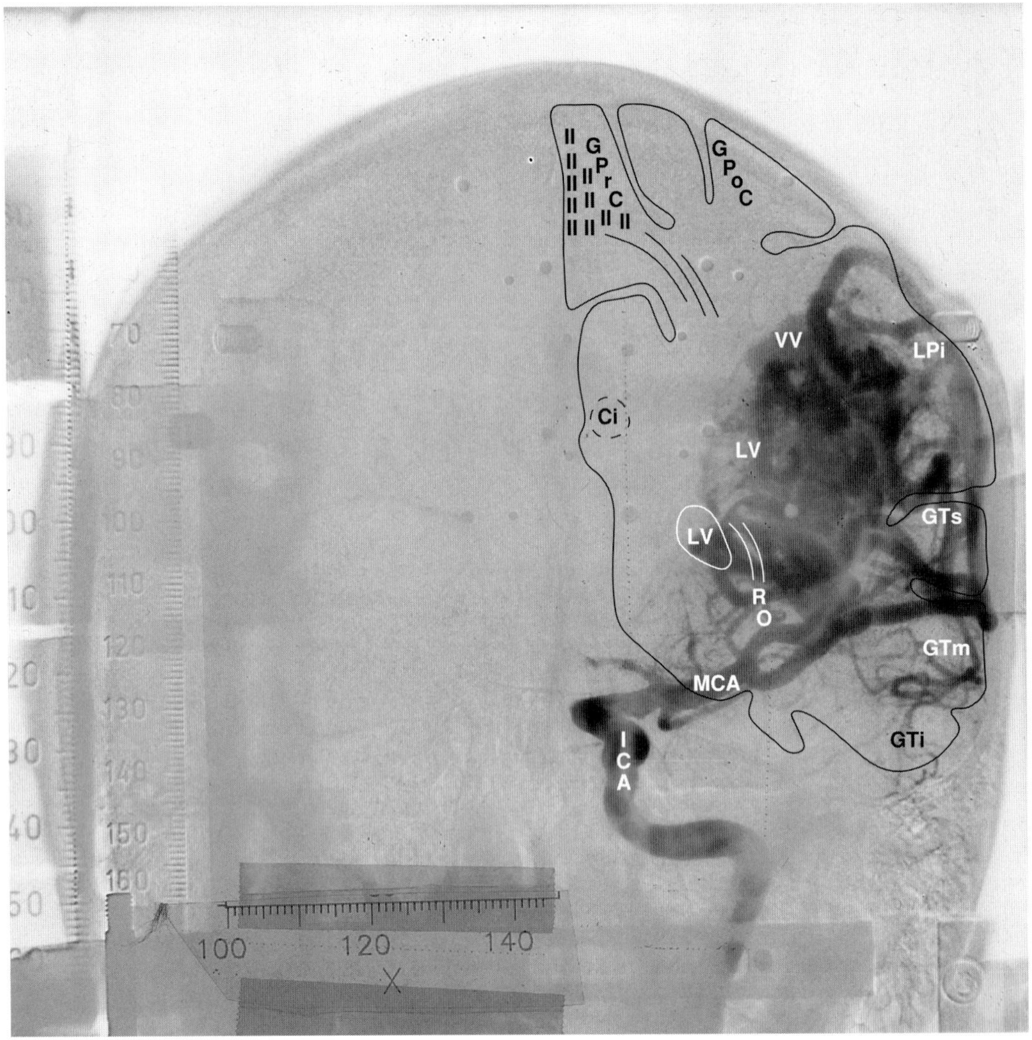
GPrC
GPoC
VV
LPi
Ci
LV
LV
GTs
RO
GTm
MCA
ICA
GTi
70
80
90
100
110
120
130
140
150
160
100
120
140
X

FIG. 4-5A.

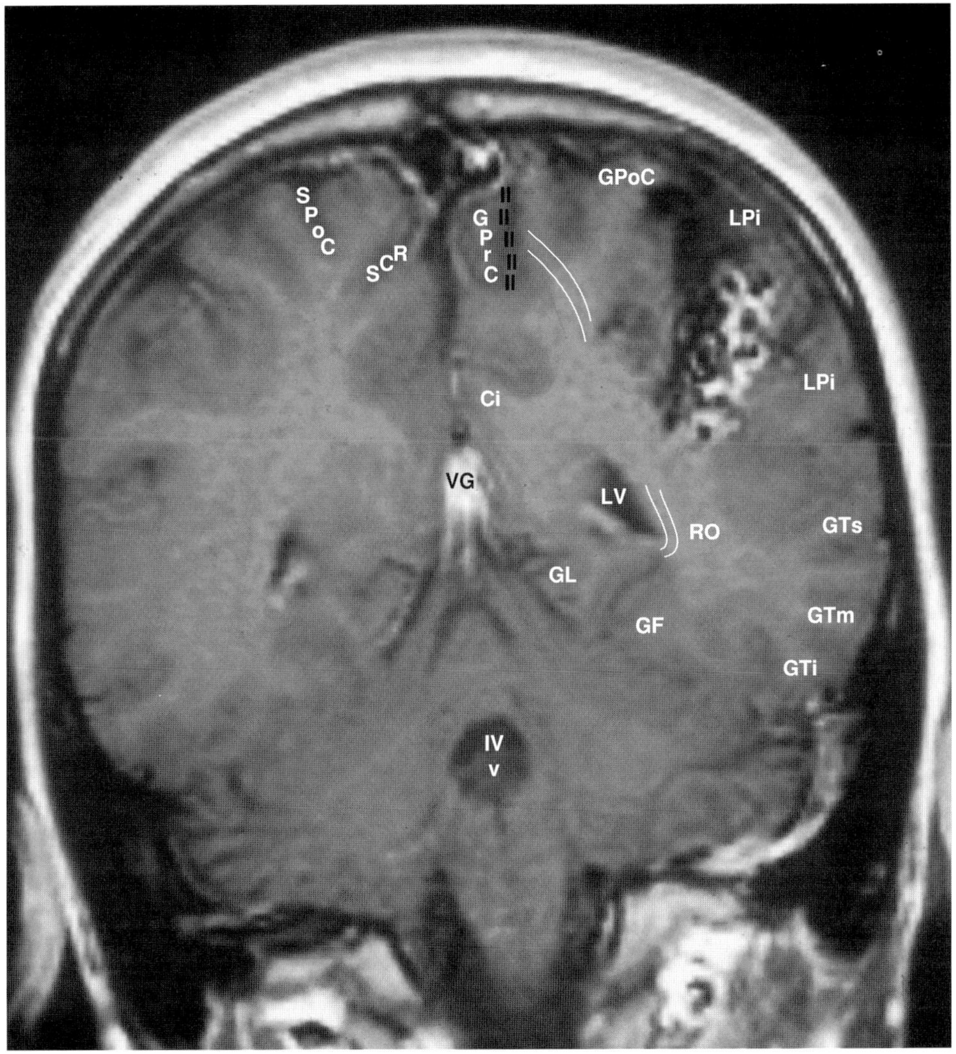

FIG. 4-5B.

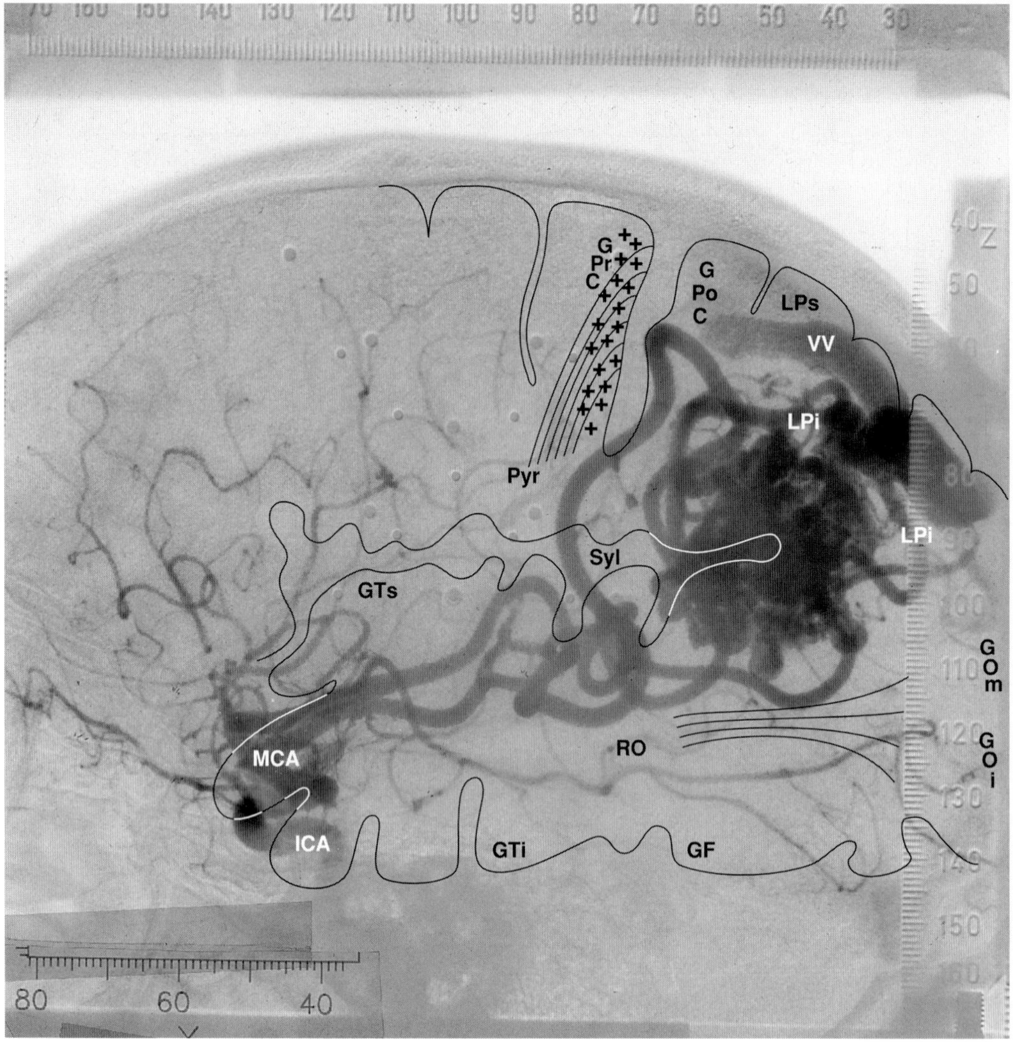

FIG. 4-5C.

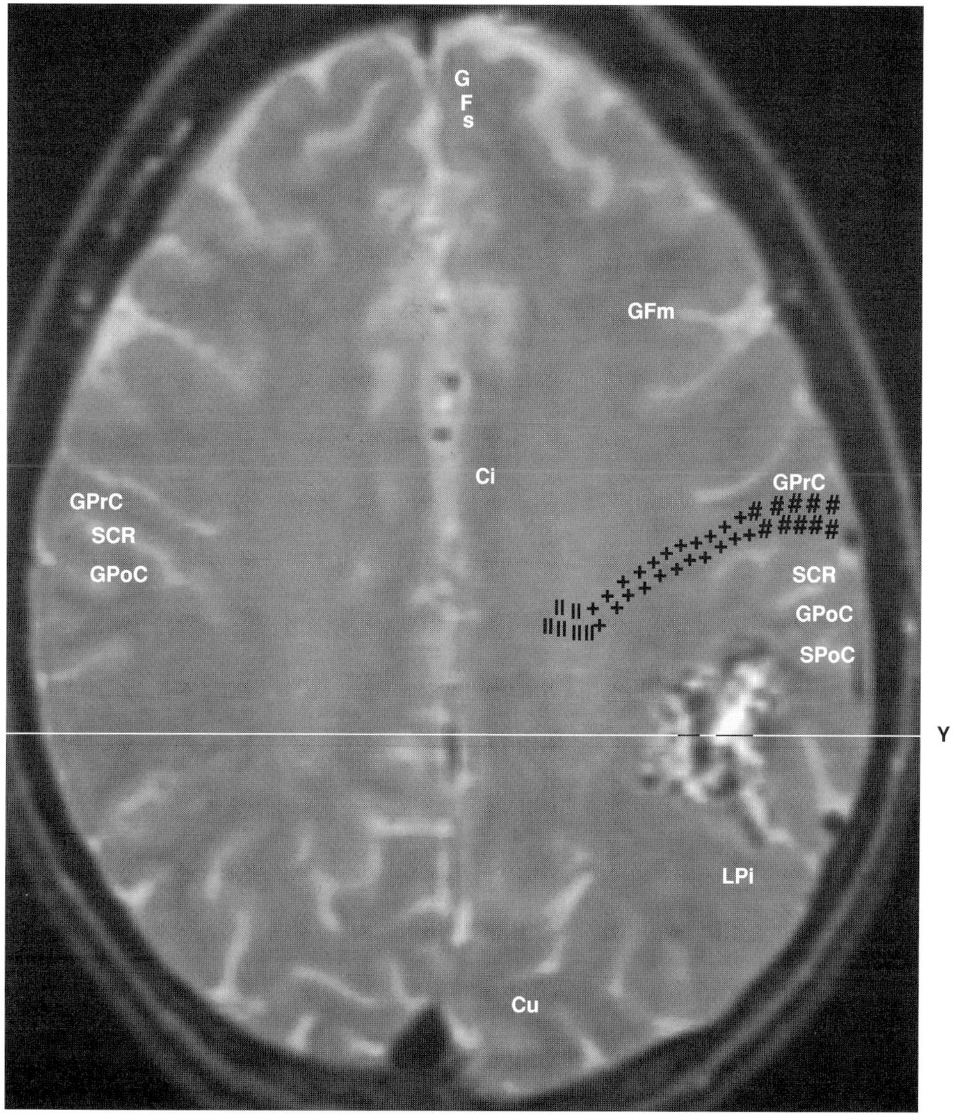

FIG. 4-5D.

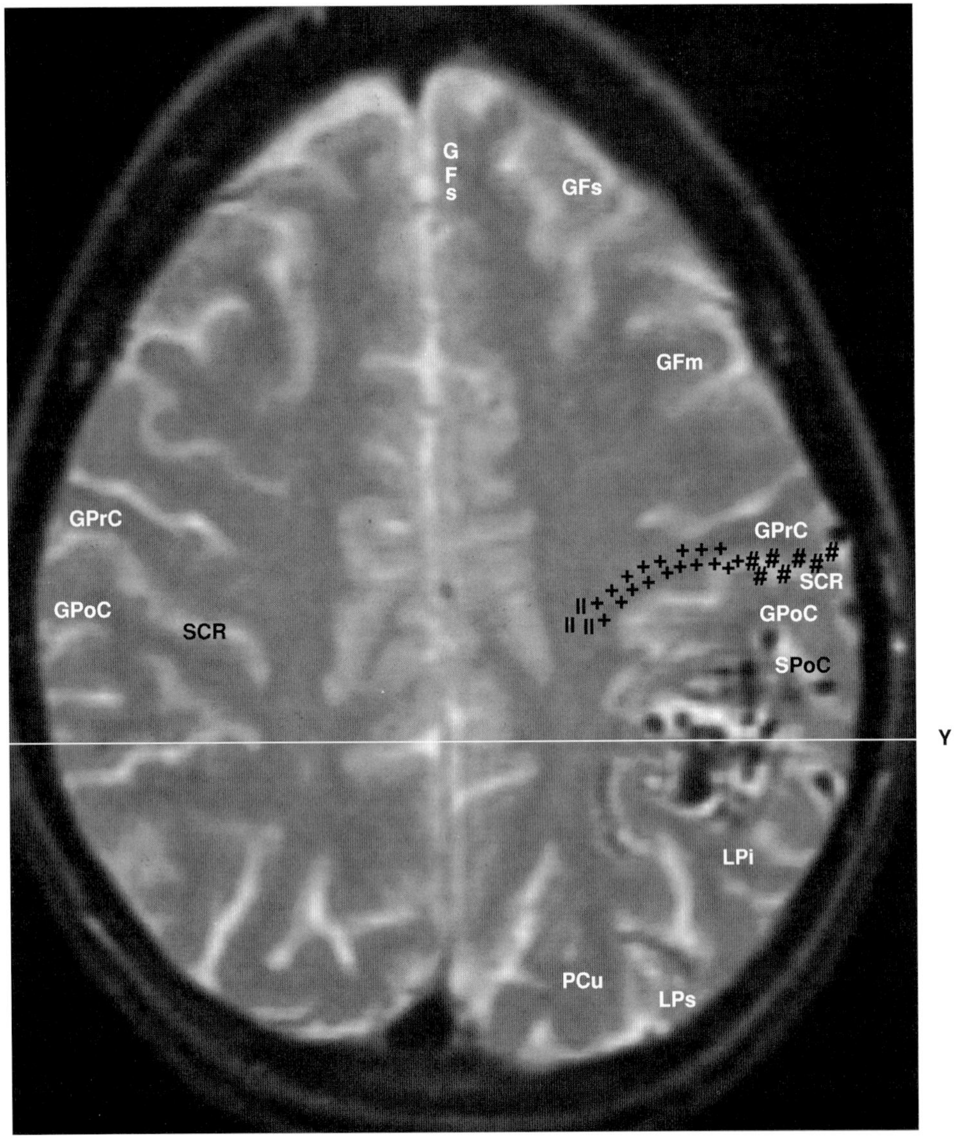

FIG. 4-5E.

FIG. 4-6. Arteriovenous malformation of the deep left posterior frontal/anterior parietal lobe junction with large associated variceal venous drainage, PA and lateral left carotid stereotactic angiogram films (**A and B**) and stereotactic T_1-weighted axial MRIs separated by 12 mm from inferior to superior, respectively (**C and D**). The axial planes in **C** and **D** correspond to lines Z_1 and Z_2 on the angiographic images, respectively. The AVM is fed by enlarged left middle cerebral artery (MCA) branches that enter the nidus around its inferior (lenticulostriate branch territory), lateral, and, to a lesser extent, superior margins. No large vessels appear to enter or exit the malformation along the medial (deep) margin, possibly because of poor anterior cerebral artery filling on this injection. An enormously dilated variceal complex (VV, **B**) that appears partially thrombosed (VVX, **C**), lies posterior, lateral, and inferior to the compact portion of the nidus. In fact, this variceal complex occupies a larger volume of the parietal lobe than does the nidus. Ultimately, the varix drains superficially into the veins of Trolard and Labbé. A small amount of deep venous drainage also may be present along the ependyma of the lateral ventricle (LV).

The nidus lies deep within the corona radiata beneath the pre- and postcentral gyri (GPrC, GPoC) and inferior parietal lobule (LPi). Telangiectatic feeding vessels distort and displace the precentral gyrus, whereas the anterior portion of the varix almost completely obscures parts of the postcentral gyrus. Pyramidal motor fibers and thalamocortical primary sensory radiations appear to percolate around and/or through the anterolateral edge of the compact portion of the nidus. The deep edge of the nidus reaches the cingulate gyrus (Ci) superiorly and the superolateral margin of the lateral ventricle inferiorly. In doing so, the AVM crosses the most posterior part of the posterior limb of the internal capsule (CPIP). Although the dorsolateral margin of the thalamus is displaced slightly in an anteromedial direction by the mass of this malformation, the AVM remains confined within the telencephalon.

The most serious neurologic risks associated with treatment of this AVM would be a contralateral (right) hemiplegia and hemisensory loss from injury to the sensorimotor cortex, corona radiata, and/or internal capsule. Damage to the inferior parietal lobule (at the posteroinferior margin of the AVM) also could cause a partial or complete Gerstmann's syndrome. *(Figure continued on following pages.)*

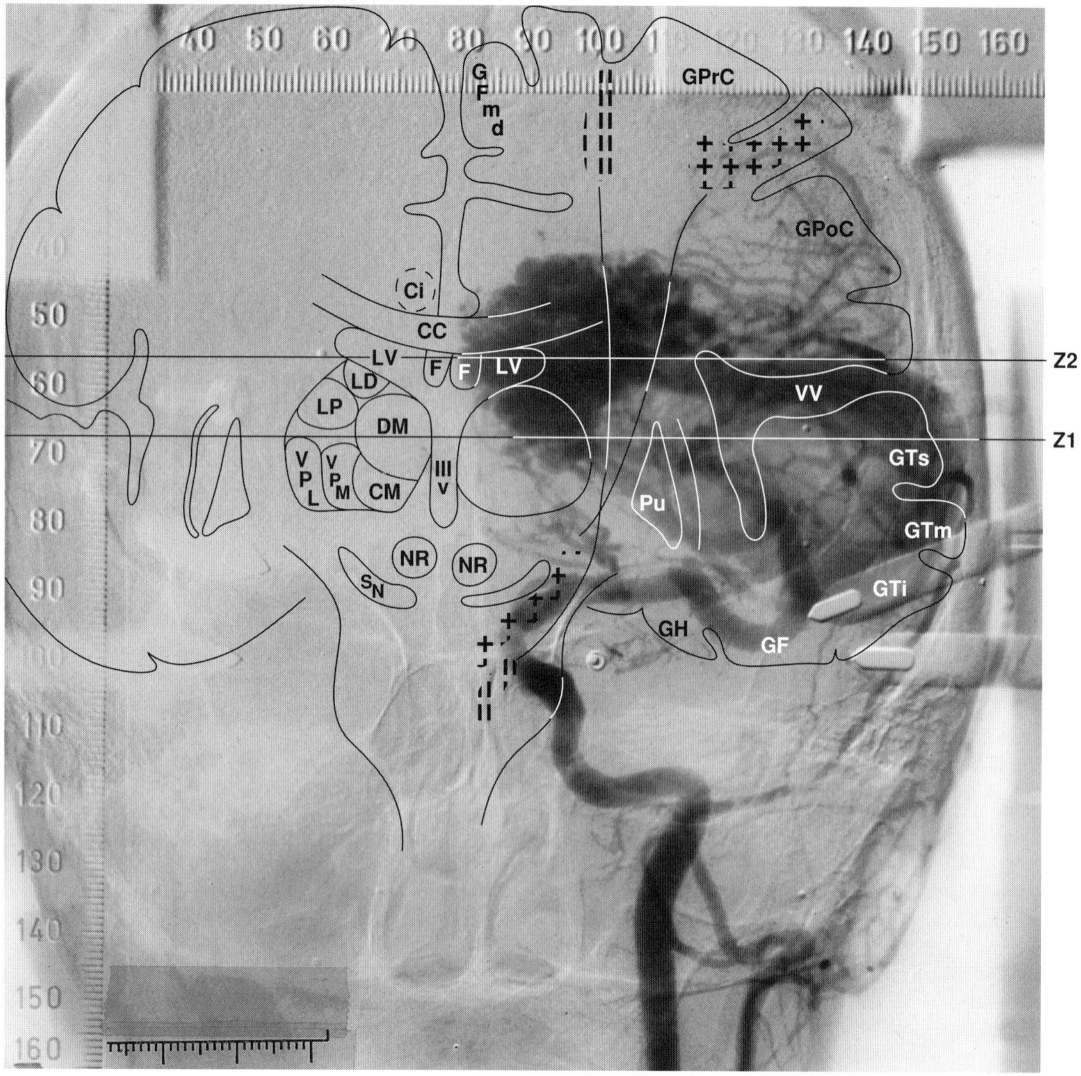

GFmd
GPrC
GPoC
Ci
CC
LV
F
F
LV
Z2
VV
LD
LP
DM
Z1
V P L
V P M
CM
III v
GTs
Pu
GTm
NR
NR
SN
GTi
GH
GF

FIG. 4-6A.

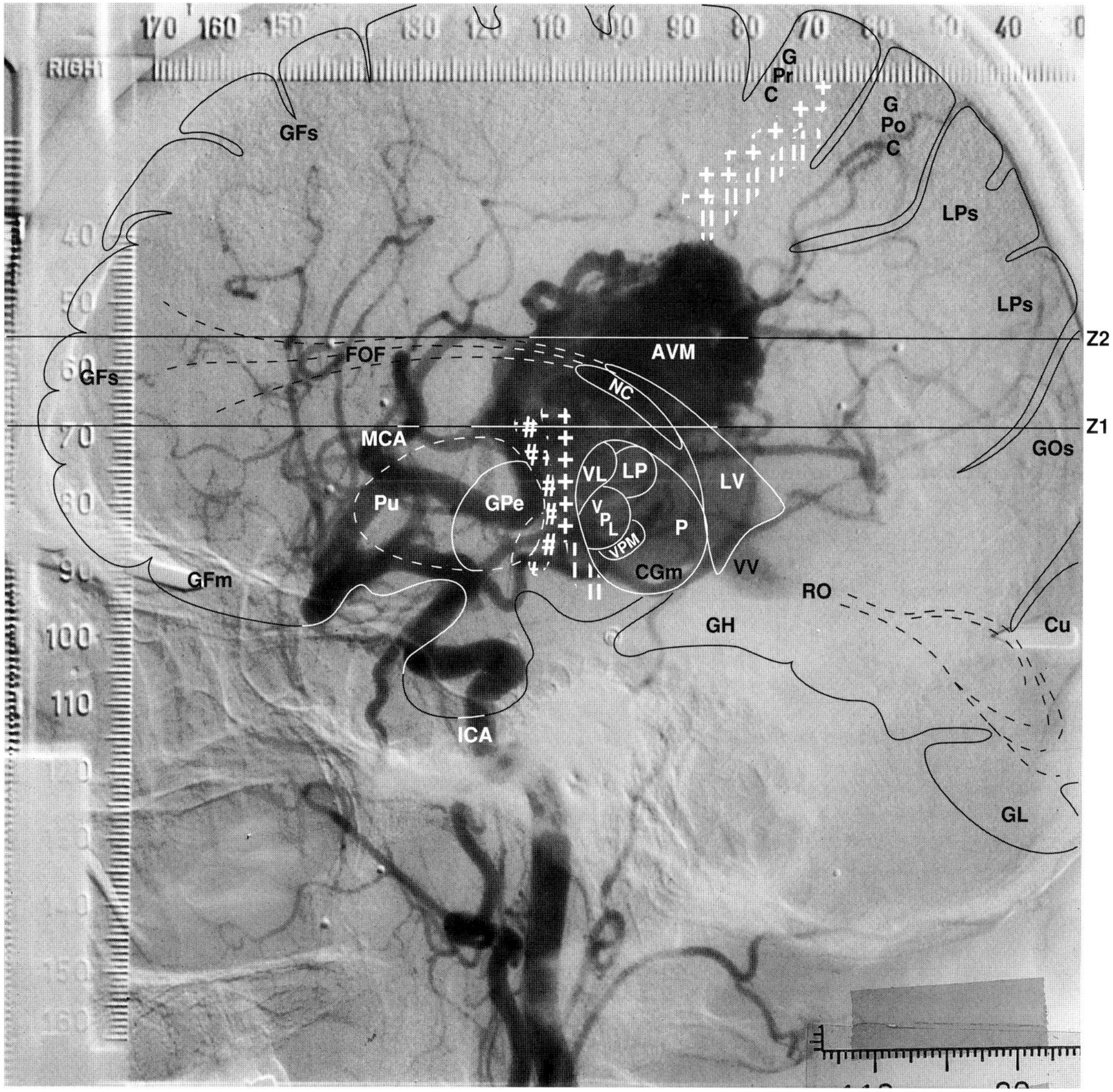
RIGHT
GFs
G
Pr
C
G
Po
C
LPs
LPs
Z2
FOF
AVM
GFs
NC
Z1
MCA
VL
LP
LV
GOs
Pu
GPe
V
P
L
VPM
P
CGm
VV
GFm
RO
GH
Cu
ICA
GL

FIG. 4-6B.

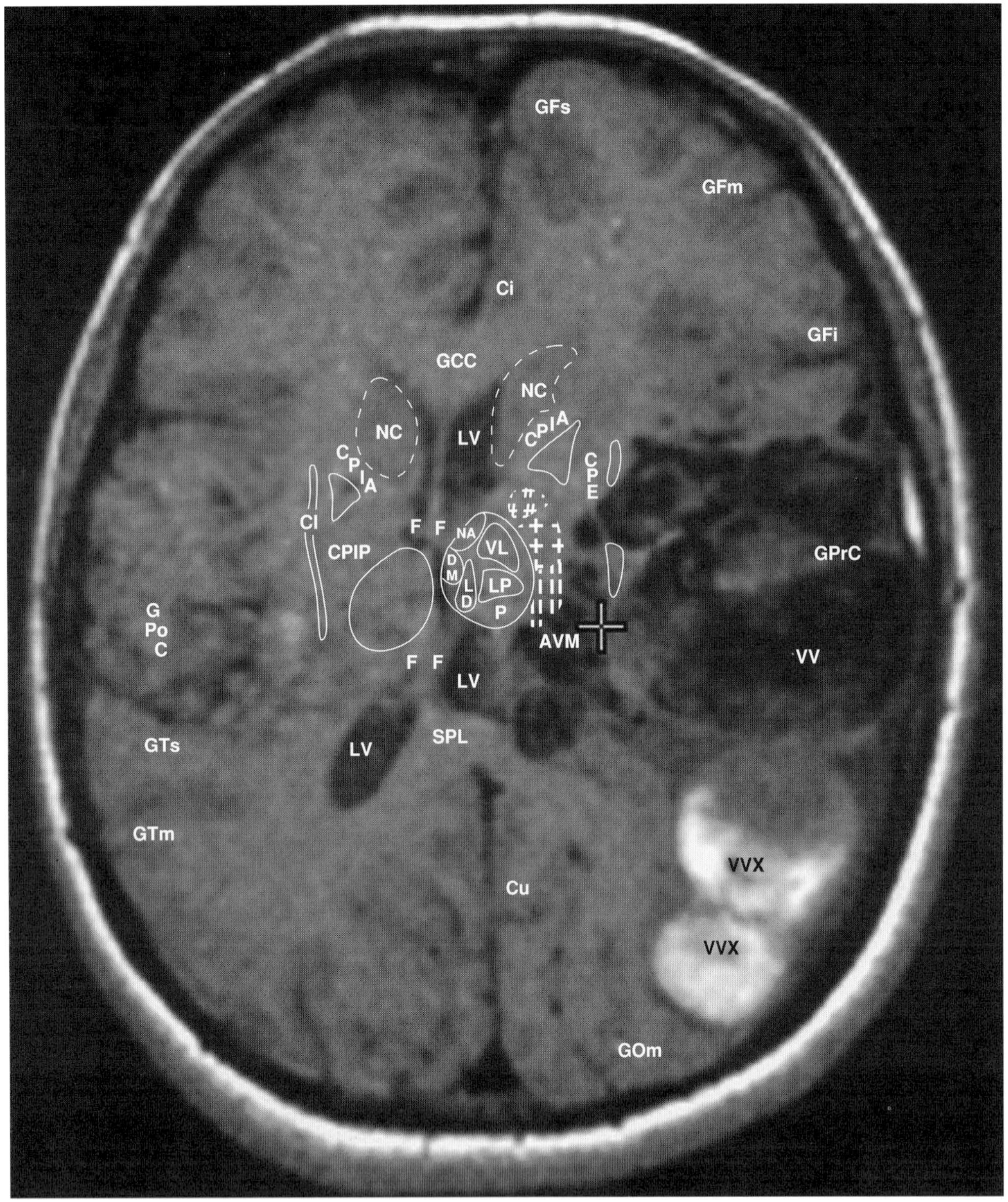
GFs
GFm
Ci
GFi
GCC
NC
NC
LV
CPIA
CPIA
CPE
CI
CPIP
F F
NA
VL
DM
LD
LP
P
GPrC
G
Po
C
AVM
F F
LV
VV
GTs
LV
SPL
GTm
VVX
Cu
VVX
GOm

FIG. 4-6C.

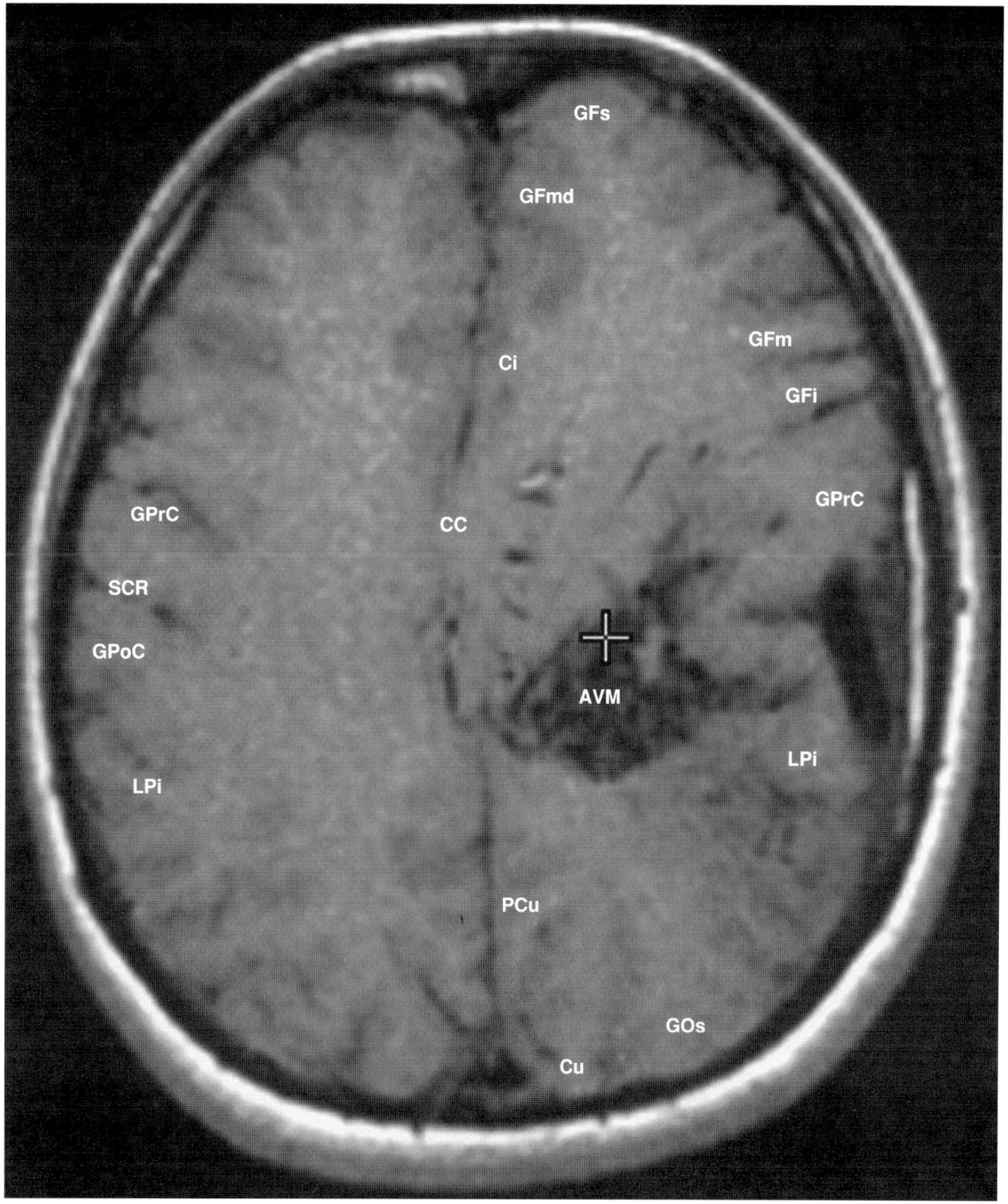

FIG. 4-6D.

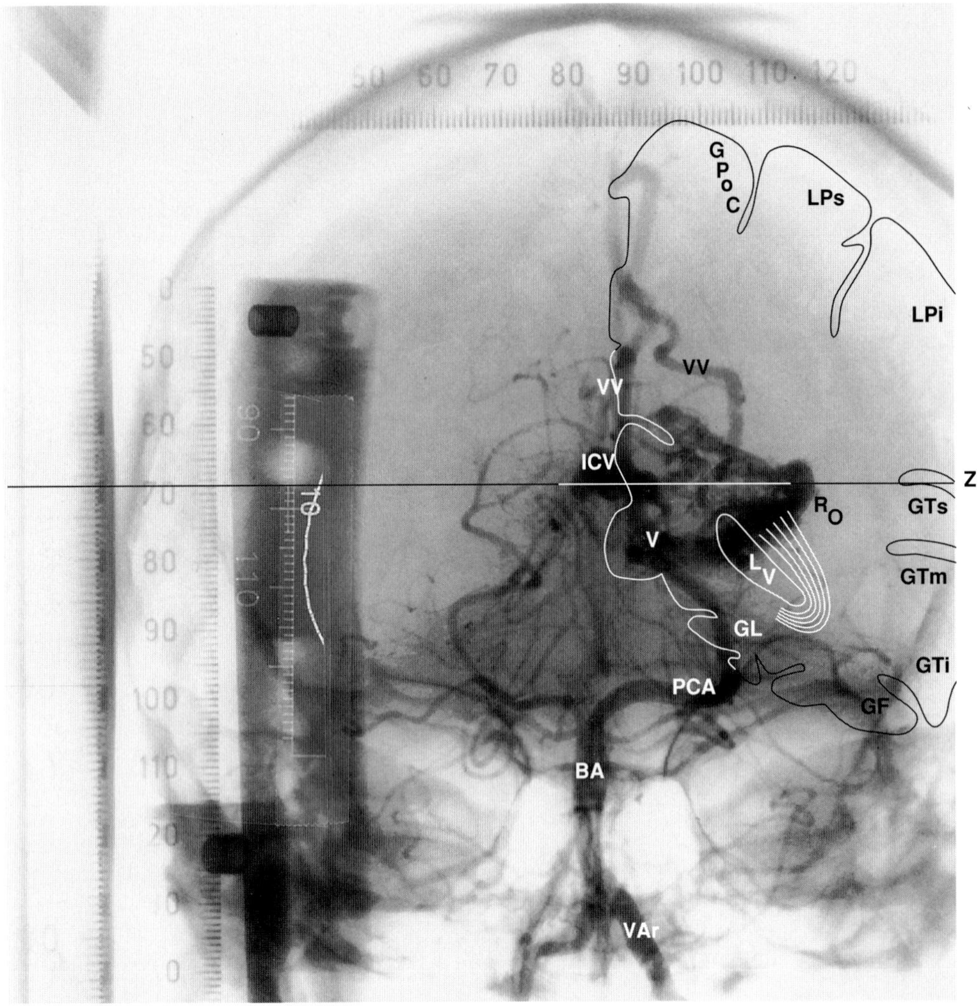

FIG. 4-7A.

FIG. 4-7. Arteriovenous malformation of the left calcarine sulcus, atrium, and occipital horn of the lateral ventricle (LV), PA and lateral stereotactic left vertebral angiogram films (**A and B**) and stereotactic T_1-weighted MRI (**C**) at the axial level of line Z in **A**. Feeding arteries include parieto-occipital branches of the posterior cerebral artery within the anterior calcarine sulcus (AA), and possibly a contribution from the lateral posterior choroidal artery, where an anterolateral appendage of the nidus appears to involve the choroid plexus (ChP) in the atrium of the lateral ventricle (LV). Venous drainage includes both the superficial and deep venous system. Superficial drainage is via two enlarged veins (vv) that exit the nidus at its posterior superior margin and posterior pole to course along the interhemispheric fissure and enter the superior sagittal sinus. The deep venous drainage (v) passes in an anteromedial direction from the anterior margin of the nidus to join the internal cerebral vein (ICV)/vein of Galen complex. Retrograde blood flow within the basal vein of Rosenthal (BVR) is seen in **B** projected posterior, and then superior, to the posterior cerebral arteries (PCA), respectively, in the posterior to anterior direction.

The densest portion of the nidus is shaped like a small sausage with both ends turned upward and is oriented along a posterolateral to anteromedial axis. The posterolateral margin involves the lateral ventricle and may displace a portion of the occipital horn in the inferolateral direction. The anteromedial edge of the nidus reaches the interhemispheric fissure along the course of the deep draining vein. The forceps major of the corpus callosum crosses above the anterior portion of the AVM, whereas the white matter of the lingual and hippocampal gyri (GL, H) lie beneath it. The optic radiation immediately abuts the AVM along its lateral margin for a substantial portion of its course between the lateral geniculate body (CGl, the top of which is seen in **C**) and the calcarine cortex. Surgical removal or radiosurgical treatment of this AVM carries the risk of causing a right-sided visual field defect from injury to the optic radiation or blood supply to that pathway and/or the primary visual cortex. *(Figure continued on following pages.)*

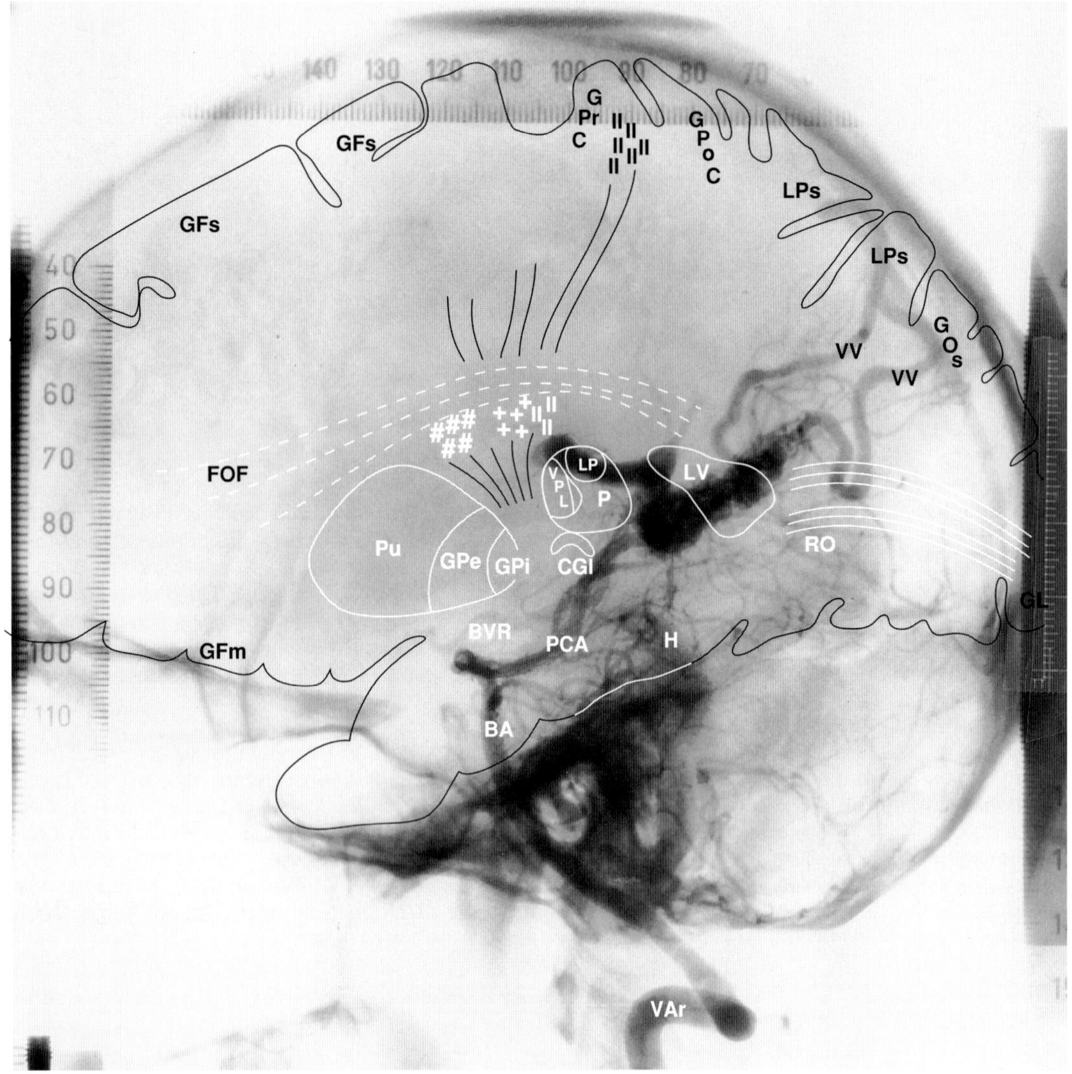
GFs
GFs
G Pr C
G P o C
LPs
LPs
G O s
VV
VV
FOF
LP
V P L
P
LV
Pu
GPe
GPi
CGl
RO
GL
GFm
BVR
PCA
H
BA
VAr
40
50
60
70
80
90
100
110
140
130
120
110
100
90
80
70

FIG. 4-7B.

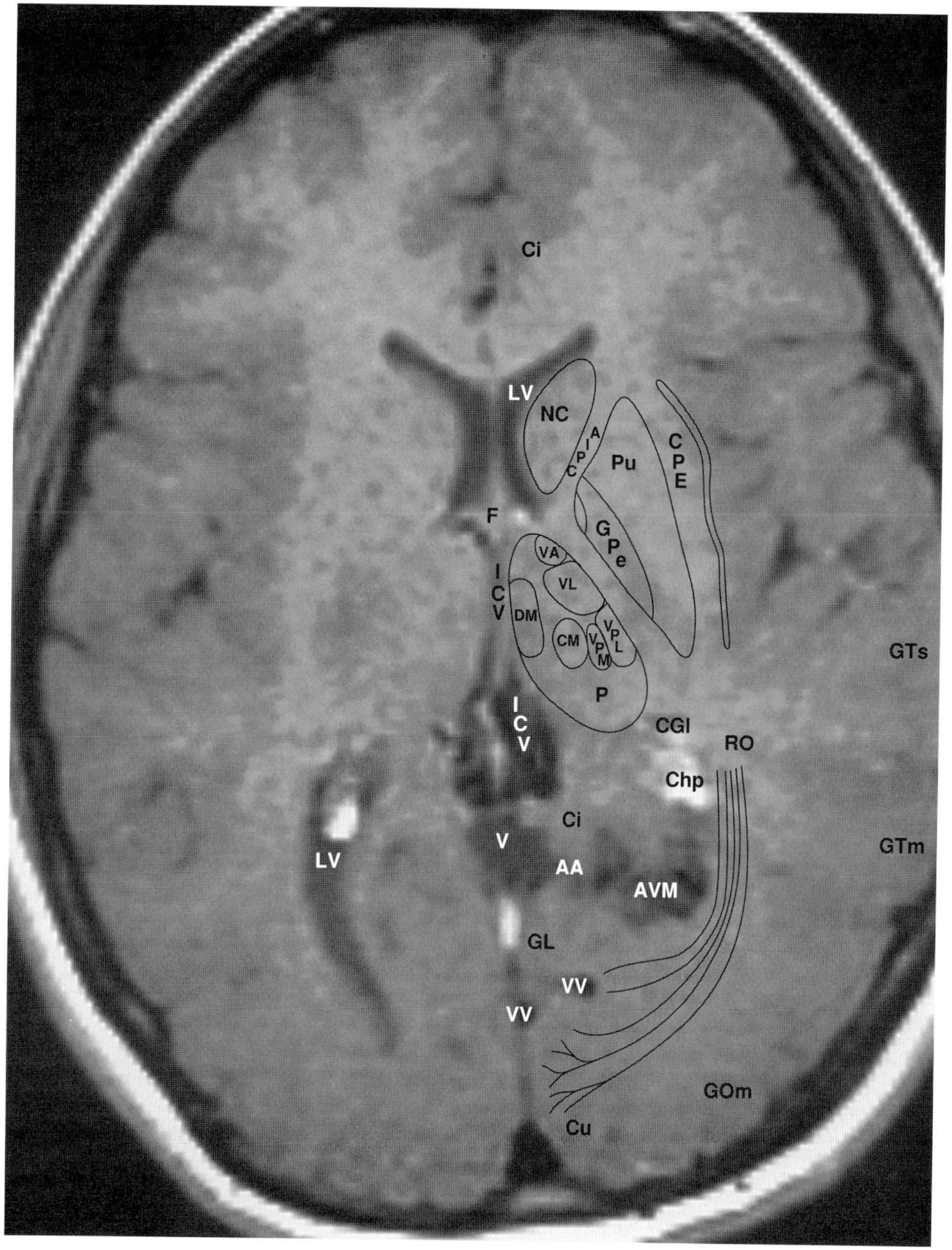
Ci
LV
NC
A
I
P
C
Pu
C
P
E
F
G
P
e
VA
VL
I
C
V
DM
CM
V
P
M
V
P
L
P
GTs
I
C
V
CGl
RO
Chp
Ci
V
LV
AA
AVM
GTm
GL
VV
VV
GOm
Cu

FIG. 4-7C.

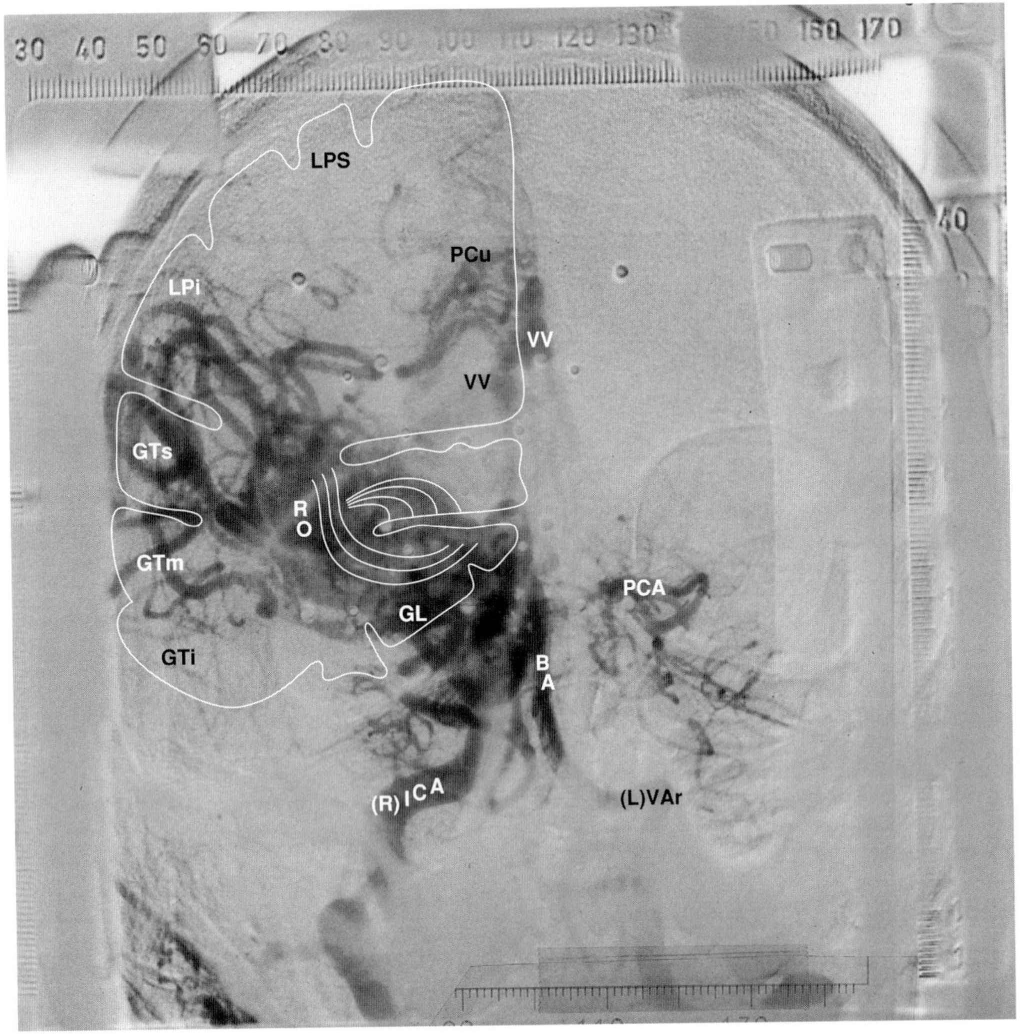

FIG. 4-8A.

FIG. 4-8. Large arteriovenous malformation occupying a substantial portion of the right occipital lobe, superimposed PA and lateral right carotid and left vertebral stereotactic angiogram films (**A and B**), and nonstereotactic sagittal T_1-weighted (**C**) and axial T_2-weighted (**D**) MRIs, respectively. Arterial phase films from the carotid and vertebral artery injection series having exactly the same magnification factor are combined to illustrate the entire AVM nidus because neither injection alone filled both vascular compartments adequately. Feeding arteries include branches of all three major vessels to the right cerebral hemisphere. The pericallosal branch of the anterior cerebral artery (ACA) feeds the anteromedial-superior portion of the nidus. The posterior parietal and angular branches of the middle cerebral artery (MCA) enter the anterolateral-superior portion of the nidus, and the parieto-occipital branch of the posterior cerebral artery supplies the entire inferior compartment of the nidus. The AVM appears to be centered within or near the parieto-occipital sulcus (SPO) and extends from the surface of the superior occipital gyrus (GOs) posteriorly to the back edge of the splenium of the corpus callosum (SPL) anteriorly. The mediolateral dimension of the nidus extends from the interhemispheric surface of the cuneate and precuneate gyri (Cu, PCu) to the subcortical white matter of the middle occipital gyrus (GOm) laterally.

The superior edge of the optic radiation (RO) probably is displaced downward to pass around or through the inferior margin of the AVM. The inferolateral AVM margin lies deep to the white matter of the inferior parietal lobule (LPi), whereas the superolateral-posterior margin involves the white matter of the superior parietal lobule (LPs). Thus, neurologic deficits that could occur as a result of surgery or radiosurgical treatment (or rupture) of this AVM include a left-sided partial (inferior) or complete homonymous hemianopsia (optic radiation, calcarine cortex), and/or disorders of higher cortical function, including apraxia (superior parietal lobule). Cortical sensory loss or hemisensory neglect from damage to the thalamocortical radiations (to the postcentral gyrus region) also could occur but would be less likely for this posteriorly located malformation. *(Figure continued on following pages.)*

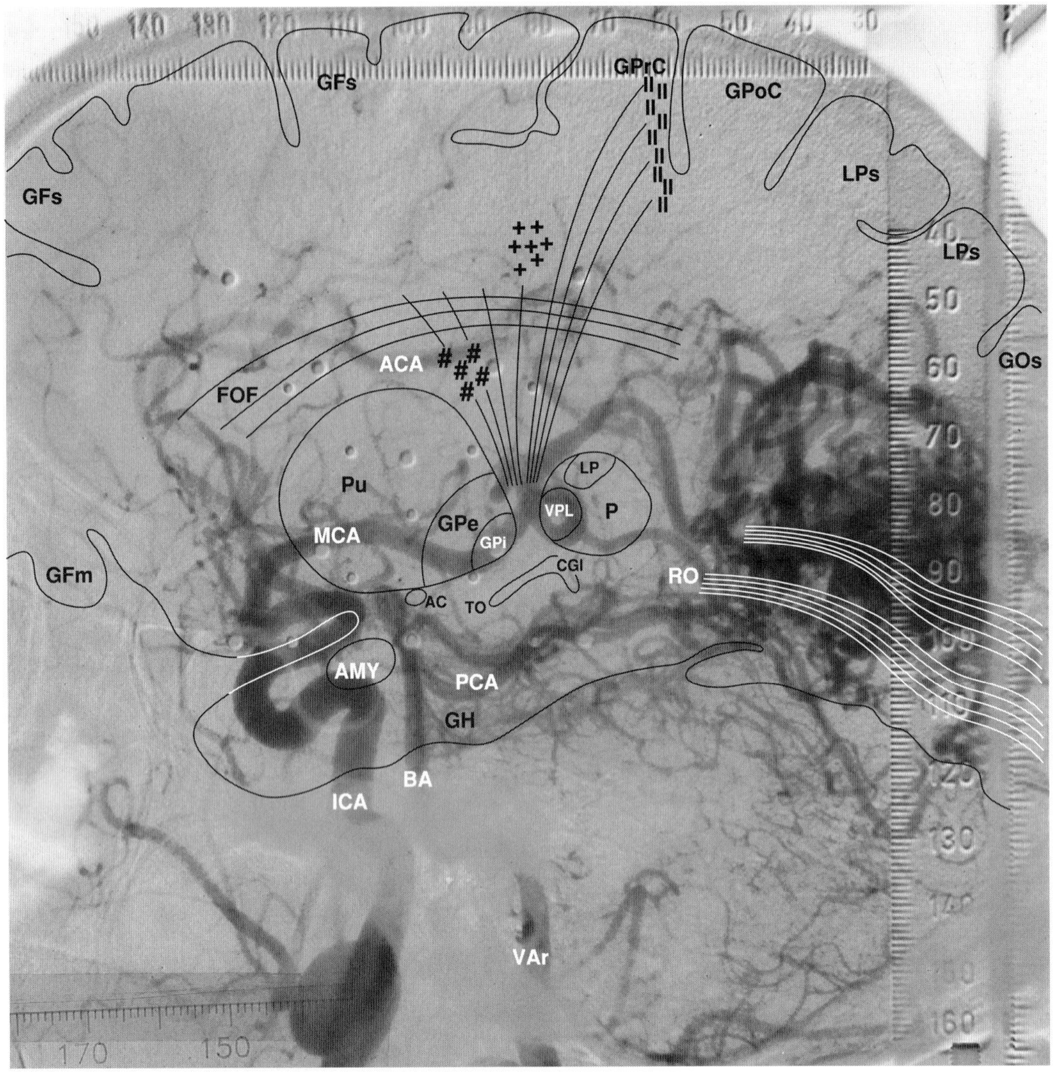
GFs
GPrC
GPoC
GFs
LPs
LPs
GOs
ACA
FOF
Pu
LP
VPL
P
GPe
GPi
MCA
CGI
RO
GFm
AC
TO
AMY
PCA
GH
BA
ICA
VAr

FIG. 4-8B.

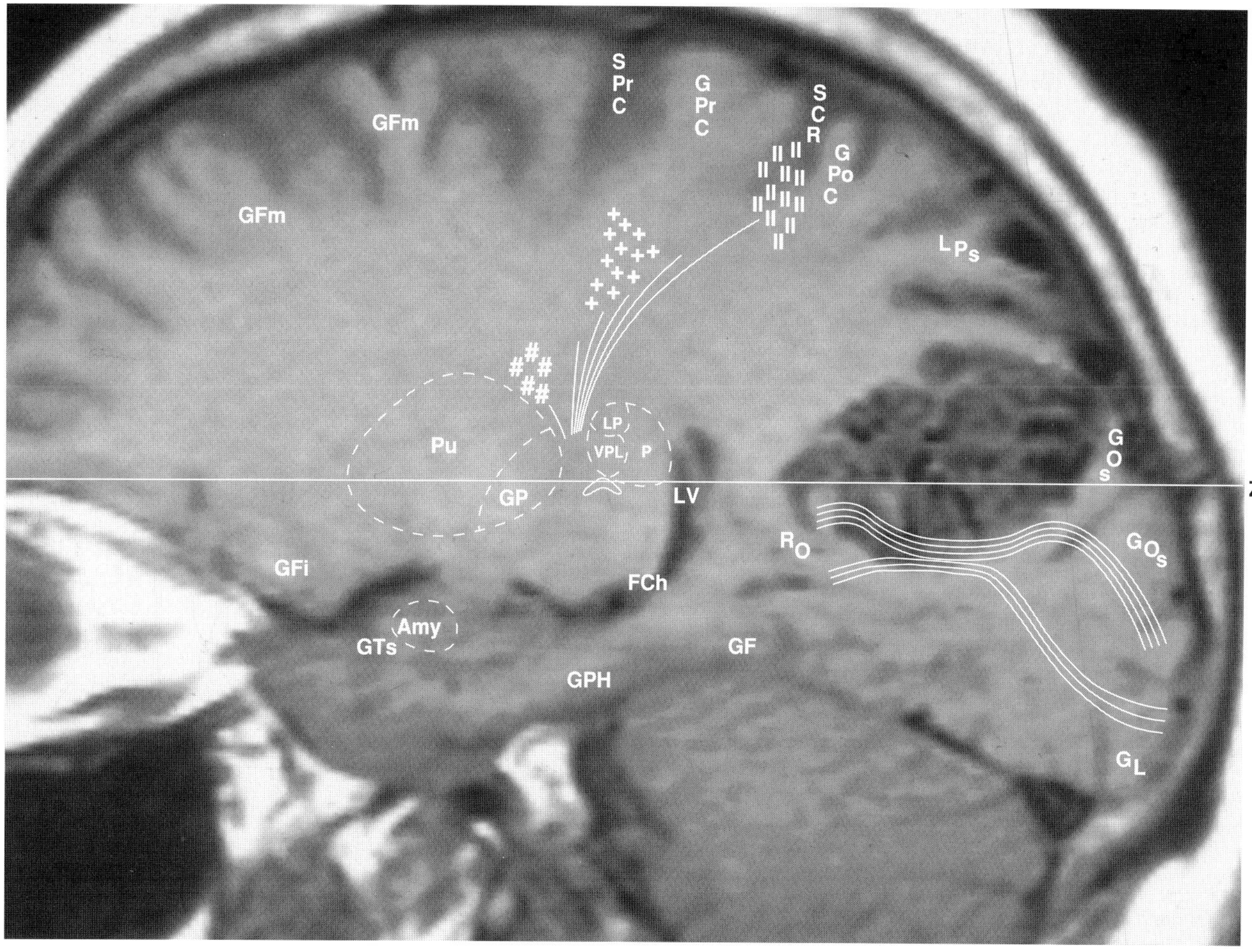
S
Pr
C
G
Pr
C
S
C
R
G
Po
C
GFm
GFm
LPs
Pu
LP
VPL
P
GP
LV
GOs
Z
RO
GOs
GFi
FCh
Amy
GTs
GF
GPH
GL

FIG. 4-8C.

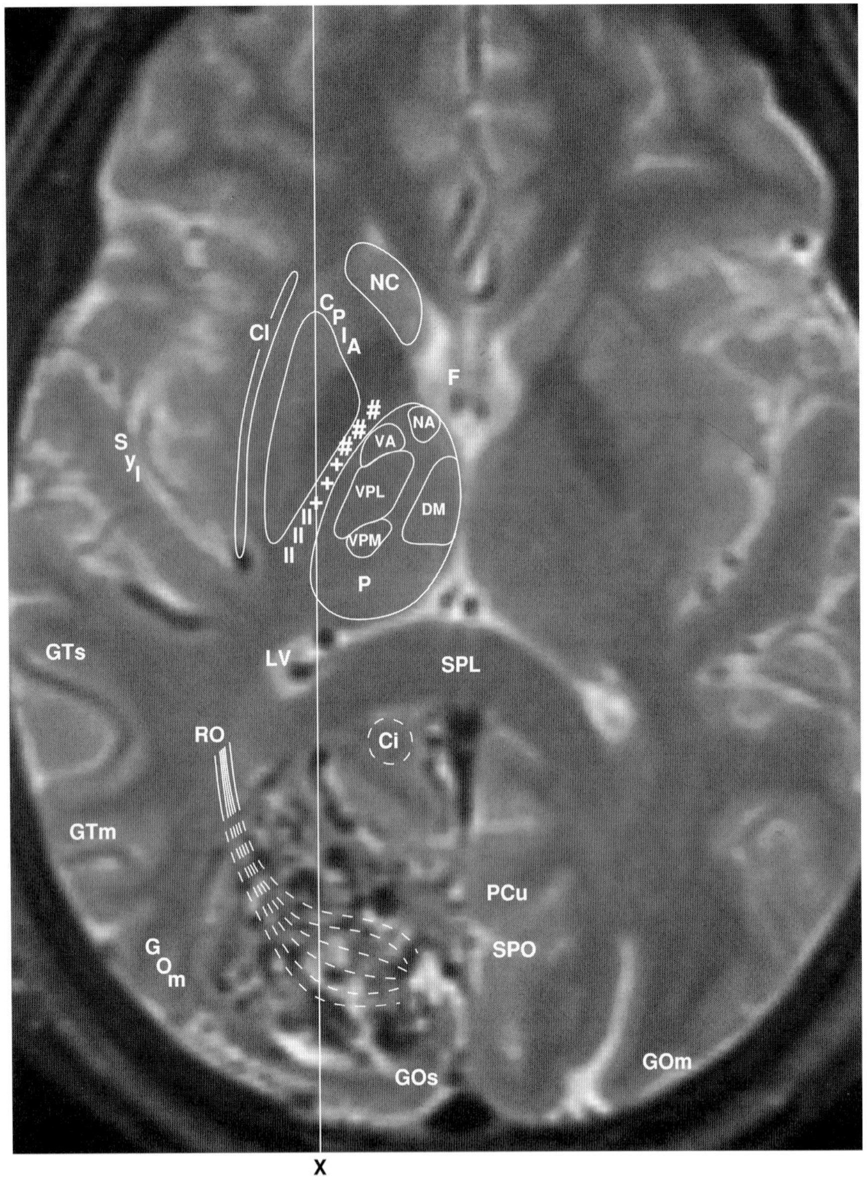

NC
C
P
I
A
Cl
F
S
y
l
NA
VA
VPL
DM
VPM
P
GTs
LV
SPL
RO
Ci
GTm
PCu
G
O
m
SPO
GOs
GOm
X

FIG. 4-8D.

FIG. 4-9. Arteriovenous malformation of the right cingulate gyrus, PA and lateral stereotactic right carotid angiogram films (**A and C**) and nonstereotactic T_1-weighted, contrast-enhanced coronal (**B**) and noncontrast sagittal (**D**) MRIs. The cavity seen in **D** within the paracentral lobule is the result of previous surgery to remove a hematoma that was located superior to the remaining AVM nidus (AVM). The coronal plane of **B** passes through the AVM nidus (anterior to the surgical defect) and through the hypothalamus–mid-brain junction at the caudal edge of the mammillary bodies (cm). This AVM is fed by the pericallosal and callosomarginal branches of the anterior cerebral artery (ACA). Venous drainage is on the deep (inferior) side of the AVM (vv), through the internal cerebral veins (ICV) toward the vein of Galen (VG).

The AVM nidus occupies the right cingulate gyrus, cingulum bundle (Ci), and superior edge of the corpus callosum at the level of the dorsomedial nucleus of the thalamus (DM). The draining vein passes inferiorly and laterally around the lateral ventricle (LV) to reach the internal cerebral vein. The superior (superficial) margin of the nidus reaches the cingulate sulcus (SC) and the deepest edge of the precentral and postcentral gyri (GPrC, GPoC). Previous hemorrhage and surgery have distorted the anatomy of the postcentral gyrus and sulcus.

The neurologic risks associated with treatment of this AVM might include contralateral leg weakness due to injury of the precentral gyrus or corticospinal (Pyr) tract. Additional cortical sensory loss from further injury to the postcentral gyrus also is possible. *(Figure continued on following pages.)*

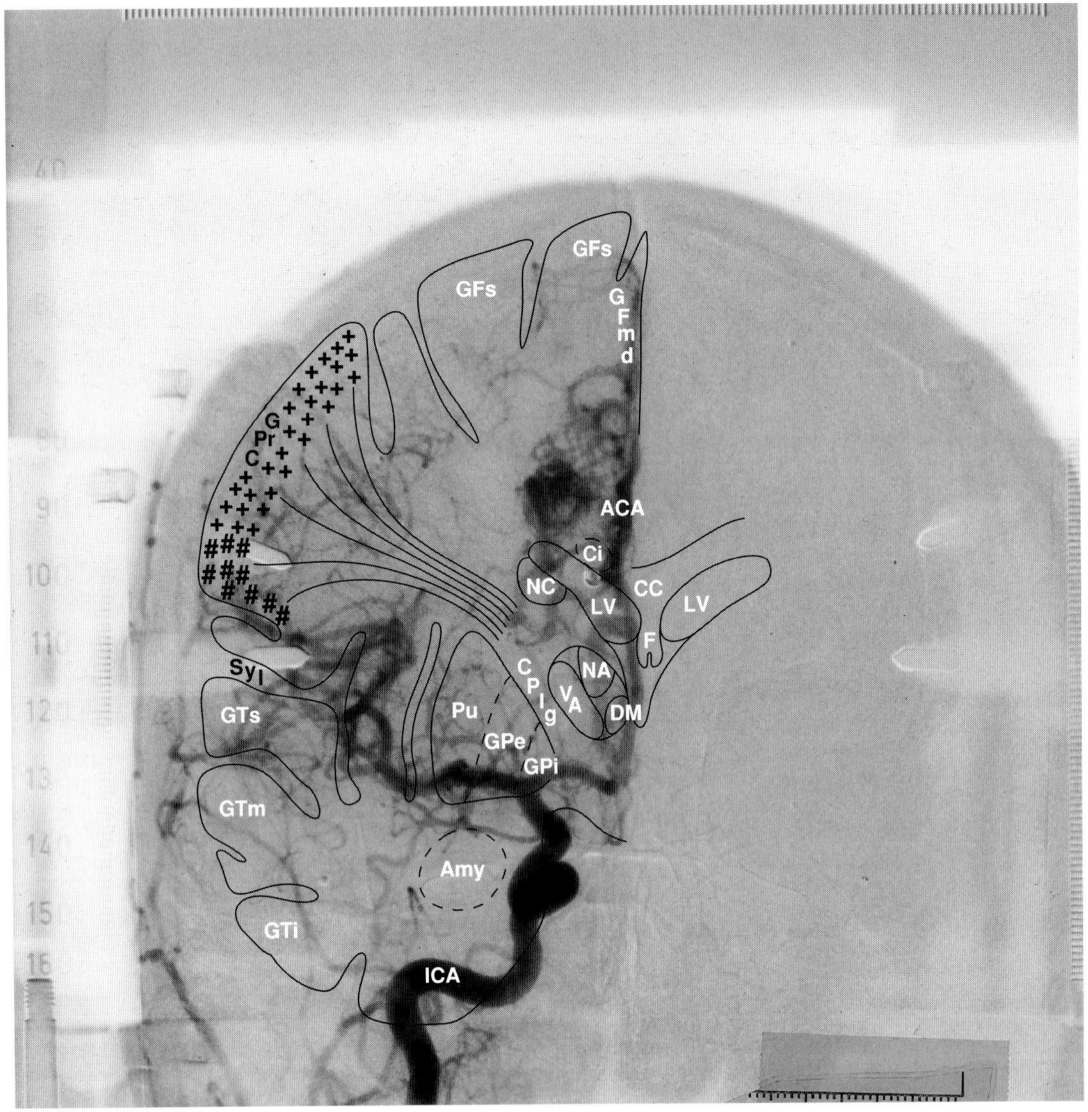
GFs
GFs
G
F
m
d
G
Pr
C
ACA
Ci
NC
CC
LV
LV
F
Syl
C
P
I
g
NA
V
A
DM
GTs
Pu
GPe
GPi
GTm
Amy
GTi
ICA

FIG. 4-9A.

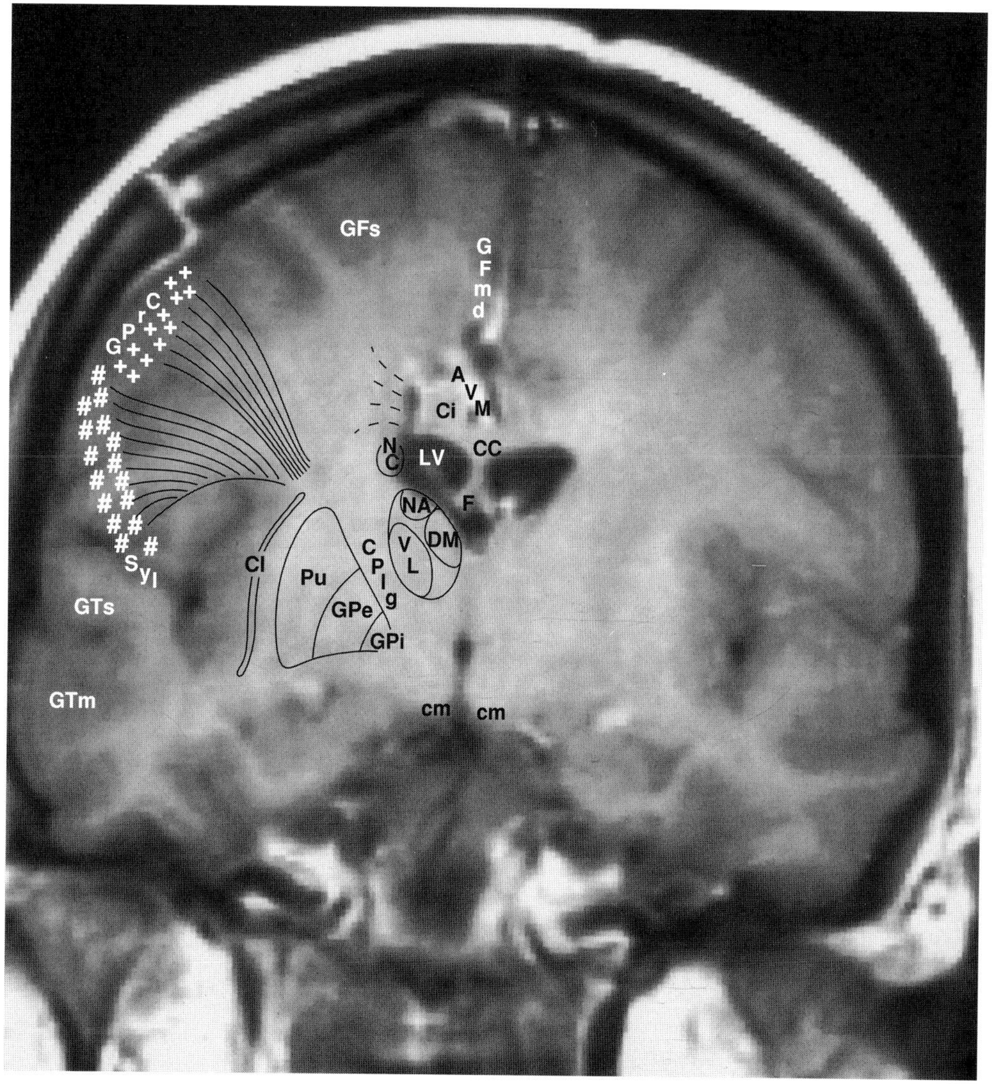
GFs
GFmd
GPrC
AVM
Ci
CC
NC
LV
NA
F
DM
VL
CPIg
Cl
Pu
GPe
GPi
Syl
GTs
GTm
cm
cm

FIG. 4-9B.

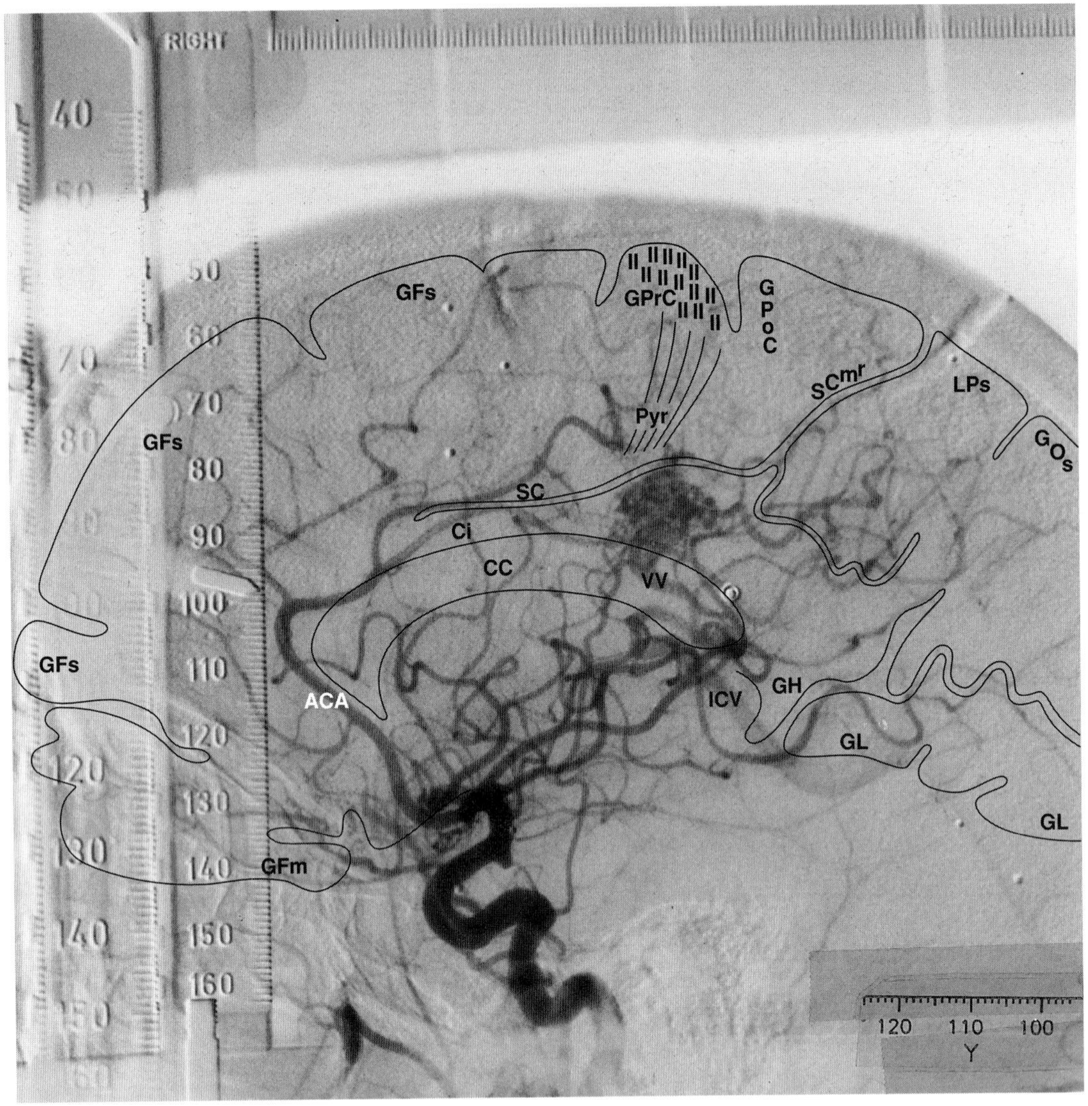
RIGHT
GFs
GPrC
GPoC
Pyr
SCmr
LPs
GOs
SC
Ci
CC
VV
GH
ICV
ACA
GL
GFm
120 110 100
Y

FIG. 4-9C.

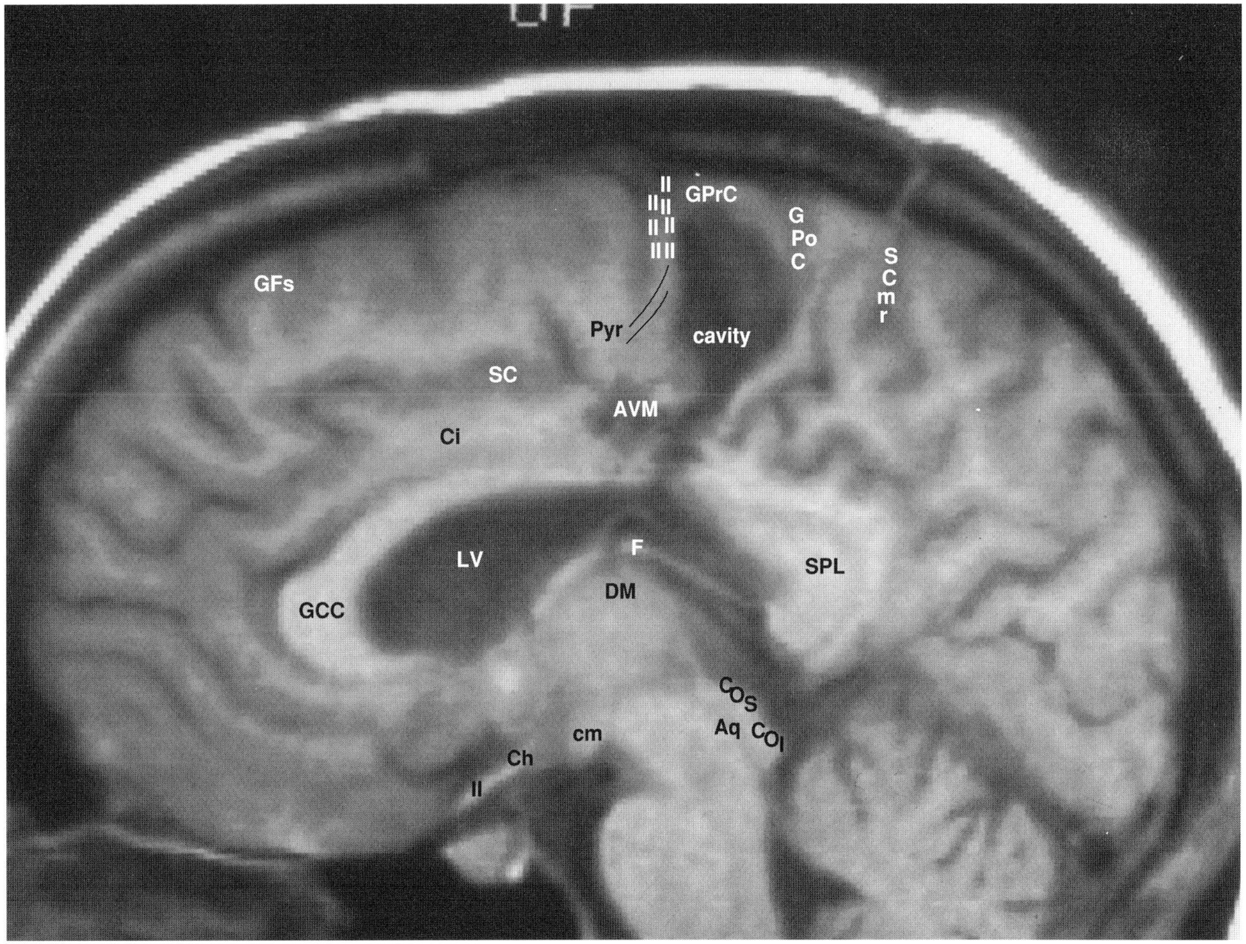
GPrC
G
Po
C
S
C
m
r
GFs
Pyr
cavity
SC
AVM
Ci
F
LV
SPL
DM
GCC
COS
Aq
COI
cm
Ch
II

FIG. 4-9D.

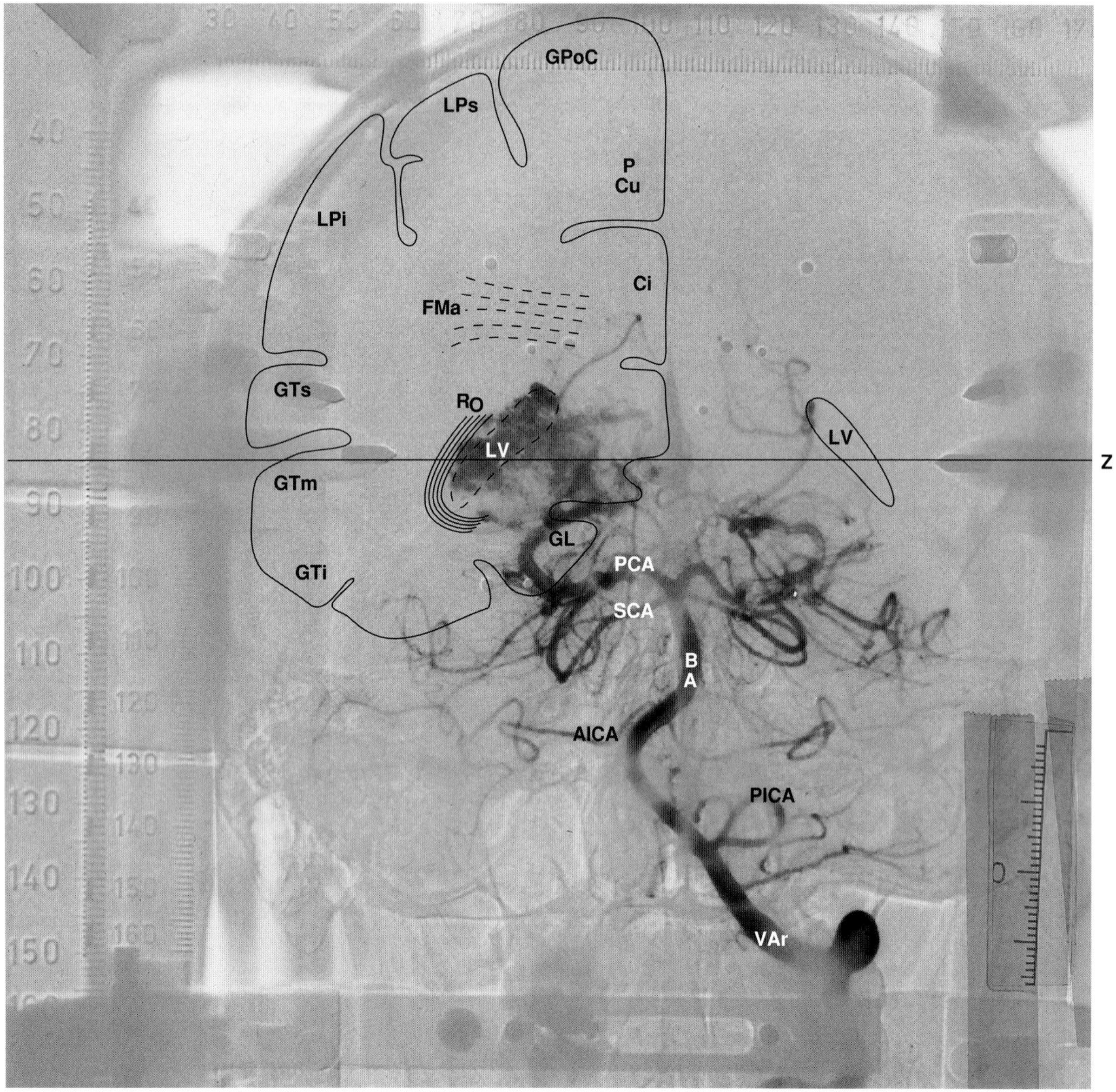
GPoC
LPs
P
Cu
LPi
Ci
FMa
GTs
RO
LV
LV
Z
GTm
GL
GTi
PCA
SCA
B
A
AICA
PICA
VAr

FIG. 4-10A.

FIG. 4-10. Previously ruptured arteriovenous malformation of the right mesial (paraventricular) parieto-occipital junction, PA and lateral stereotactic vertebral angiogram films (**A and B**) and nonstereotactic axial proton density MRI (**C**). The AVM is fed principally by an enlarged right posterior cerebral artery (PCA) including the calcarine branch(es). Venous drainage (vv), best seen in **C**, is via the deep venous system and courses through the retropulvinaric cistern anterior to the atrium of the lateral ventricle (LV) and fasciolar gyrus (GFa) to join the internal cerebral vein (ICV) before it enters the vein of Galen complex. The AVM nidus lies within the anterior calcarine sulcus and posteromedial wall of the atrium and occipital horn of the lateral ventricle. Feeding arteries also appear to traverse the parieto-occipital sulcus to enter the posteromedial margin of the nidus. The cuneate gyrus (Cu) forms the medial margin of the AVM, whereas the white matter deep to the middle occipital gyrus forms the lateral margin. The lingual gyrus (GL) lies inferior (and posterior) to the nidus; the forceps major (FMa) of the corpus callosum passes above the nidus.

The angiograms and MRIs illustrate that the optic radiation (RO) passes immediately through or adjacent to the lateral edge of the AVM along a considerable distance as that pathway skirts the margin of the lateral ventricle. Accordingly, the most likely neurologic risk associated with surgical removal or radiosurgery of this AVM would be a left homonymous visual field deficit, possibly a complete hemanopsia. *(Figure continued on following pages.)*

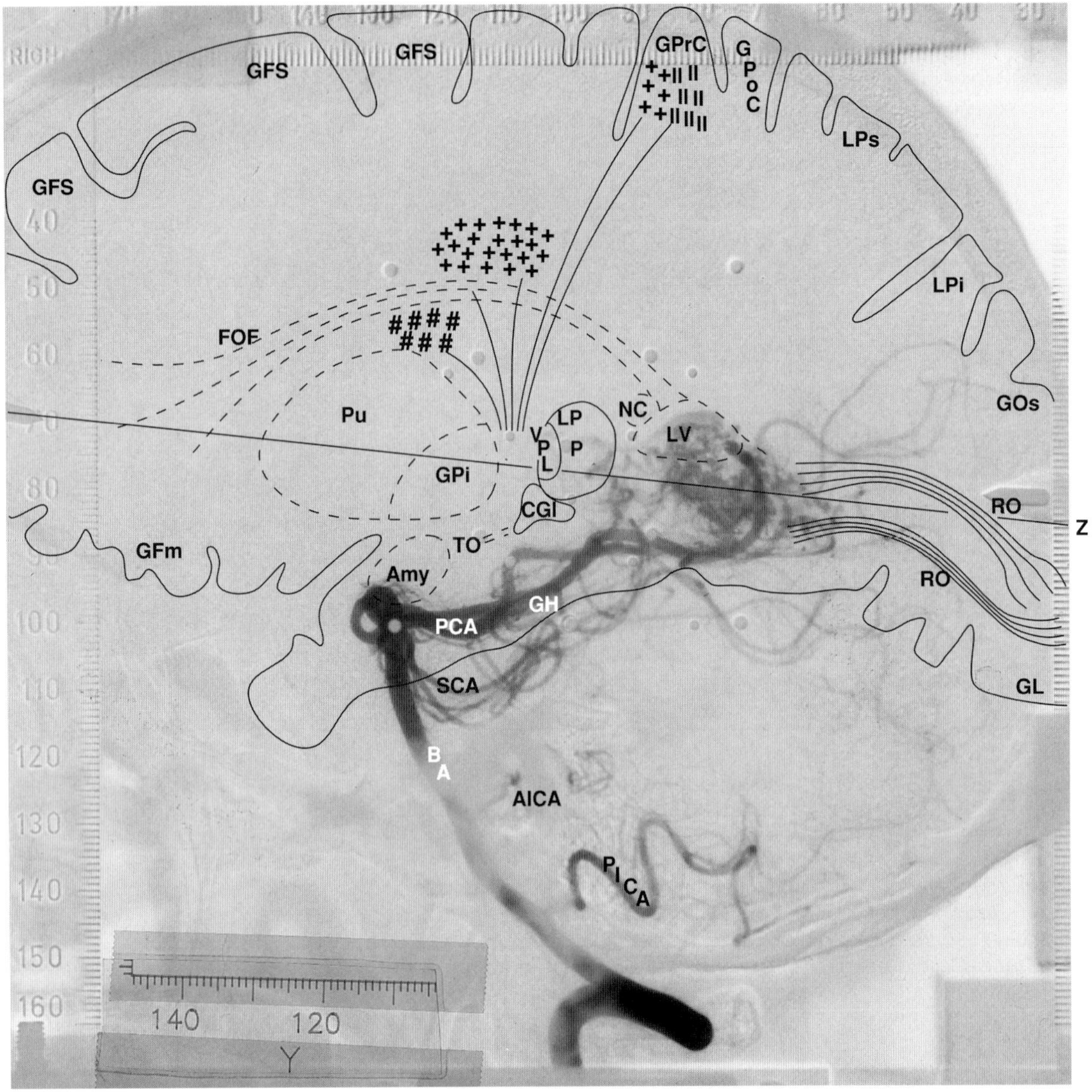
GFS
GFS
GFS
GPrC
GPoC
LPs
LPi
GOs
FOF
Pu
GPi
VPL
LP
P
NC
LV
CGl
TO
Amy
GFm
GH
PCA
SCA
BA
AICA
PICA
RO
RO
Z
GL
140
120
Y

FIG. 4-10B.

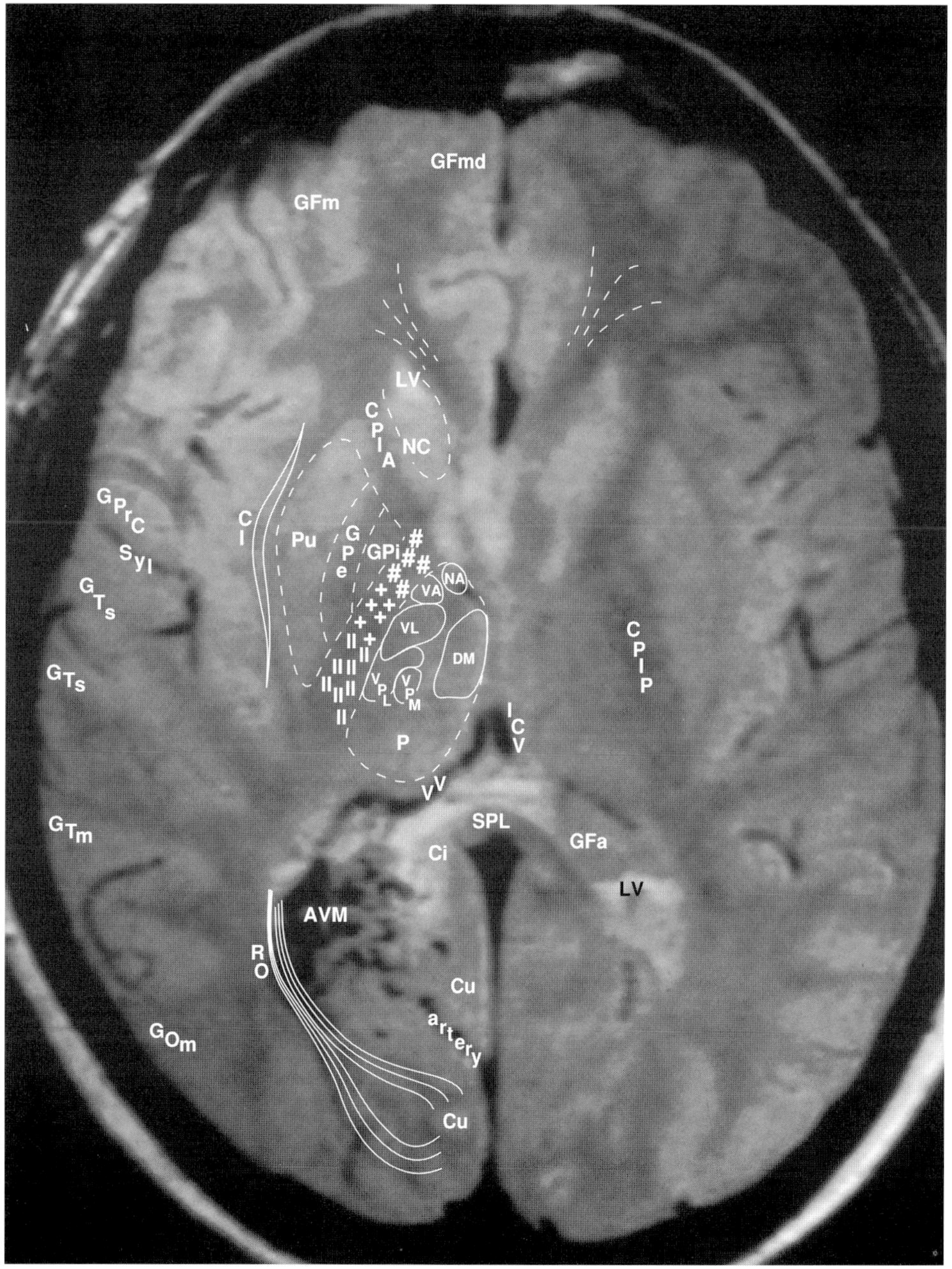

GFmd
GFm
LV
C P I A
NC
GPrC
SyI
GTs
GTs
C I
Pu
G P e
GPi
NA
VA
VL
DM
V P L
V P M
P
I C V
C P I P
V V
SPL
GTm
Ci
GFa
LV
AVM
R O
Cu
artery
GOm
Cu

FIG. 4-10C.

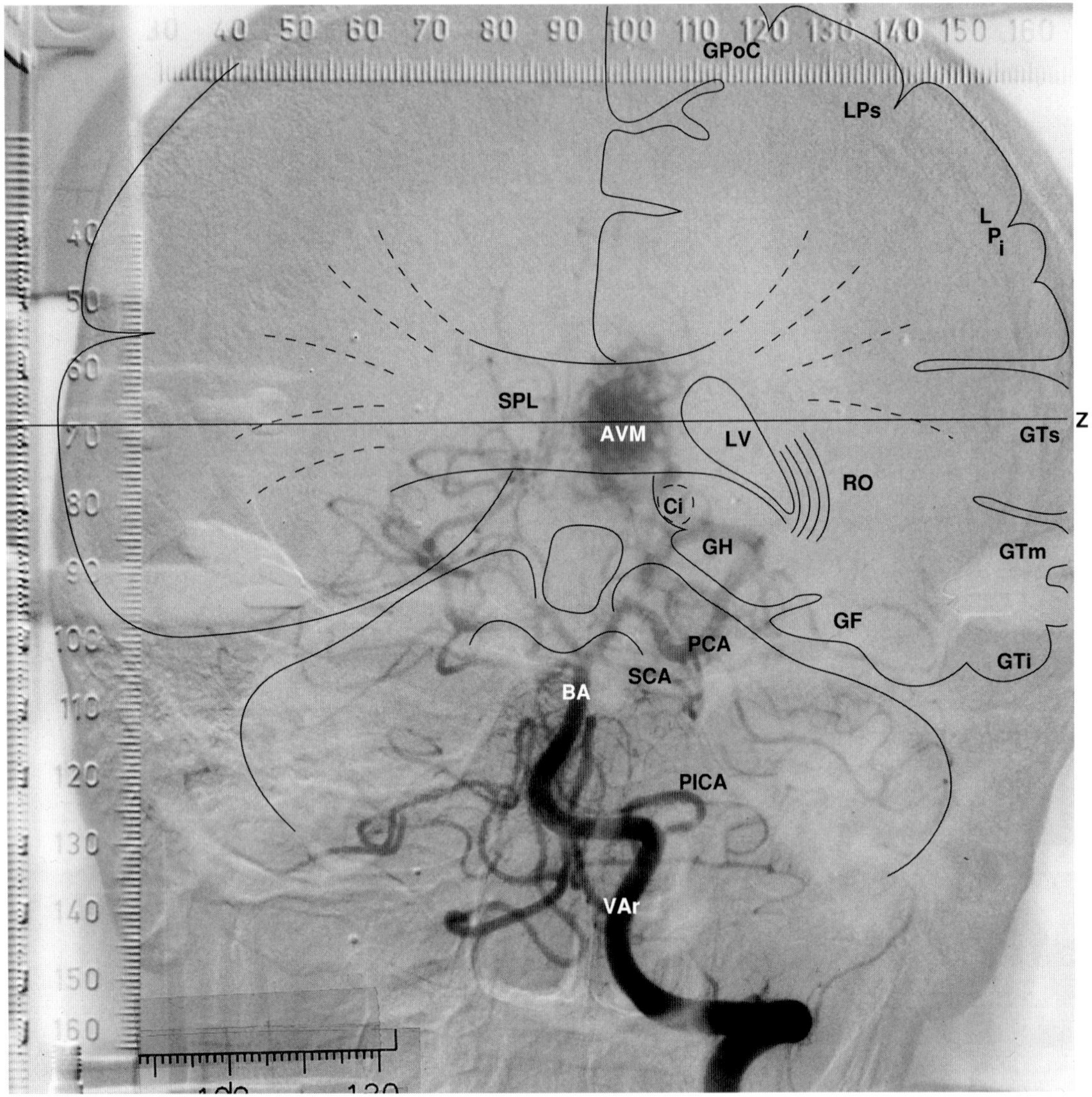
GPoC
LPs
L
P
i
SPL
AVM
LV
Z
GTs
RO
Ci
GH
GTm
GF
PCA
GTi
SCA
BA
PICA
VAr

FIG. 4-11A.

FIG. 4-11. Arteriovenous malformation of the left side of the splenium of the corpus callosum (Spl) and cistern of the velum interpositum, PA and lateral stereotactic left vertebral angiogram films (**A and B**) and nonstereotactic proton density MRI (**C**) at the axial level of plane Z indicated on the angiographic images. Feeding arteries include branches of the hypertrophied left posterior cerebral artery (PCA), which include the posterior medial choroidal and posterior pericallosal artery branches (not labeled). Venous drainage is through the dilated left internal cerebral vein (vv on the left, ICV on the normal right side in **C**).

The nidus appears to traverse the substance of the splenium to enter the cistern of the velum interpositum along the dorsal and posterior segment of the internal cerebral vein. **B** and **C** illustrate the thalamic nuclei immediately adjacent to the lateral margin of the nidus and its venous drainage. The posterior margin of the AVM ocupies or, most likely, displaces the retrosplenial portion of the cingulate gyrus and white matter bundle (Ci). The crus of the fornix on the left side is obscured completely by the AVM.

Neurologic complications of surgery (and possibly radiosurgery, but less likely so) could include interruption of the internal cerebral vein or other elements of the deep venous system with subsequent venous infarction of the left diencephalon. Other neurologic sequelae that are possible, but less likely, might include deficits of verbal memory from damage to the fornix, a partial callosal disconnection syndrome, or even alexia without agraphia if the splenium and left visual cortex both were damaged directly or by a vascular insult. *(Figure continued on following pages.)*

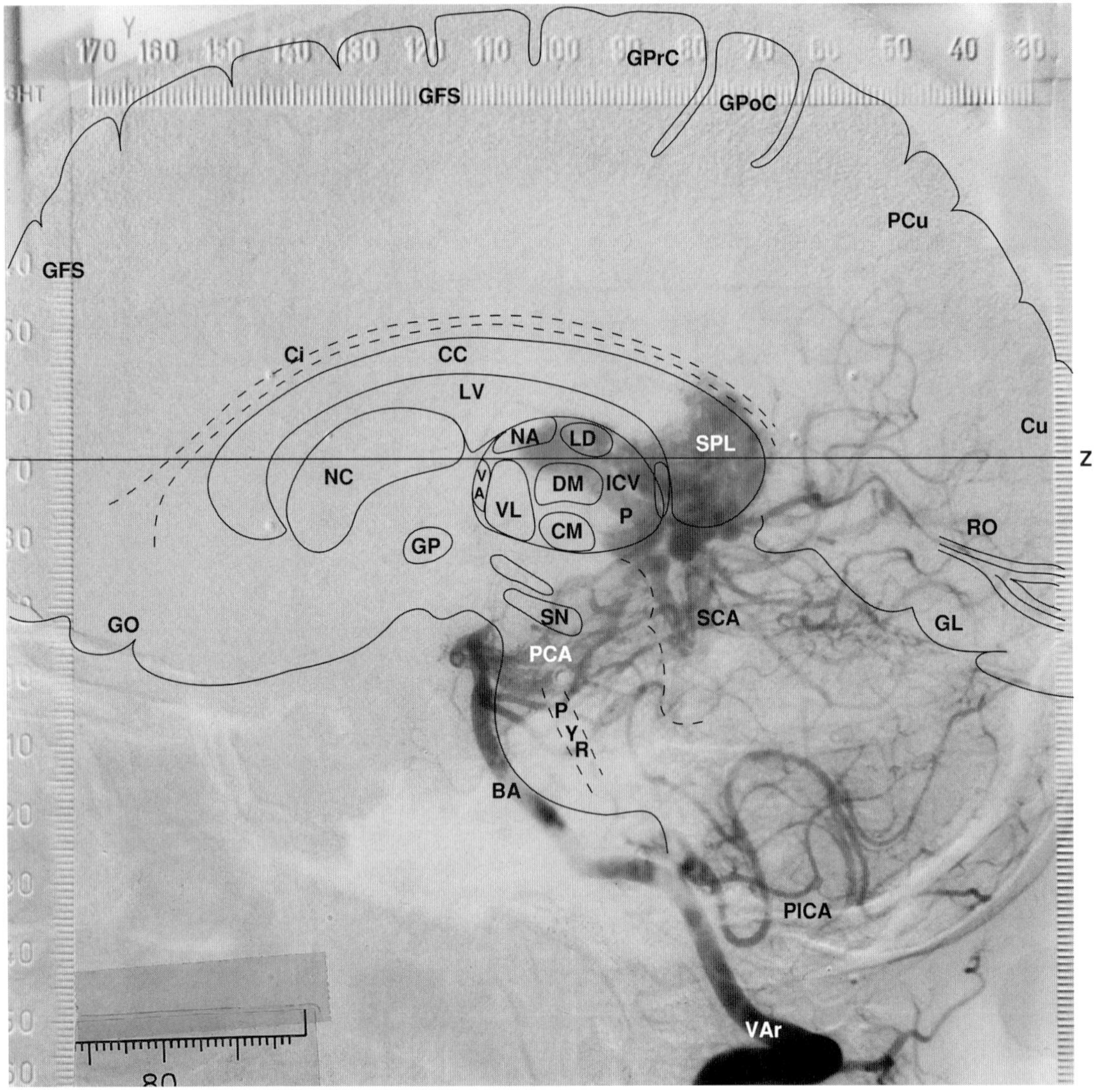
GFS
GPrC
GPoC
PCu
GFS
Ci
CC
LV
NA
LD
SPL
Cu
Z
NC
V
A
DM
ICV
VL
P
CM
GP
RO
SN
SCA
GO
GL
PCA
P
Y
R
BA
PICA
VAr

FIG. 4-11B.

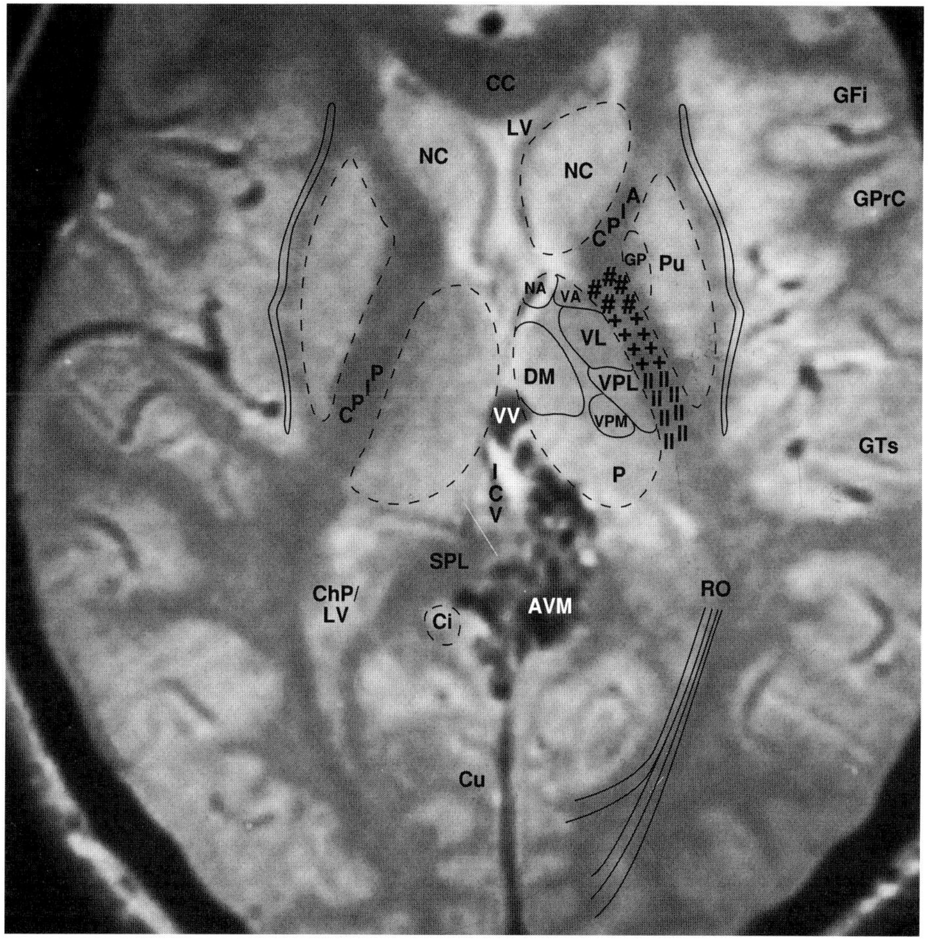
CC
LV
NC
NC
GFi
GPrC
A
P
C
GP
Pu
NA
VA
VL
DM
VPL
VPM
VV
P
C
P
GTs
I
C
V
P
SPL
ChP/
LV
Ci
AVM
RO
Cu

FIG. 4-11C.

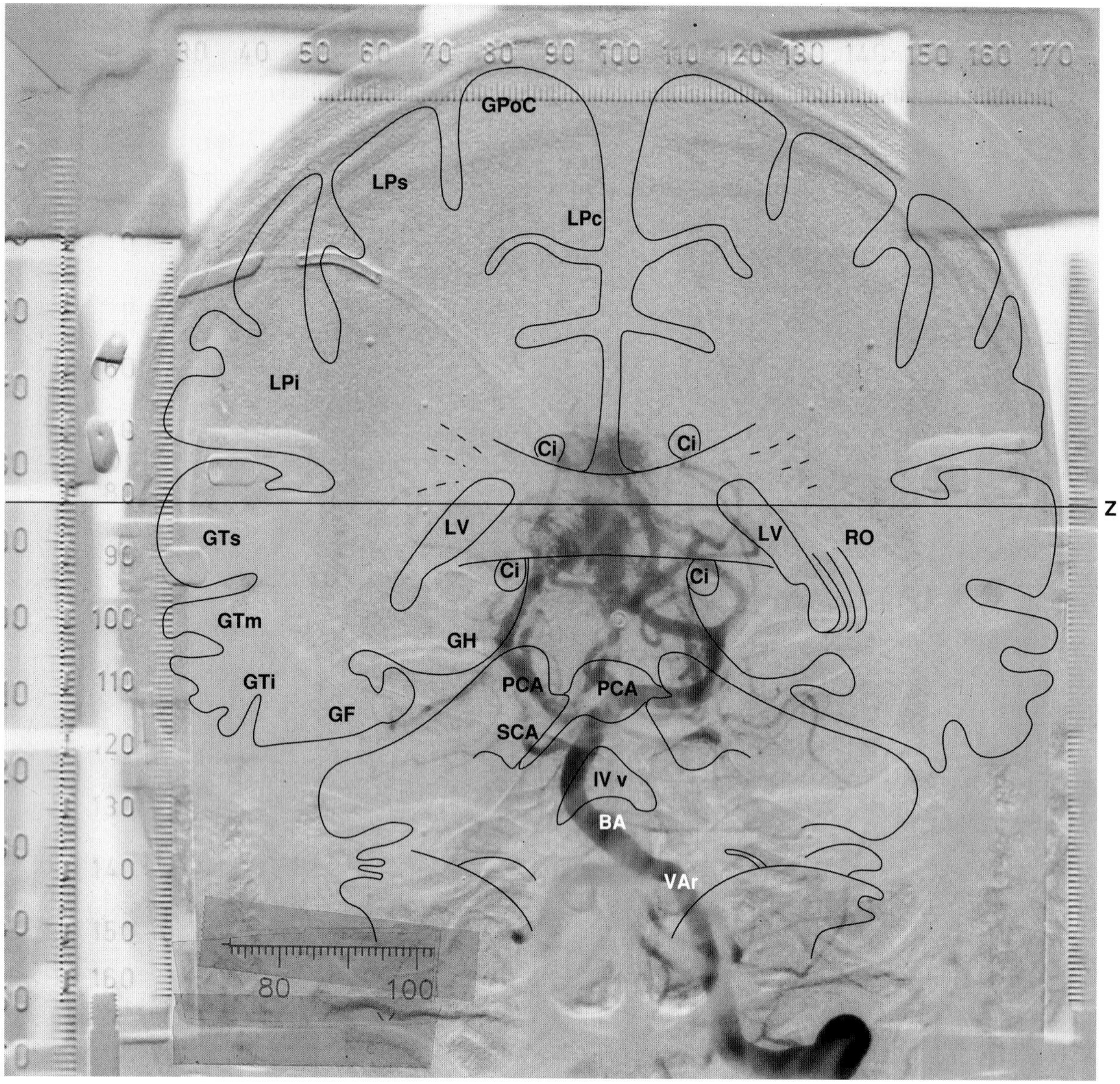

GPoC
LPs
LPc
LPi
Ci
Ci
Z
LV
LV
RO
GTs
Ci
Ci
GTm
GH
GTi
PCA
PCA
GF
SCA
IV v
BA
VAr

FIG. 4-12A.

FIG. 4-12. Arteriovenous malformation of the posterior third ventricle, pineal region, and splenium of the corpus callosum (SPL), PA, and lateral stereotactic left vertebral angiogram films (**A and B**) and stereotactic T_1-weighted MRI (**C**) in the axial plane of line Z on the angiographic images. A right frontal ventriculoperitoneal shunt is in place with a portion of the valve projected over the superior compartment of the AVM in **B** and causing metallic artifact in **C**. Feeding arteries arise from branches of both posterior cerebral arteries (PCA) and include enlarged thalamoperforator arteries, posterior lateral choroidal arteries, posterior medial choroidal arteries, and posterior pericallosal arteries. Venous drainage is entirely through the deep system, especially the basal vein of Rosenthal (BVR), which is partially superimposed over the posterior cerebral arteries in **B**. A deep vein (vv) that is seen more faintly may enter the vein of Galen complex directly.

The nidus appears to have two interconnected compartments, with the larger inferior one located predominantly below the splenium and the smaller more dorsal compartment centered at and to the right of the mid-line and involving the right cingulate gyrus (Ci). In fact, the posterolateral edge of the inferior nidus compartment also resides eccentrically toward the right retropulvinaric cistern and indents and displaces the tail of the right hippocampus (GH) and isthmus of the cingulate gyrus (Ci). The anterior margin of the nidus reaches as far forward in the third ventricle and cistern of the velum interpositum at the level of the dorsomedian nucleus of the thalamus (DM). The inferior edge of the nidus just reaches the level of the superior colliculi (COS) and posterior commissure in the mid-line.

Neurologic risks associated with surgical or radiosurgical treatment of this AVM include vascular or direct tissue injury to the posterior cingulate gyri, splenium of the corpus callosum, hippocampal-forniceal system, and dorsal thalamus, the consequence of which would be a variety of intellectual, emotional, and/or memory disorders. Injury to the collicular plate and posterior commissure region also could cause disorders of extraocular motion, especially vertical gaze and convergence functions. *(Figure continued on following pages.)*

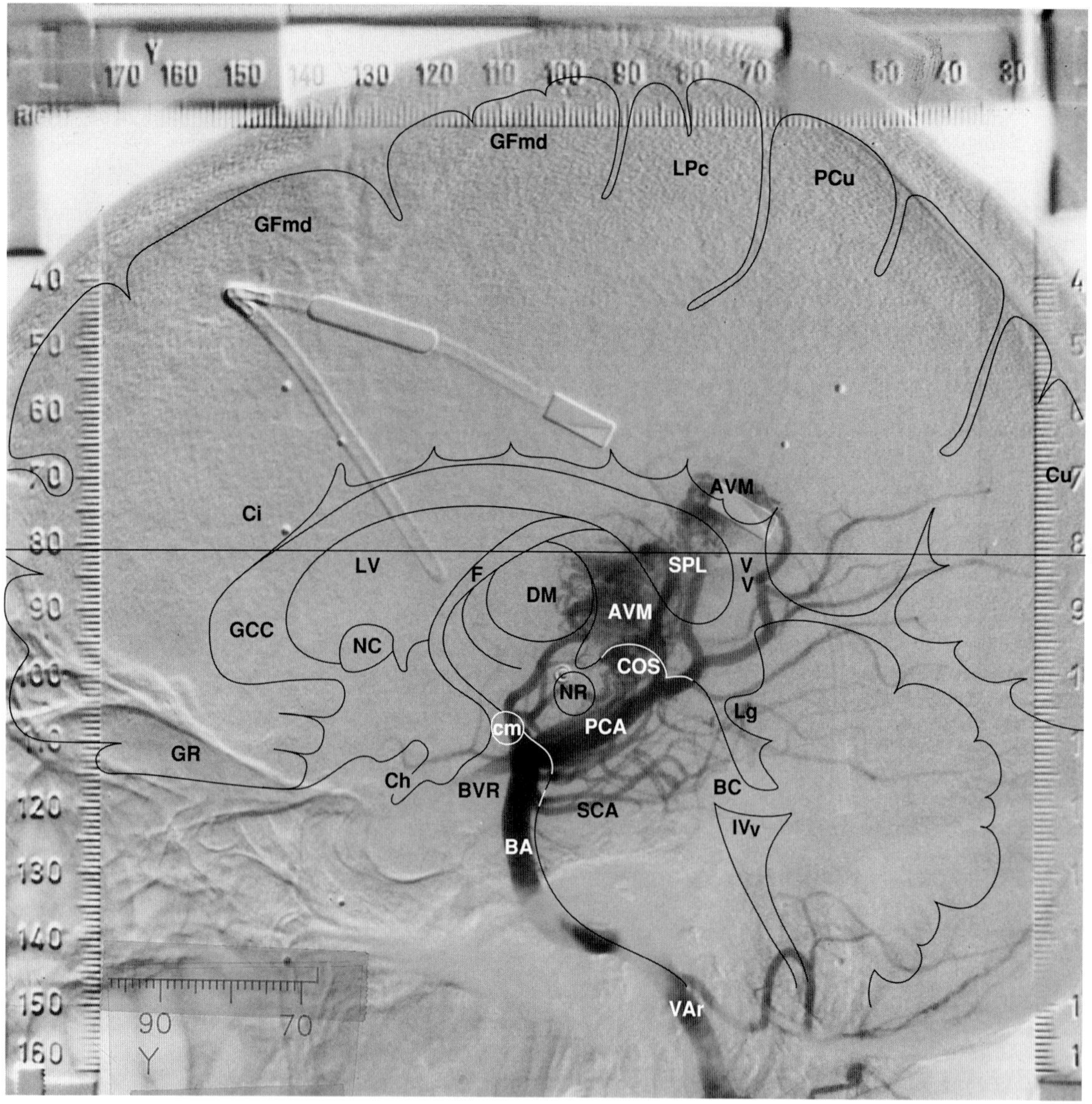
GFmd
GFmd
LPc
PCu
Ci
LV
F
DM
AVM
AVM
SPL
V
V
Z
Cu
GCC
NC
COS
NR
Lg
cm
PCA
GR
Ch
BVR
SCA
BC
IVv
BA
VAr
Y

FIG. 4-12B.

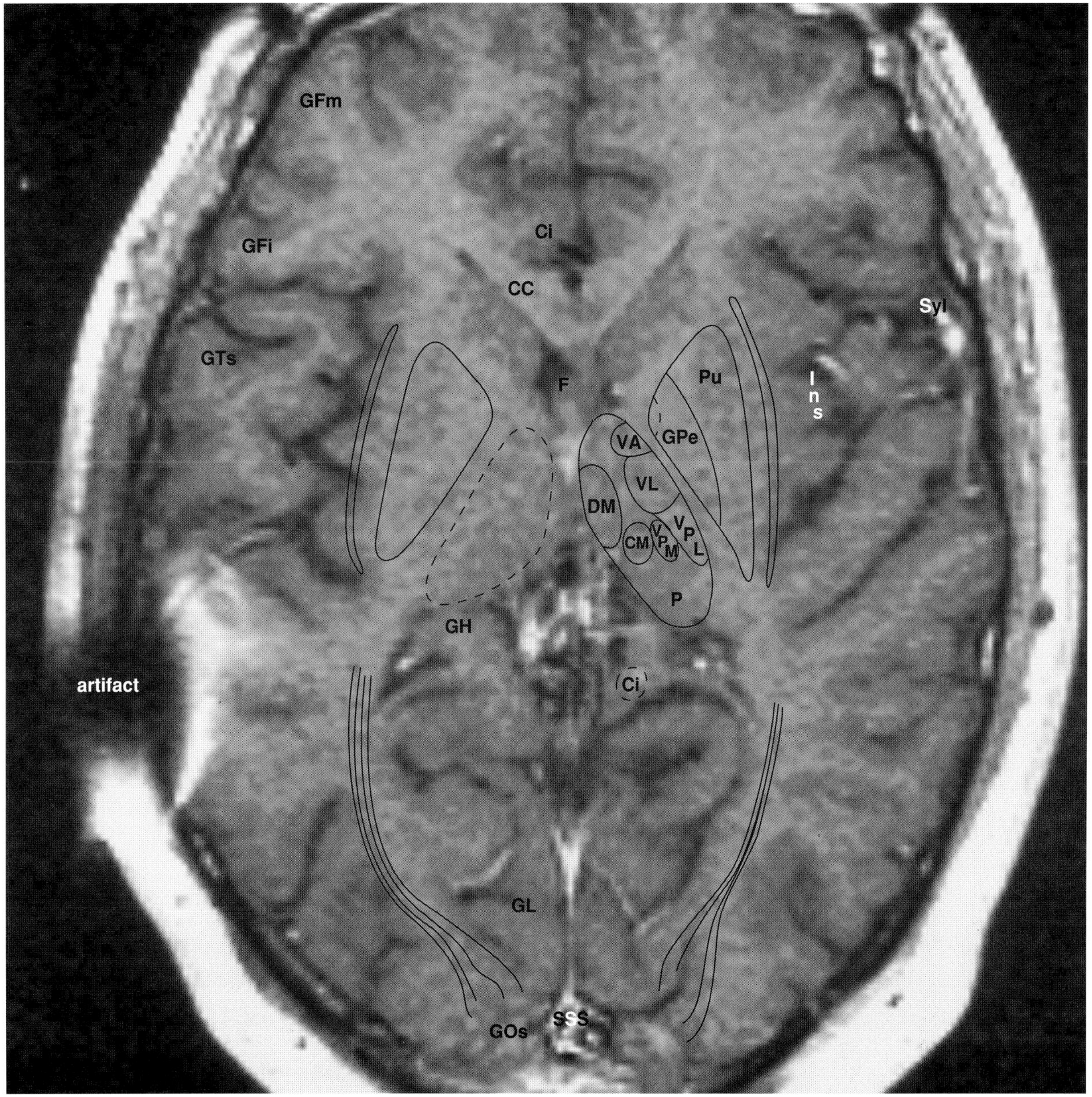
GFm
Ci
GFi
CC
Syl
GTs
F
Pu
I
n
s
VA
GPe
VL
DM
V
P
L
CM
V
P
M
P
GH
artifact
Ci
GL
GOs
SSS

FIG. 4-12C.

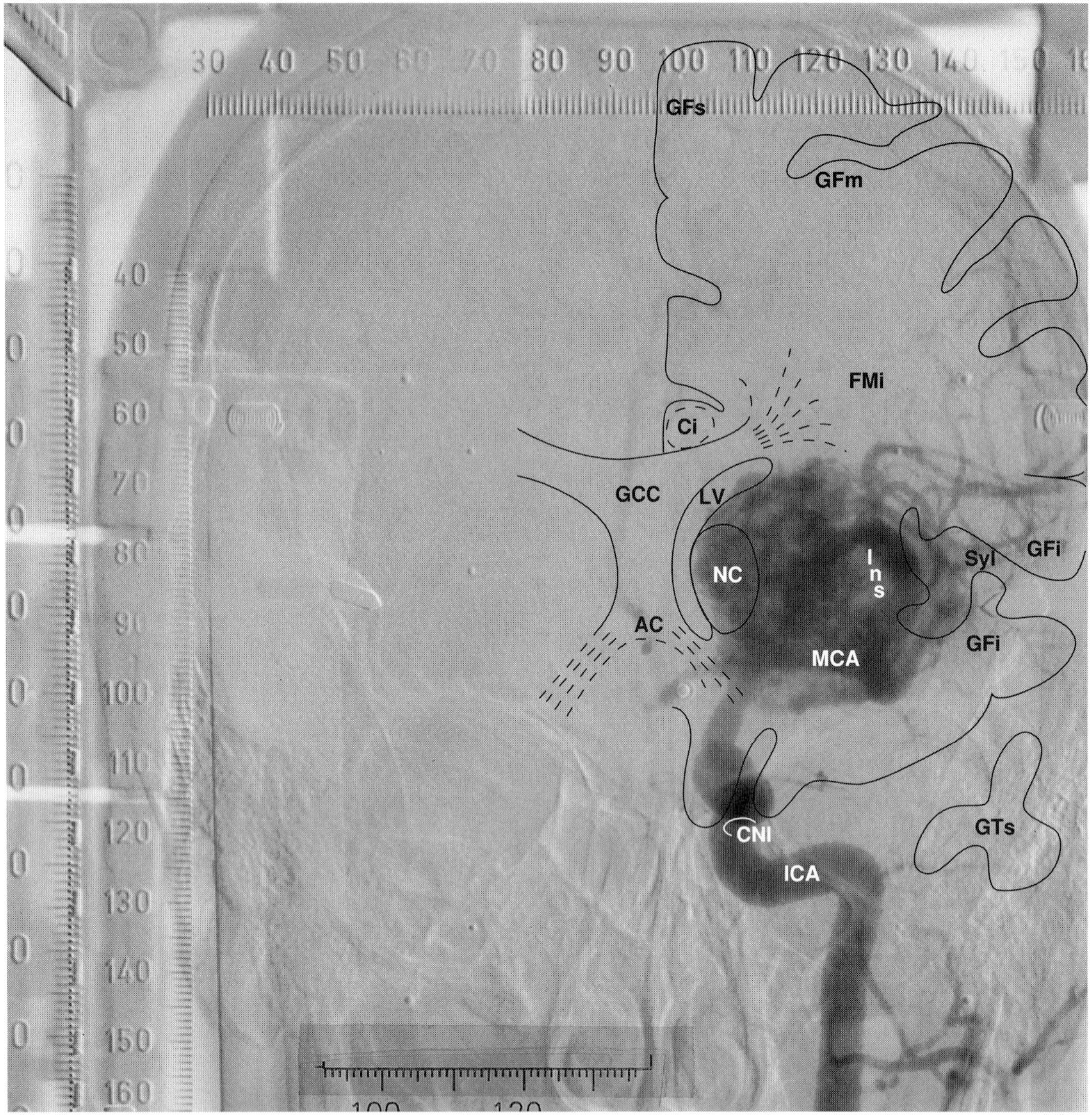

FIG. 4-13A.

FIG. 4-13. Arteriovenous malformation of the left frontal lobe, opercular region and basal ganglia, PA and lateral stereotactic left carotid angiogram films (**A and B**) and nonstereotactic T_2-weighted axial MRI (**C**) through the center of the AVM at the level of the inferior edge of the foramen of Monro. Feeding vessels to the nidus include frontal opercular branches and lenticulostriate branches of the middle cerebral artery (MCA). The venous drainage consists of dilated varices that communicate with superficial cortical veins (seen on later films of the angiographic series). Although major feeding arteries and draining veins occupy a superficial location within the sylvian fissure (Syl) and frontal operculum, the actual AVM nidus extends all the way to the head of the caudate nucleus (NC) and frontal horn of the lateral ventricle (LV), which is compressed from lateral to medial by the AVM. The anterolateral AVM margin is surrounded by the inferior frontal gyrus (GFi) and is separated from the temporal lobe (GTs) by the sylvian fissure. The posterior margin of the AVM encroaches upon the anterior edge of the insula (Ins), extreme capsule (CPEx), claustrum (Cl), external capsule (CPE), putamen (Pu), and anterior limb of the internal capsule (CPIA), from lateral to medial, respectively, before reaching the caudate nucleus and frontal horn. The superior margin of the nidus lies just below the forceps minor of the corpus callosum (FMi), whereas the inferior margin of the nidus lies within the white matter of the inferior frontal gyrus. The genu and posterior limb of the internal capsule (CPIg, CPIP) lie approximately 16 mm medial and posterior to the most medial extent of the AVM.

The neurologic risks associated with treatment of this AVM could include a language disorder from injury to Broca's area or the underlying white matter of the dominant frontal opercular region. Other risks could include an involuntary movement disorder or deficits in the initiation of voluntary movements as a consequence of injury to the basal ganglia. *(Figure continued on following pages.)*

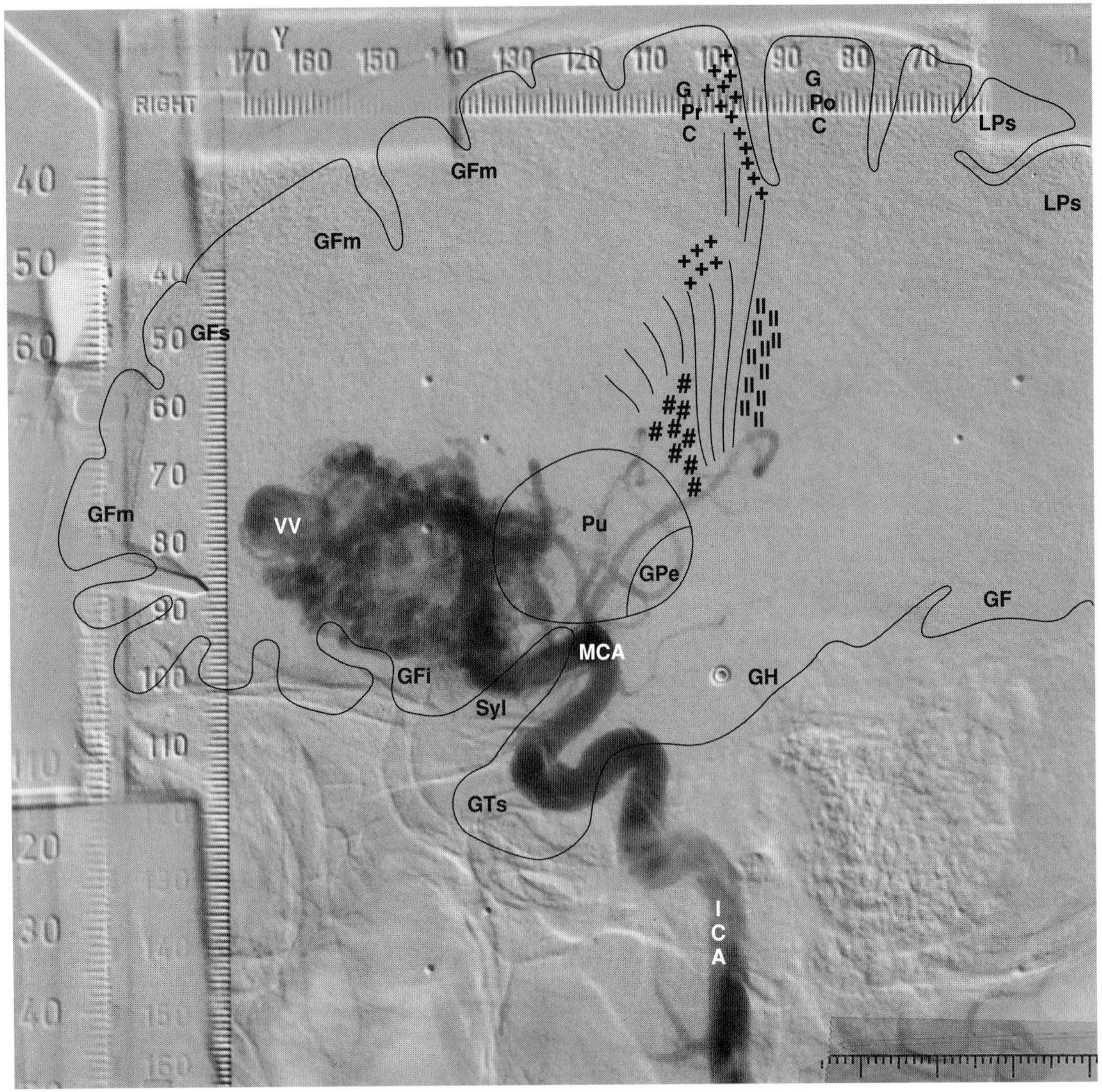
RIGHT
G
Pr
C
G
Po
C
LPs
LPs
GFm
GFm
GFs
GFm
VV
Pu
GPe
GF
MCA
GH
GFi
Syl
GTs
I
C
A

FIG. 4-13B.

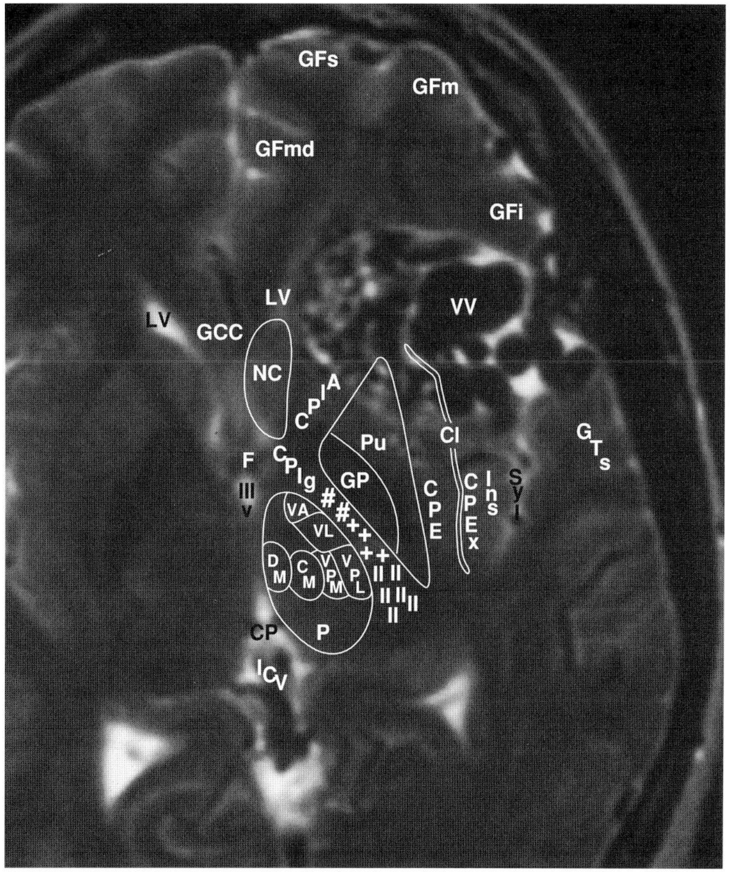
GFs
GFm
GFmd
GFi
LV
LV
GCC
VV
NC
CPIA
Pu
Cl
GTs
F
CPIg
GP
III v
CPE
CPEx
Ins
Syl
VA
VL
DM
CM
VPM
VPL
CP
P
ICV

FIG. 4-13C.

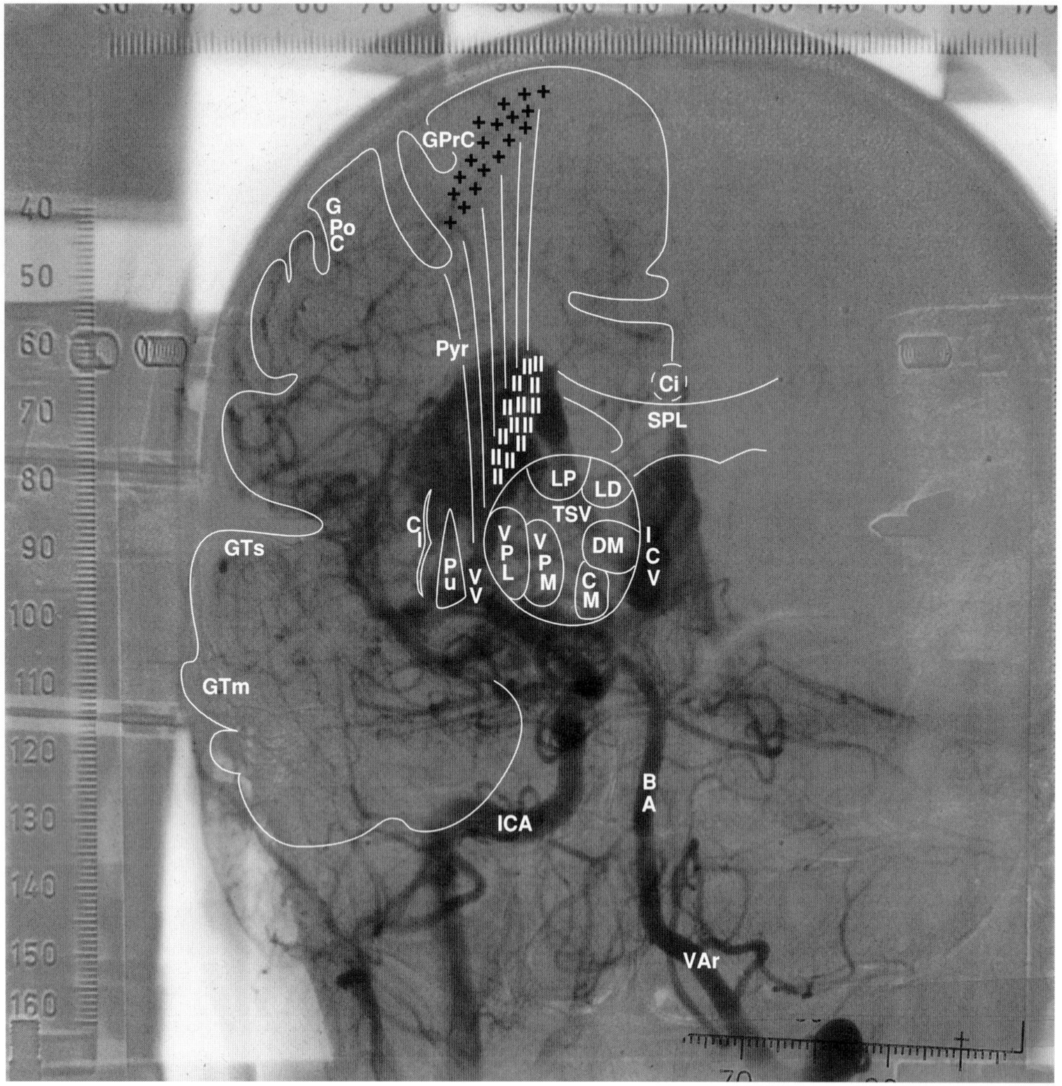
GPrC
G
Po
C
Pyr
Ci
SPL
LP
LD
TSV
C
I
GTs
V
P
L
V
P
M
DM
I
C
V
P
u
V
V
C
M
GTm
B
A
ICA
VAr

FIG. 4-14A.

FIG. 4-14. Arteriovenous malformation of the right internal capsule, basal ganglia, and lateral ventricle, PA and lateral stereotactic angiogram films with superimposition of right carotid and left vertebral artery injections (**A and B**), and stereotactic T_1-weighted axial MRIs (**C and D**) separated by 6 mm from inferior to superior. Feeding arteries include branches of the middle cerebral artery (MCA), anterior choroidal artery (AChA), and posterolateral choroidal branches of the posterior cerebral artery (PChA, PCA). Venous drainage is exclusively through the deep venous system via two principal conduits: the thalamostriate to internal cerebral vein route (TSV, ICV) and a lateral atrial vein (vv) to basal vein of Rosenthal (BVR) route.

The AVM nidus has a racemose configuration that percolates through the entire posterior limb of the internal capsule (CPIP), and all but the most anterior corner of the putamen (Pu). The lateral margin of the nidus reaches the gray matter–white matter junction of the insula (Ins), whereas the medial margin reaches the thalamocapsular border (**C**) and even extends into the atrium and body of the lateral ventricle (LV) caudal and superior to the thalamus (**C and D**). Corticospinal tract (Pyr) fibers pass through and/or anteromedial to the AVM from the level of the corona radiata to the thalamus–mid-brain junction. The borders of the nidus appear to respect the boundary between telencephalic structures (which are involved) and the diencephalon (which is spared).

Neurologic risks associated with treatment of this AVM include contralateral hemiplegia and hemisensory loss from injury to the internal capsule and putamen. Damage or thrombosis of the deep venous system could cause infarction of the thalamus and basal ganglia. *(Figure continued on following pages.)*

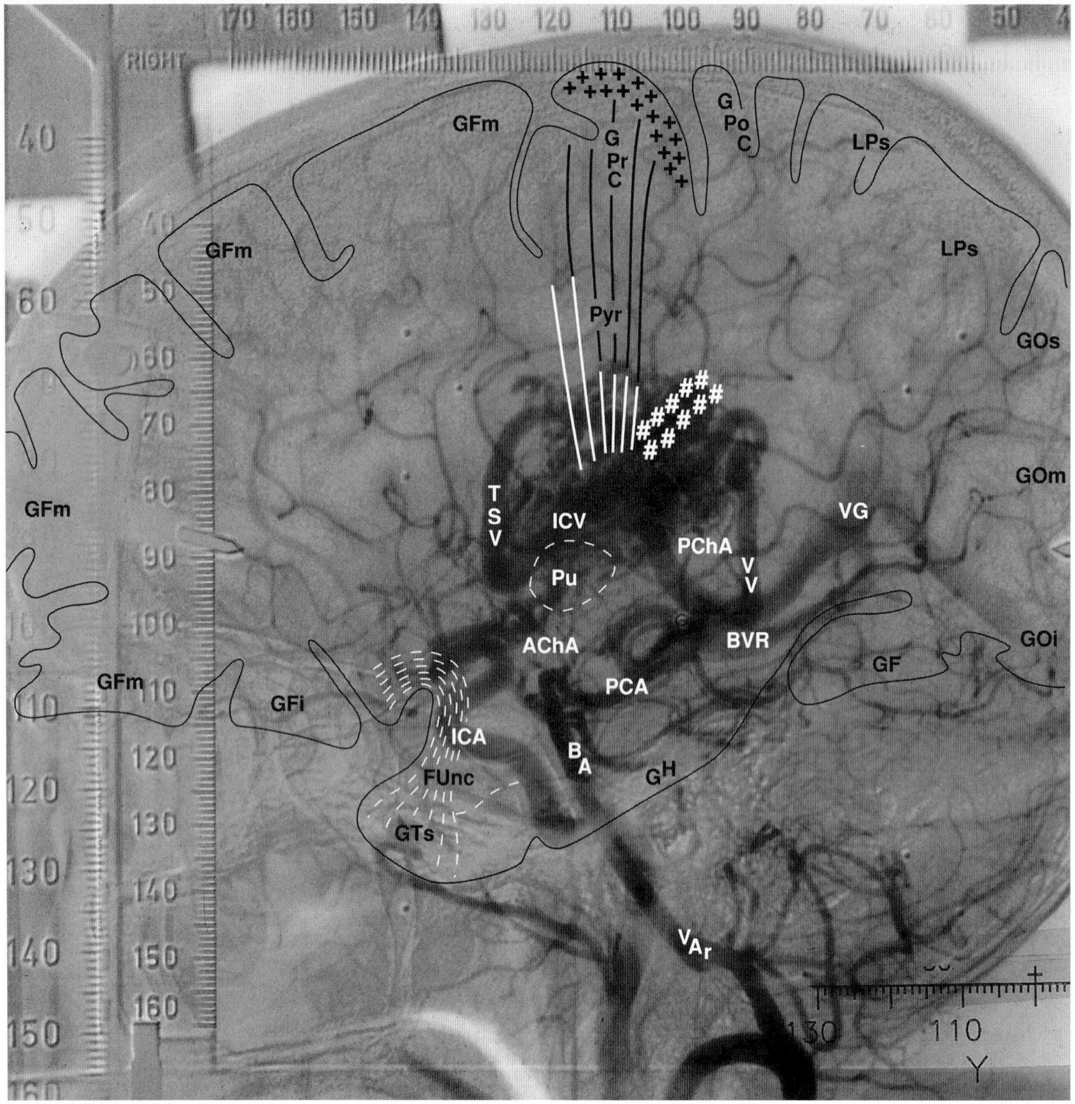
GFm
G
Pr
C
G
Po
C
LPs
GFm
LPs
Pyr
GOs
GOm
T
S
V
ICV
VG
GFm
PChA
V
V
Pu
BVR
AChA
GOi
GF
GFm
PCA
GFi
ICA
B
A
G
H
FUnc
GTs
V
Ar
Y

FIG. 4-14B.

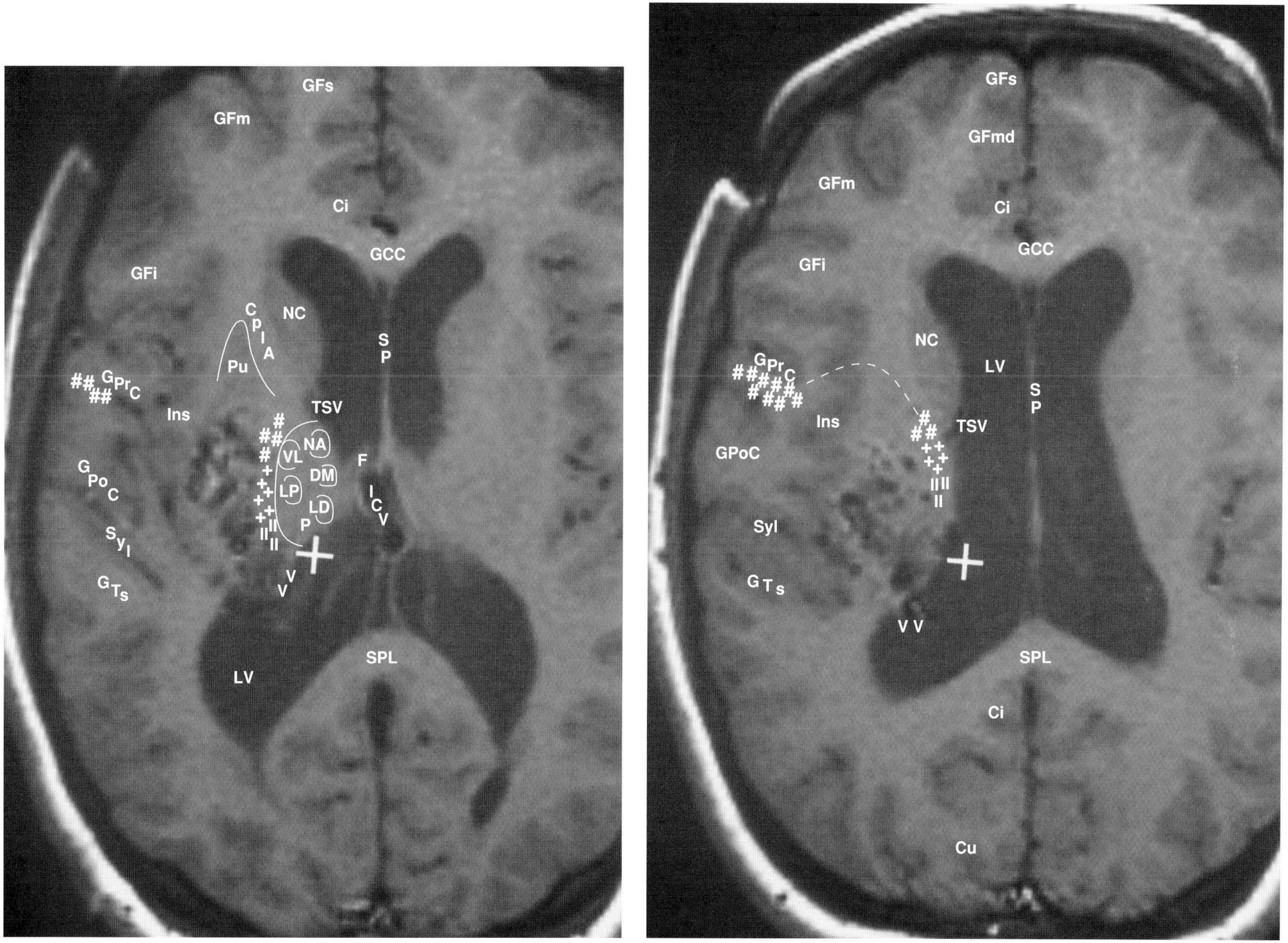

FIG. 4-14C and D.

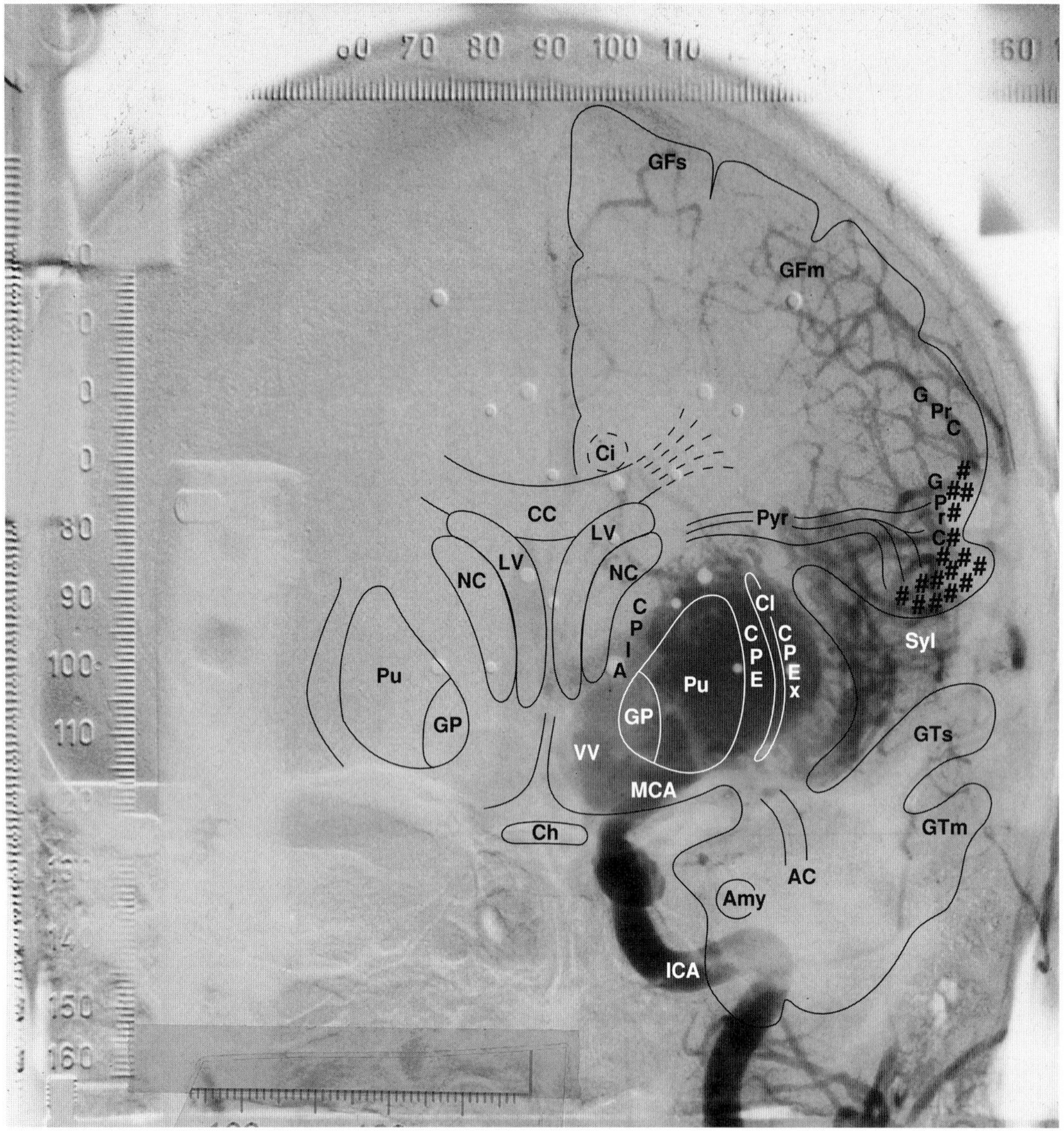
GFs
GFm
G Pr C
G P r C
Ci
CC
LV
LV
NC
NC
Pyr
C P I A
Cl
C P E
C P E x
Syl
Pu
GP
Pu
GP
VV
MCA
GTs
GTm
Ch
AC
Amy
ICA

FIG. 4-15A.

FIG. 4-15. Arteriovenous malformation of the left basal ganglia and anterior limb of the internal capsule (CPIA) at the level of the anterior commissure (AC), PA, and lateral stereotactic left carotid angiogram films (**A and D**), and stereotactic T_1-weighted coronal MRIs (**B and C**) separated by 9 mm from posterior to anterior. The nidus is fed by lenticulostriate branches and innumerable twigs off the candelabra of the middle cerebral artery (MCA). Venous drainage is through a varix that empties into the deep venous system via the basal vein of Rosenthal (BVR). From lateral to medial, this AVM occupies the region of the extreme capsule (CPEx), claustrum (Cl), external capsule (CPE), putamen (Pu), globus pallidus (GP), and anterior limb of the internal capsule (CPIA). The most medial edge of the nidus and a few small draining venules also appear to involve the head of the caudate nucleus (NC).

The most anterior and inferior fibers of the corticospinal tract, which arise from the foot of the precentral gyrus and which subserve voluntary motion of the orofacial muscles (##), pass just superior and posterior (dorsal) to the nidus as the pyramidal tract (Pyr) approaches the genu and posterior limb of the internal capsule. The crossing fibers of the anterior commissure (AC) pass from medial to lateral, inferior, and anterior to the nidus, whereas fibers of the uncinate fasciculus (FUnc) cross the stem of the temporal lobe beneath the anterior edge of the nidus (**D**).

Neurologic risks associated with treatment of this AVM include contralateral hemiparesis or involuntary movement disorder from injury to the putamen and globus pallidus, facial weakness from injury to the pyramidal tract, and language disorder from injury to Broca's area, the white matter beneath the inferior frontal gyrus, or the blood supply to that region. *(Figure continued on following pages.)*

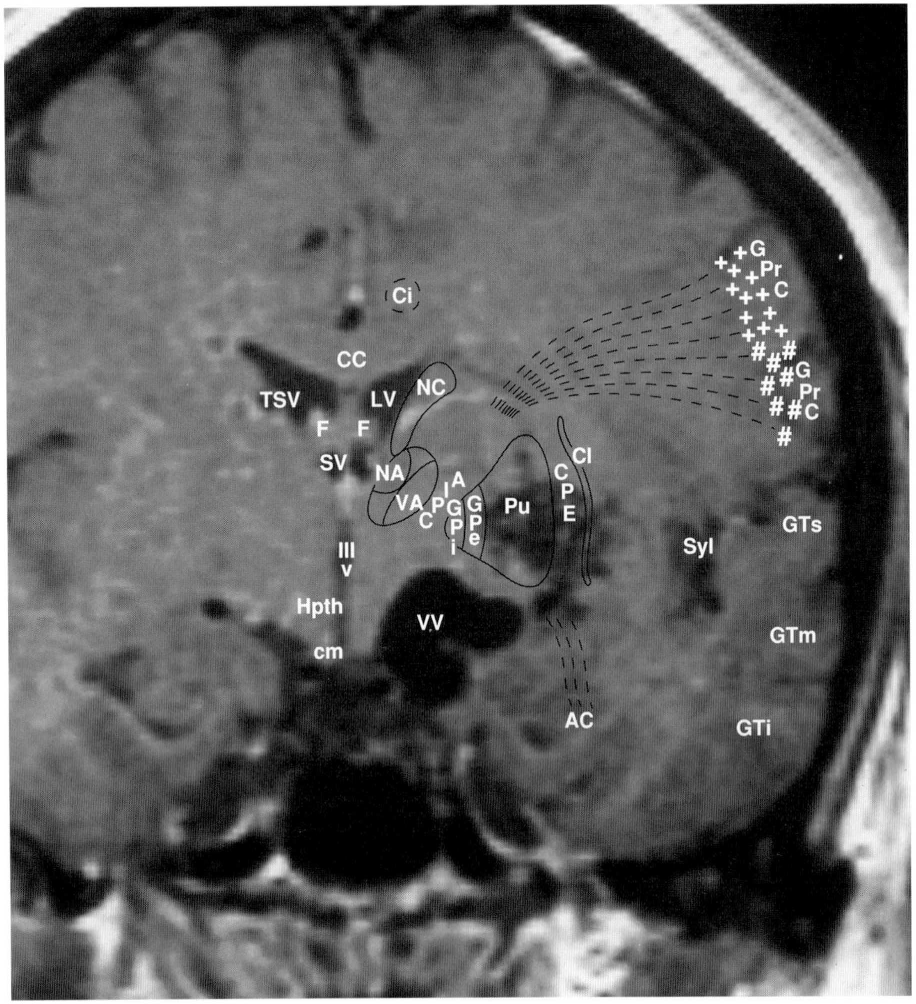
Ci
CC
TSV
LV
NC
F
F
SV
NA
VA
C
P
I
A
G
P
i
G
P
e
Pu
C
P
E
Cl
G
Pr
C
G
Pr
C
III
v
Hpth
VV
cm
Syl
GTs
GTm
GTi
AC

FIG. 4-15B.

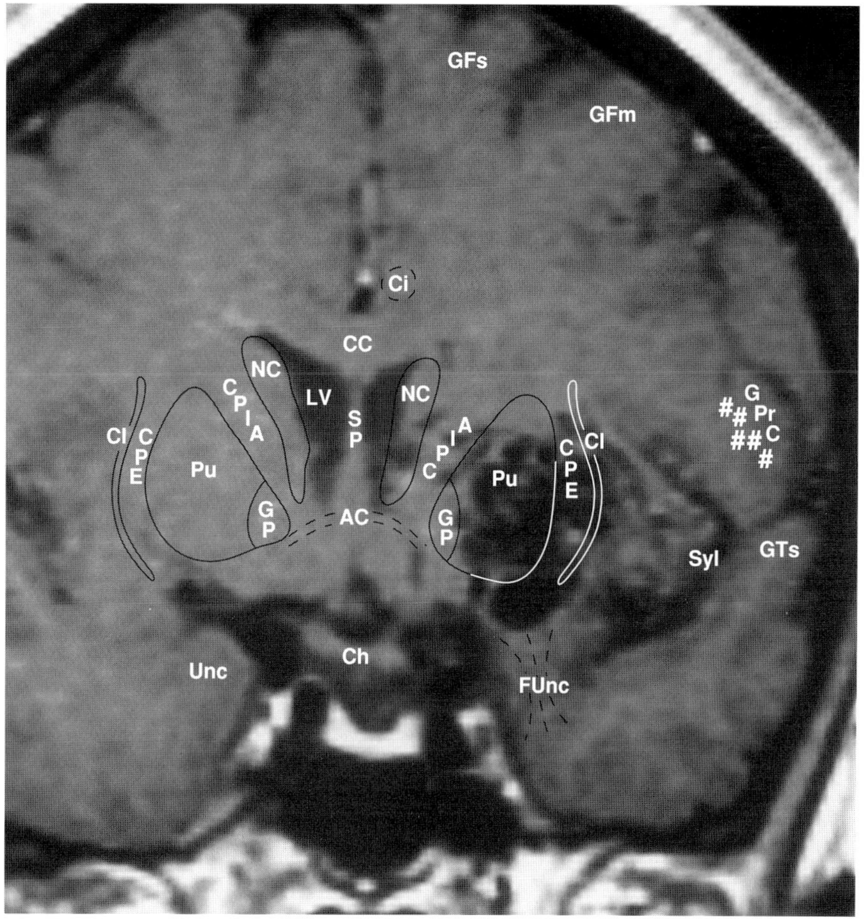
GFs
GFm
Ci
CC
NC
LV
NC
C
P
I
A
S
P
A
I
P
C
Cl
C
P
E
Pu
Pu
C
P
E
Cl
G
#
#
Pr
##
C
#
G
P
AC
G
P
Syl
GTs
Ch
Unc
FUnc

FIG. 4-15C.

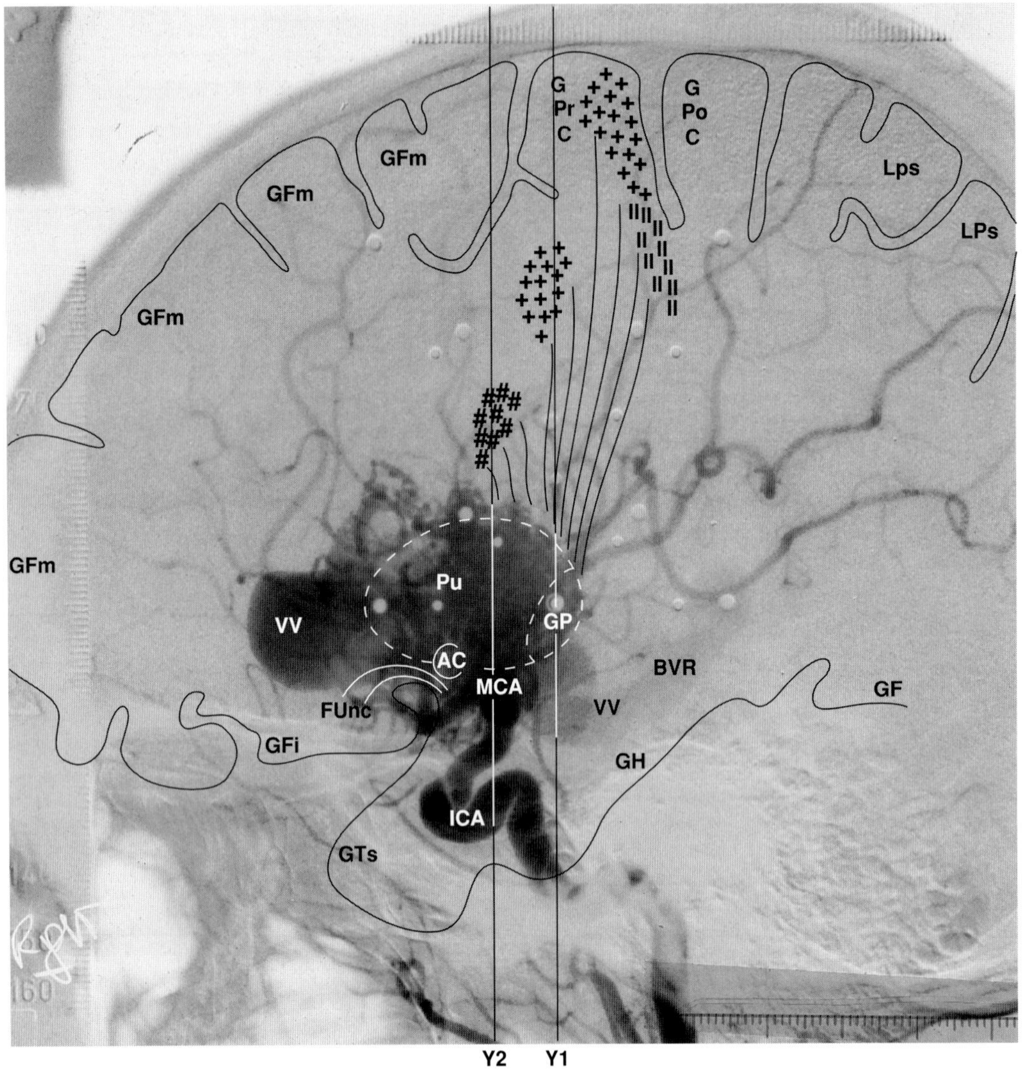
G
Pr
C
G
Po
C
GFm
GFm
GFm
Lps
LPs
GFm
GFm
Pu
VV
GP
AC
MCA
BVR
VV
GF
FUnc
GFi
GH
ICA
GTs
Y2
Y1

FIG. 4-15D.

FIG. 4-16. Arteriovenous malformation (recently ruptured) within the left thalamus and internal capsule in a 9-year-old child, PA and lateral stereotactic left vertebral angiogram films (**A and B**) and stereotactic T_1-weighted MRI (**C**) at the axial level Z indicated on the angiographic images. Feeding arteries include the posterior medial and posterior lateral choroidal branches (not labeled) of the left posterior cerebral artery (PCA), which arise from the PCA from proximal to distal, respectively. In addition, an enlarged thalamoperforating branch that arises near the basilar bifurcation also may feed the AVM nidus (**B**). Venous drainage passes almost directly from lateral to medial out of the posterior portion of the AVM (vv) through the retropulvinaric cistern (anterior to the fasciolar gyrus [GF]) to join the vein of Galen complex (VG). The relatively compact nidus occupies most of the ventral and dorsal tier of thalamic nuclei including the ventral posterior lateral and medial (VPL, VPM), centromedian (CM), lateral posterior (LP), dorsomedian (DM) nuclei, and the pulvinar (P). The medial geniculate body (CGm) lies ventral to the nidus, whereas the ependyma of the floor of the body of the lateral ventricle (LV), or roof of the thalamus, lies immediately dorsal to it. Laterally, the edge of the nidus encroaches upon the most posterior extent of the posterior limb of the internal capsule (CPIP), which contains the thalamocortical sensory radiation (posteriorly) and descending pyramidal tract fibers that subserve voluntary movement of the right leg (////). However, for all practical purposes, the AVM is contained entirely within the diencephalon.

Intraventricular rupture of the AVM 1 month before these images were obtained rendered the patient temporarily hemiplegic on the right side; she recovered completely in the interim. Neurologic complications of surgical removal or radiosurgical treatment of this AVM could include multimodality sensory loss of the right hemibody and face (VPL and VPM nuclei and/or internal capsule) and right hemiparesis or hemiplegia (internal capsule and/or more dorsally located pyramidal tract fibers). *(Figure continued on following pages.)*

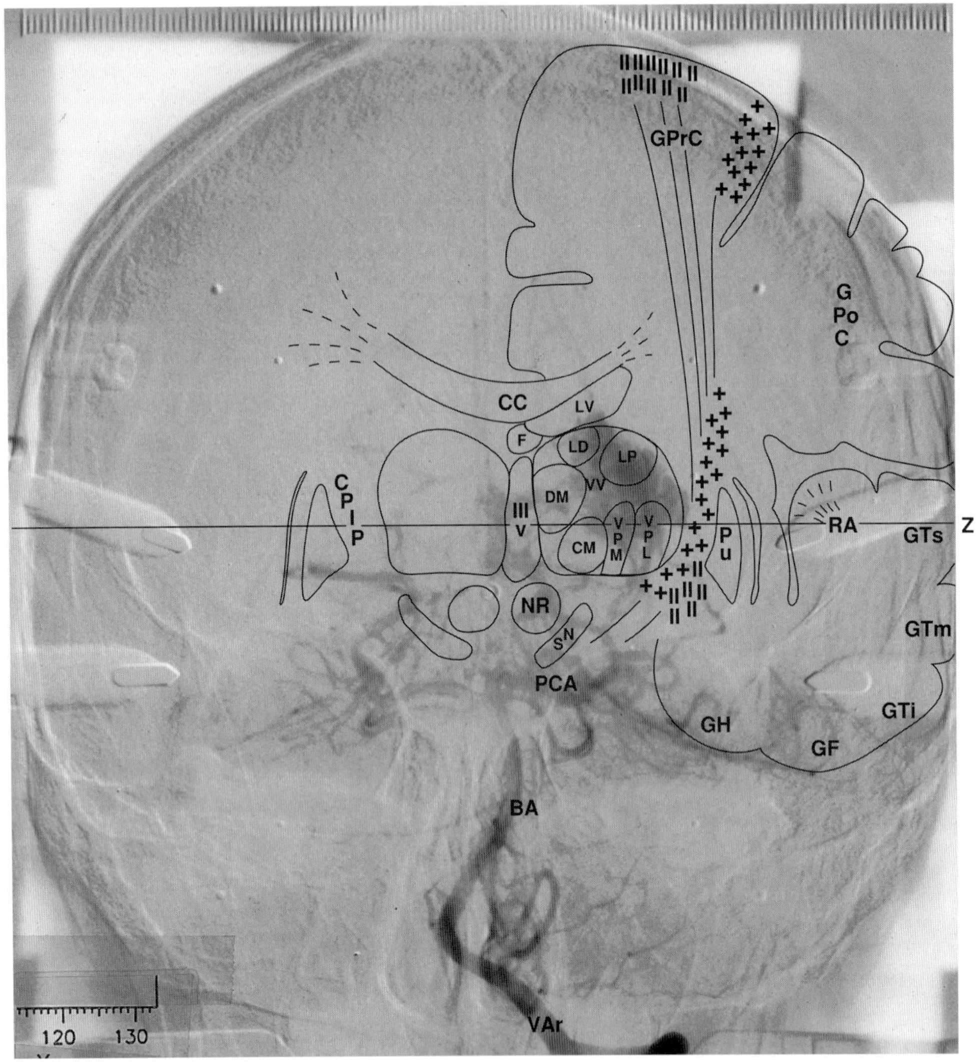
GPrC
G
Po
C
CC
LV
F
LD
LP
DM
VV
C
P
I
P
III
V
CM
V
P
M
V
P
L
P
u
RA
Z
GTs
NR
SN
PCA
GTm
GTi
GH
GF
BA
VAr
120
130

FIG. 4-16A.

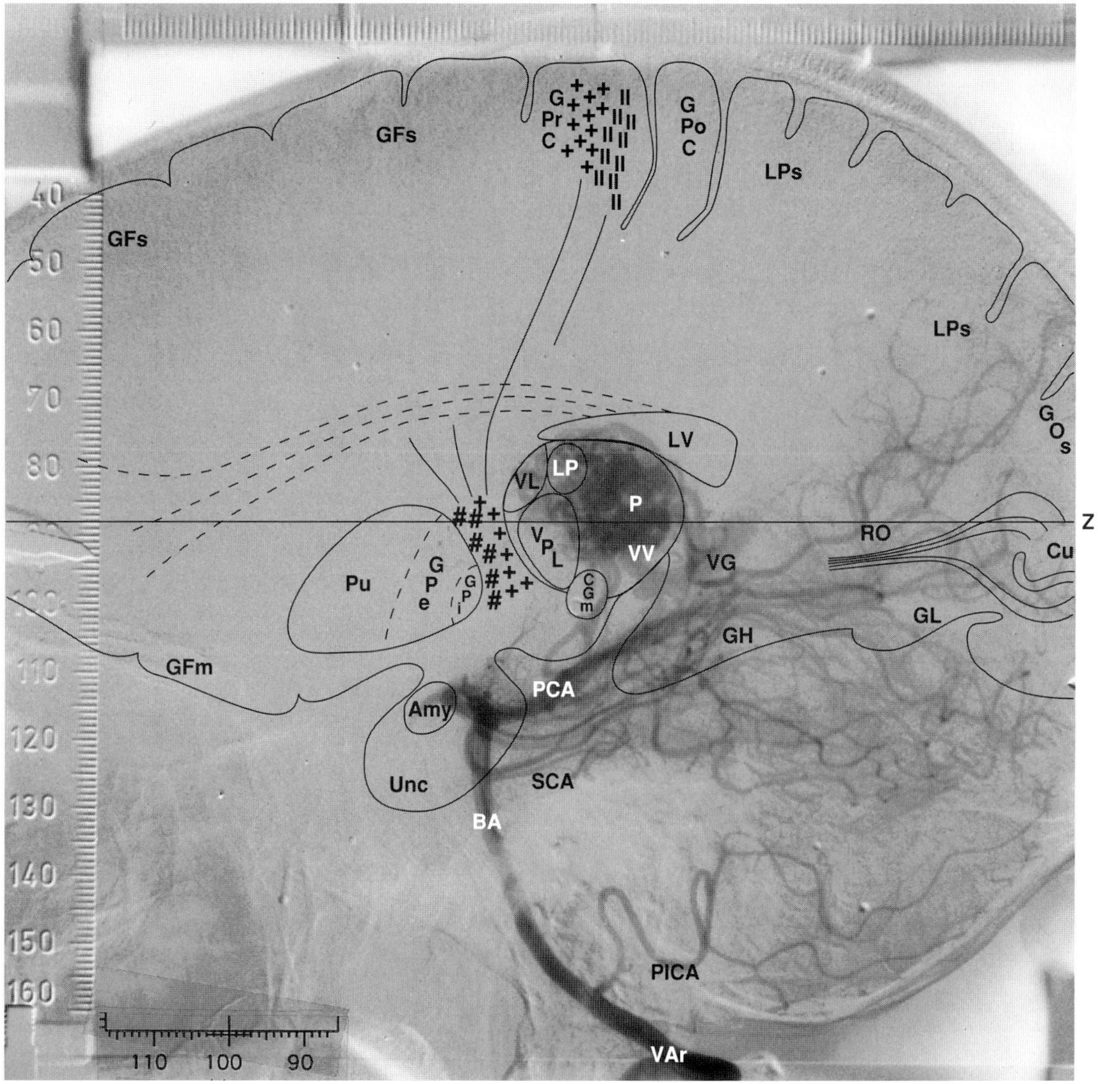
GFs
G Pr C
G Po C
LPs
GFs
LPs
G O s
LV
LP
VL
P
VPL
VV
VG
RO
Z
Cu
Pu
G P e
G P i
C G m
GL
GH
GFm
PCA
Amy
Unc
SCA
BA
PICA
VAr
40
50
60
70
80
110
120
130
140
150
160
110
100
90

FIG. 4-16B.

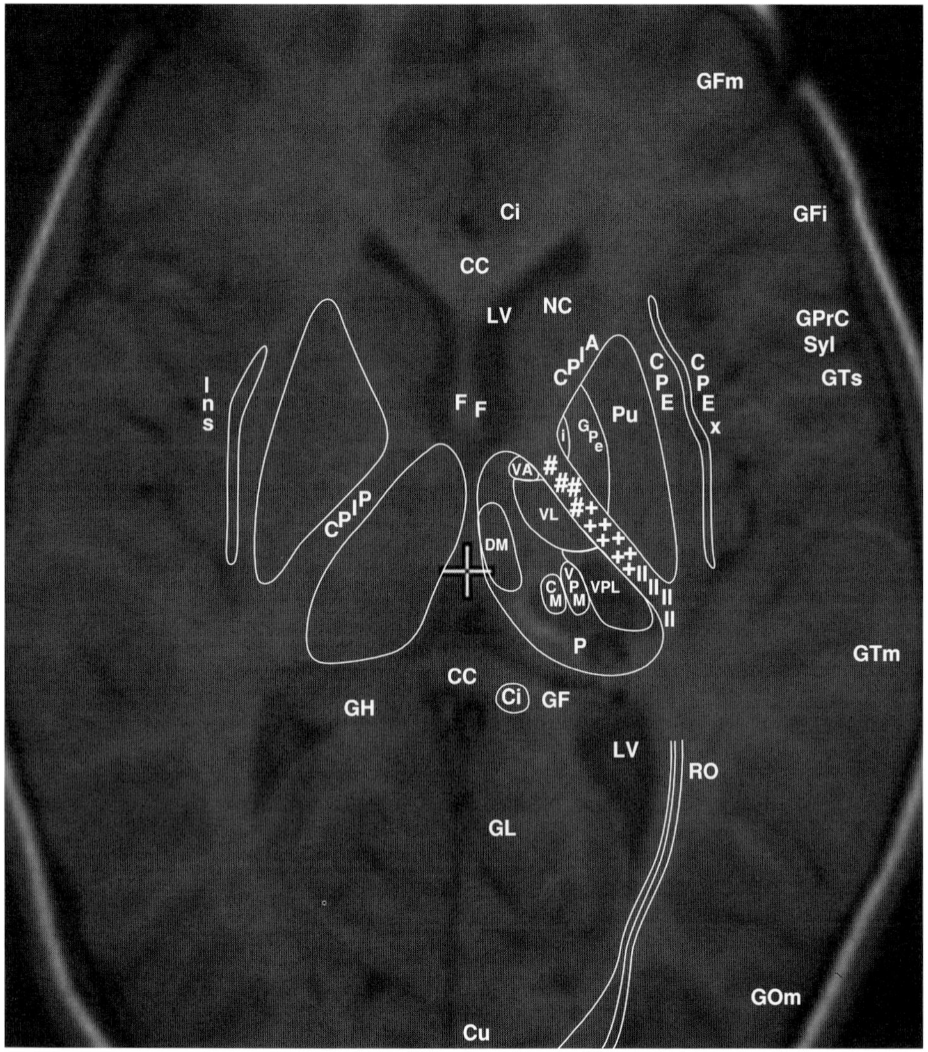
GFm
Ci
GFi
CC
LV
NC
GPrC
Syl
GTs
CPI/A
CPE
CPEx
Ins
F
F
Pu
GPe
i
VA
VL
CPI/P
DM
CM
VPM
VPL
P
GTm
CC
Ci
GF
GH
LV
RO
GL
GOm
Cu

FIG. 4-16C.

FIG. 4-17. Arteriovenous malformation of the right mid-brain and caudal thalamus, PA and lateral stereotactic vertebral angiogram films (**A and B**) and T_1-weighted stereotactic axial MRIs (**C and D**) separated by 6 mm from inferior to superior. The axial levels of **C** and **D** are indicated in **A**. Feeding arteries are difficult to identify individually but probably include thalamoperforating branches of the proximal posterior cerebral artery on the right side. The principal draining vein passes through the right cerebral peduncle to join the deep venous system, probably the basal vein of Rosenthal.

The AVM nidus occupies virtually the entire right half of the mid-brain tegmentum from the caudal extent of the red nucleus (NR) and substantia nigra (SN) up to the level of the base of the thalamus at the intercommissural (AC-PC) plane. The basal edge of the ventral posterolateral (VPL), ventral posteromedial (VPM), and centromedian (CM) thalamic nuclei sit on the superior surface of the nidus. Although a few vessels appear to bulge across the mid-line, for the most part this AVM appears to respect the mid-line plane. The posterior (dorsal) border of the nidus reaches the aqueduct of Sylvius (Aq), whereas the anterior (ventral) margin reaches the interpeduncular cistern in the mid-line and the ventral edge of the cerebral peduncle approximately 1 cm to the right of the mid-line. The medial margin of the nidus just reaches the contralateral (left) red nucleus (NR), whereas the lateral margin of the nidus leaves only a sliver of mid-brain tegmentum on the right side through which the spinothalamic and lemniscal tracts travel. The red nucleus, substantia nigra, and medial half of the cerebral peduncle on the right side are engulfed by AVM vessels. The medial and lateral geniculate bodies (CGm, CGl) lie just posterolateral to the lateral corner of the AVM in **D**.

Potential neurologic complications from treatment of this AVM could include contralateral hemiplegia as a consequence of pyramidal tract injury (cerebral peduncle), an involuntary movement disorder from injury to the red nucleus and/or substantia nigra, eye movement disorder from injury to the oculomotor complex, contralateral hemisensory loss from injury to the spinothalamic tract, altered level of consciousness from injury to the mid-line reticular activating system, and visual or binaural integrated hearing loss from injury to the lateral or medial geniculate bodies. In fact, this AVM had been irradiated using proton beam therapy at another institution 7 years before this set of imaging studies was obtained. As a consequence of that treatment, the patient developed a delayed but severe rubral tremor, dysarthria, and moderate hemiparesis involving the contralateral arm and leg. Subsequent obliteration 2.5 years after radiosurgery performed on the basis of these imaging studies resulted in no new neurologic deficits. *(Figure continued on following pages.)*

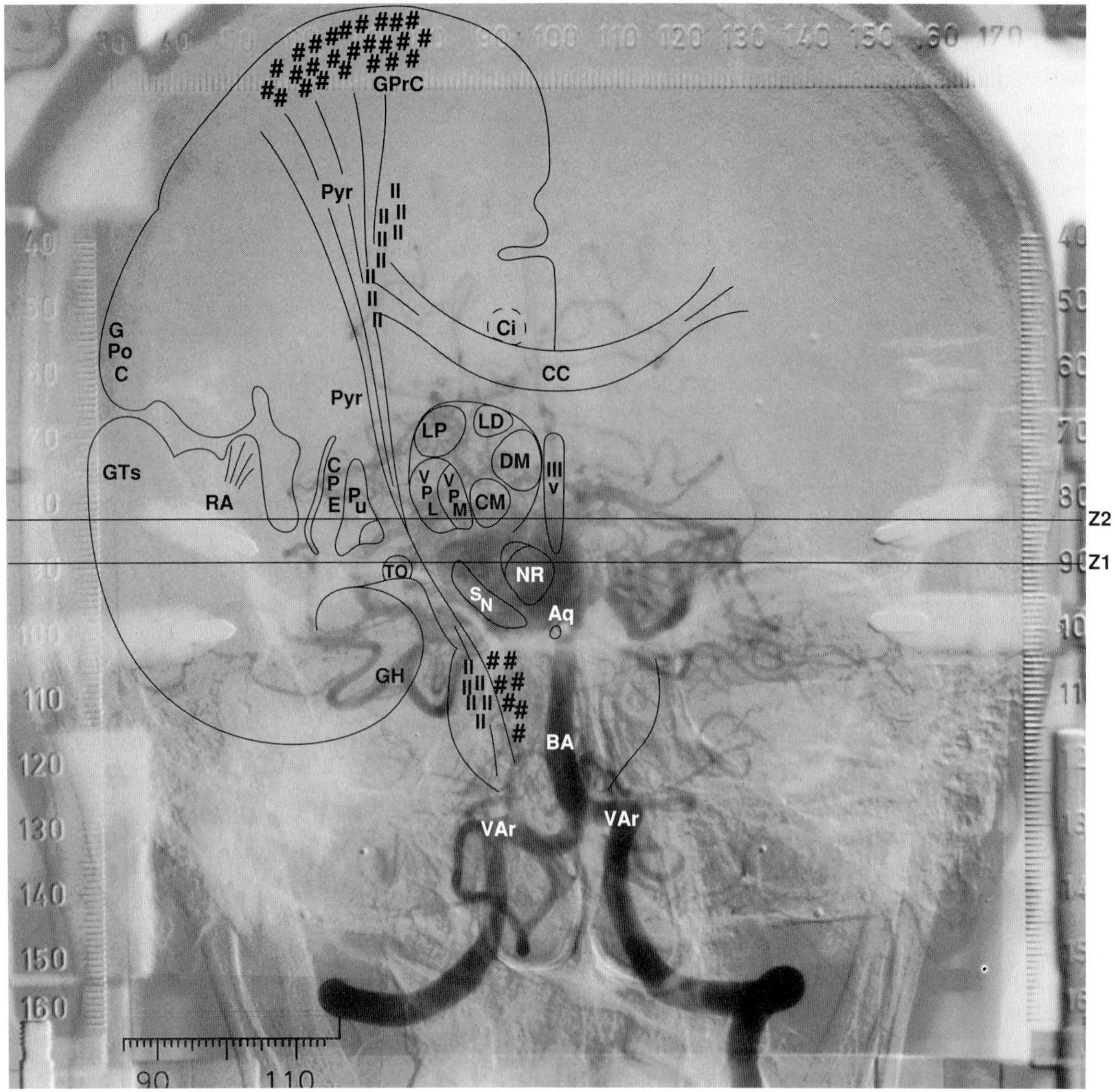
GPrC
Pyr
Pyr
Ci
CC
G
Po
C
GTs
RA
C
P
E
Pu
LP
LD
DM
V
P
L
V
P
M
CM
III
V
Z2
Z1
TO
NR
SN
Aq
GH
BA
VAr
VAr

FIG. 4-17A.

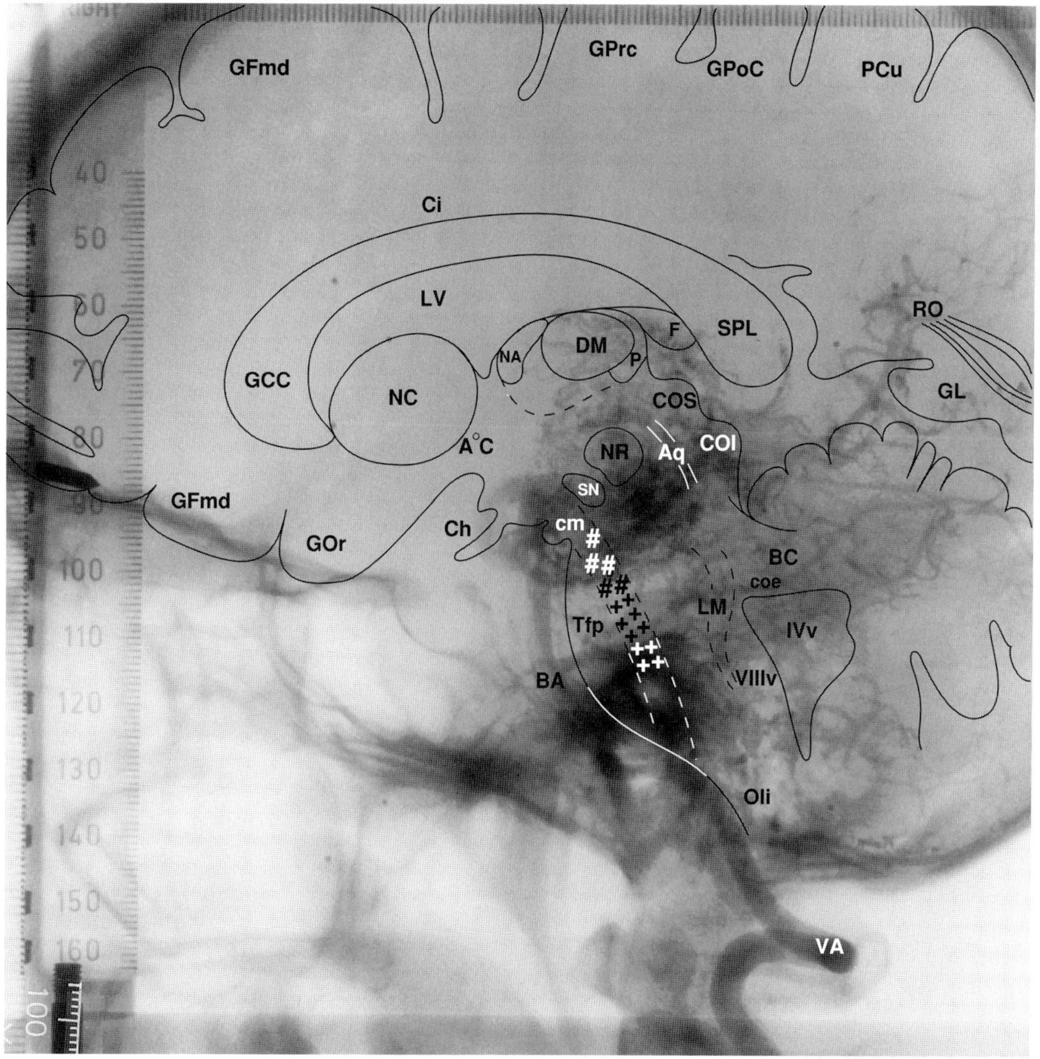
GFmd
GPrc
GPoC
PCu
Ci
LV
RO
F
SPL
DM
NA
P
GL
GCC
NC
COS
A°C
NR
Aq
COI
SN
GFmd
Ch
GOr
cm
BC
coe
LM
Tfp
IVv
BA
VIIIv
Oli
VA

FIG. 4-17B.

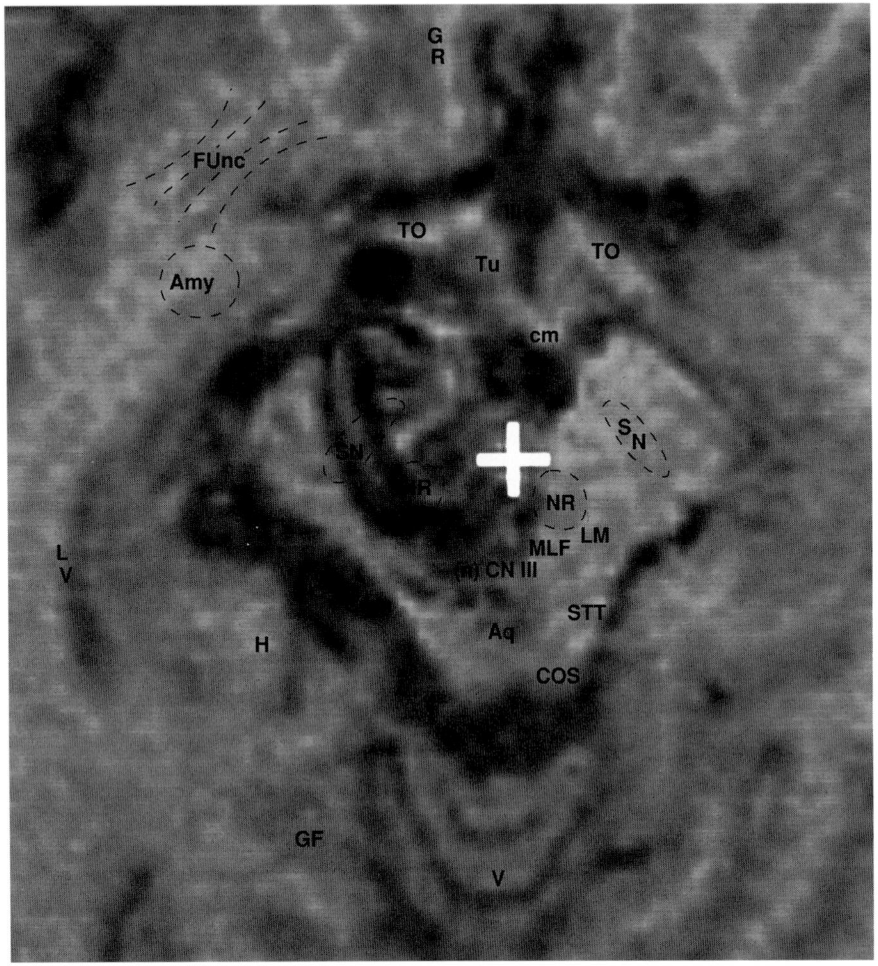

FIG. 4-17C.

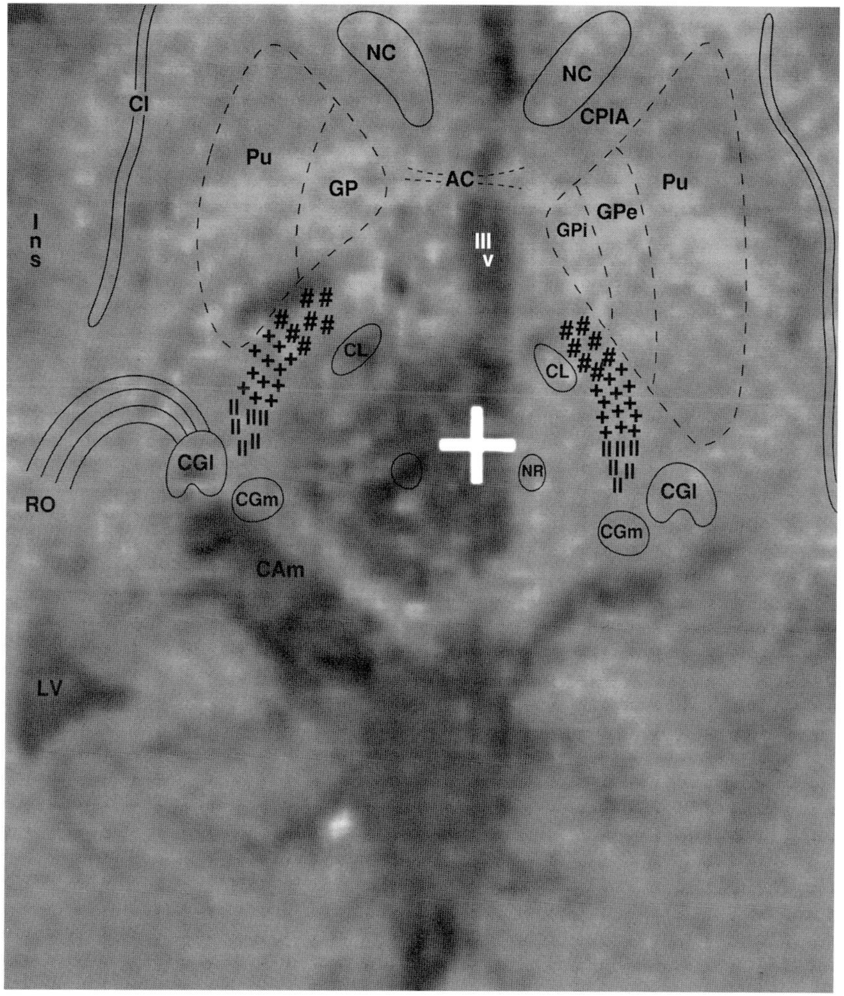
NC
NC
CI
CPIA
Pu
AC
Pu
GP
GPe
GPi
I n s
III V
CL
CL
CGl
NR
CGl
RO
CGm
CGm
CAm
LV

FIG. 4-17D.

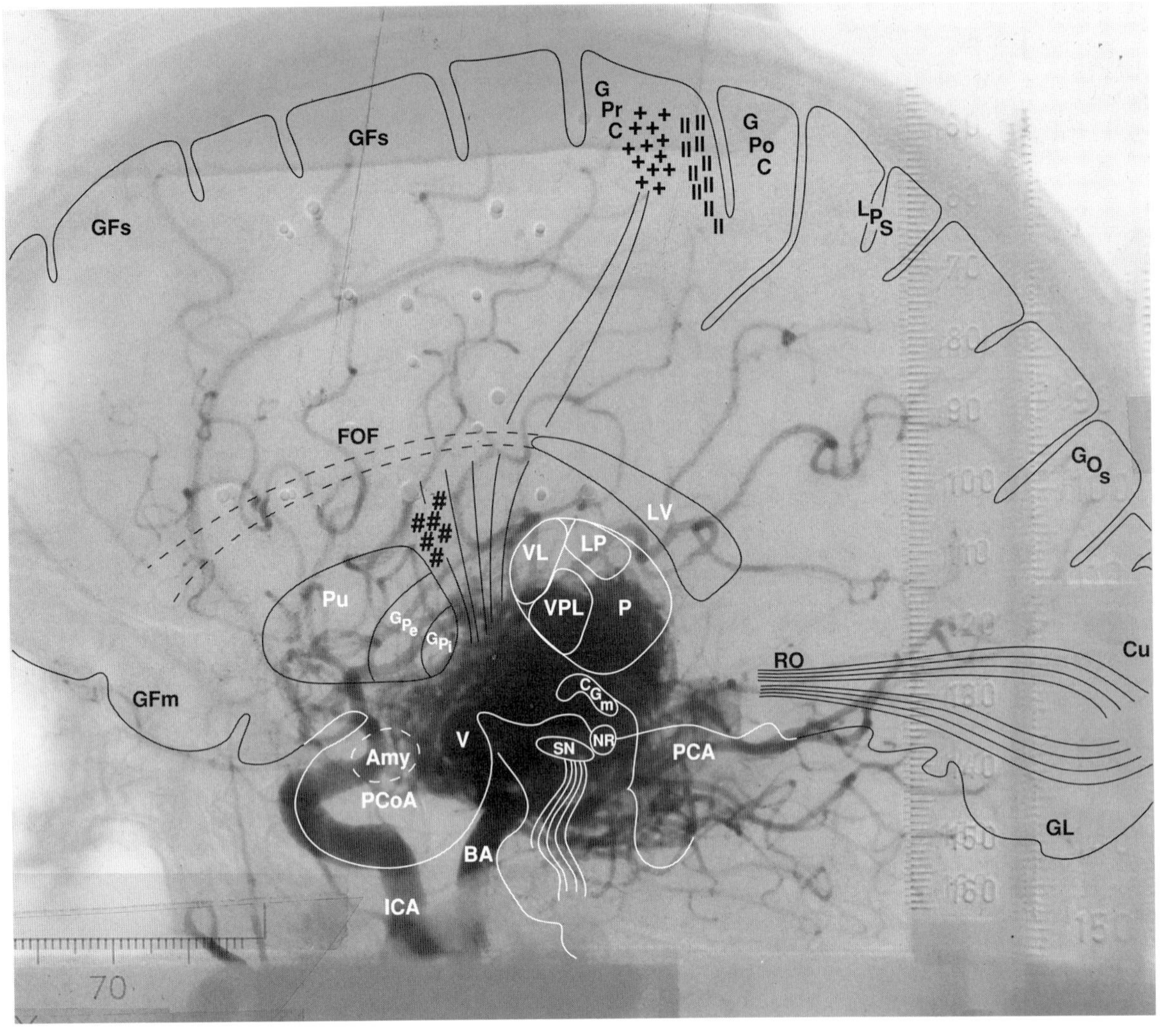
G
Pr
C
GFs
G
Po
C
GFs
LPS
FOF
GOs
LV
VL
LP
Pu
VPL
P
GPe
GPi
RO
Cu
GFm
CGm
V
Amy
SN
NR
PCA
PCoA
GL
BA
ICA
70

FIG. 4-18A.

FIG. 4-18. Large AVM (volume greater than 30 cm^3) of the right mid-brain, thalamus, hypothalamus, third ventricle, and choroidal fissure, lateral right carotid and vertebral artery stereotactic angiogram films (superimposed arterial phase projections (**A**), and contrast-enhanced, T_1-weighted coronal (**B**) and axial stereotactic MRIs (**C and D**). The Z coordinate levels of **C** and **D** are indicated in **B** and the Y coordinate level of **B** is indicated in **C** and **D**. Most of the nidus fills from the vertebral artery injection via perforating branches arising from the apex of the basilar artery (BA) and proximal segment of the right posterior cerebral artery (PCA). The anterolateral compartment of the nidus fills from the internal carotid circulation (ICA) by perforating branches of the posterior communicating artery (PCoA) and by a substantial contribution from the anterior choroidal artery (not labeled, but located just distal to PCoA on the posterior wall of the carotid artery). Venous drainage is entirely through the deep venous system, including an enlarged basal vein of Rosenthal (BVR) that is mostly hidden by the nidus but can be seen in **A** (v, projected medial to the temporal lobe and also behind the posterior edge of the AVM), as well as in **C**. An anterior knuckle of this dilated vein encroaches upon the right optic tract (TO), as does the center of the nidus itself (**C**).

The AVM displaces and/or percolates through the substance of the hypothalamus, right cerebral peduncle, mid-brain tegmentum, and basal thalamus. Feeding arteries, draining veins, and nidus vessels fill the interpeduncular cistern and choroidal fissure, whereas the bulk of the nidus exerts mass-effect upon the third ventricle, causing right to left shift of the third ventricle and contralateral (left) thalamus. In similar fashion, the lateral edge of the nidus appears to compress and obscure the right uncus, anterior portion of the hippocampal formation, and inferior margin of the basal ganglia. Between the lentiform nucleus (putamen [Pu], and globus pallidus [GPe, GPi]) and the thalamus, the AVM occupies virtually the entire posterior limb of the internal capsule (CPIP). More ventrally, the subthalamic nucleus (corpus luysii [CL]), substantia nigra (SN), and red nucleus (NR) also are obscured by the AVM. Variceal dilation of the deep venous system (vv in **C**) also distorts the mid-brain tectum bilaterally, pushing the collicular plate in an anterior and ventral direction.

Owing to the number and volume of critical structures located around this AVM, treatment of any sort could result in a host of severe, disabling, and potentially lethal neurologic deficits. In fact, radiosurgical treatment resulted in complete obliteration of the AVM after 3 years, and caused only an incomplete (incongruous) left homonymous visual field deficit and mild worsening of the patient's pre-existing left hemiparesis (18). *(Figure continued on following pages.)*

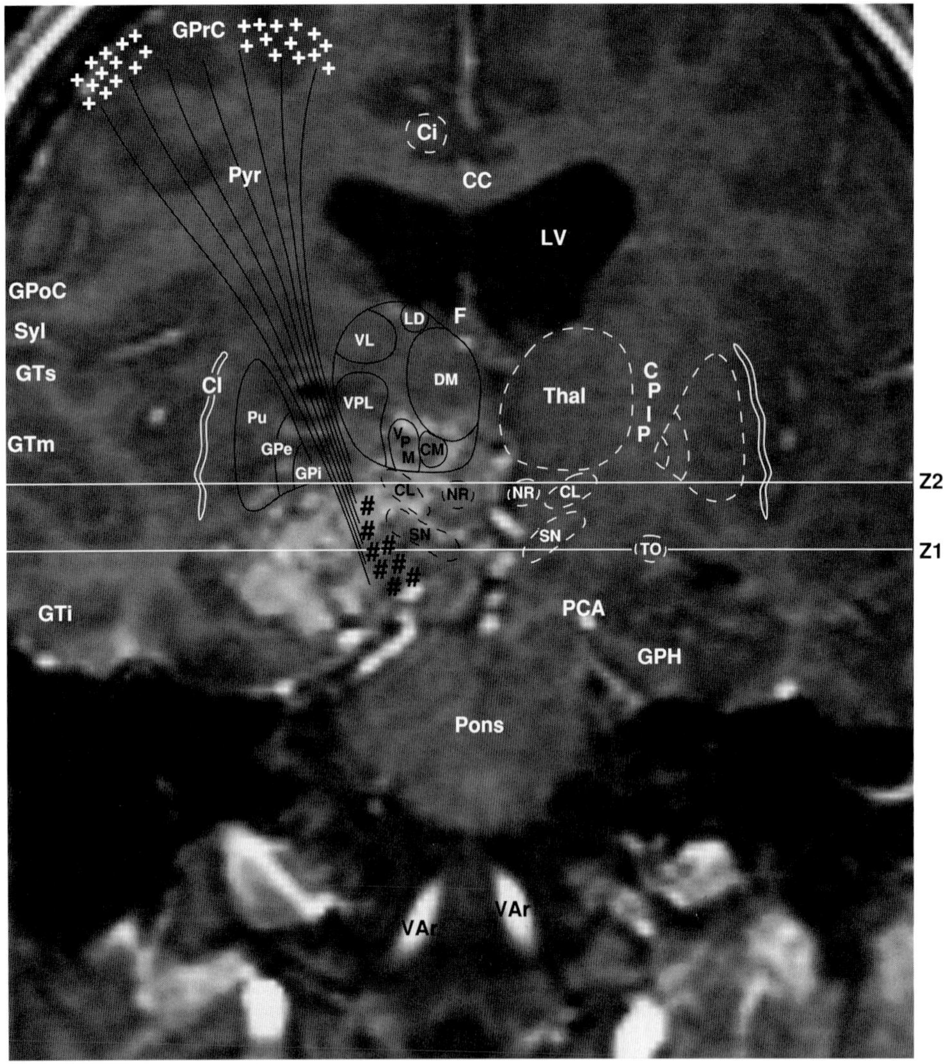
GPrC
Pyr
Ci
CC
LV
GPoC
Syl
GTs
Cl
GTm
LD
F
VL
DM
VPL
Thal
C
P
I
P
Pu
GPe
GPi
V
P
M
CM
CL
NR
NR
CL
SN
SN
TO
Z2
Z1
GTi
PCA
GPH
Pons
VAr
VAr

FIG. 4-18B.

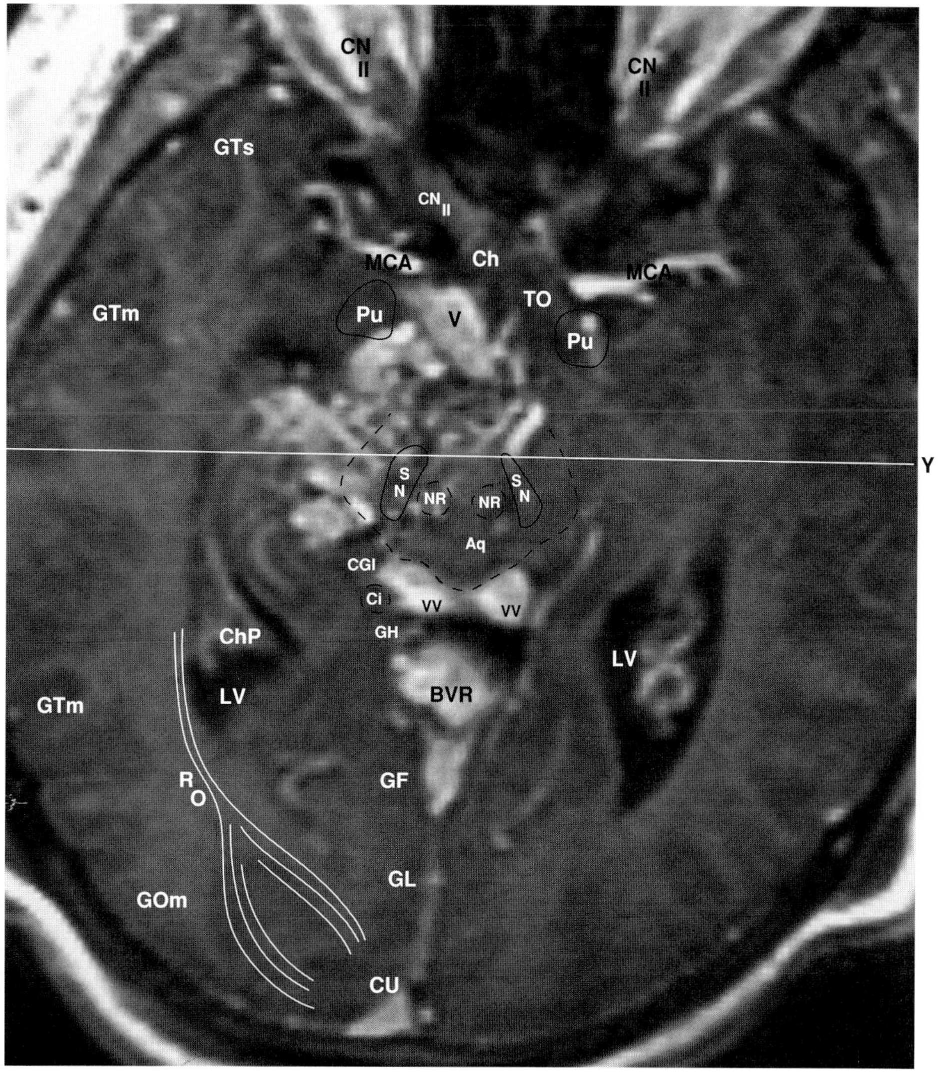
CN II
CN II
GTs
CN II
MCA
Ch
MCA
TO
GTm
Pu
V
Pu
Y
S N
NR
NR
S N
Aq
CGl
Ci
VV
VV
GH
ChP
LV
GTm
LV
BVR
R O
GF
GL
GOm
CU

FIG. 4-18C.

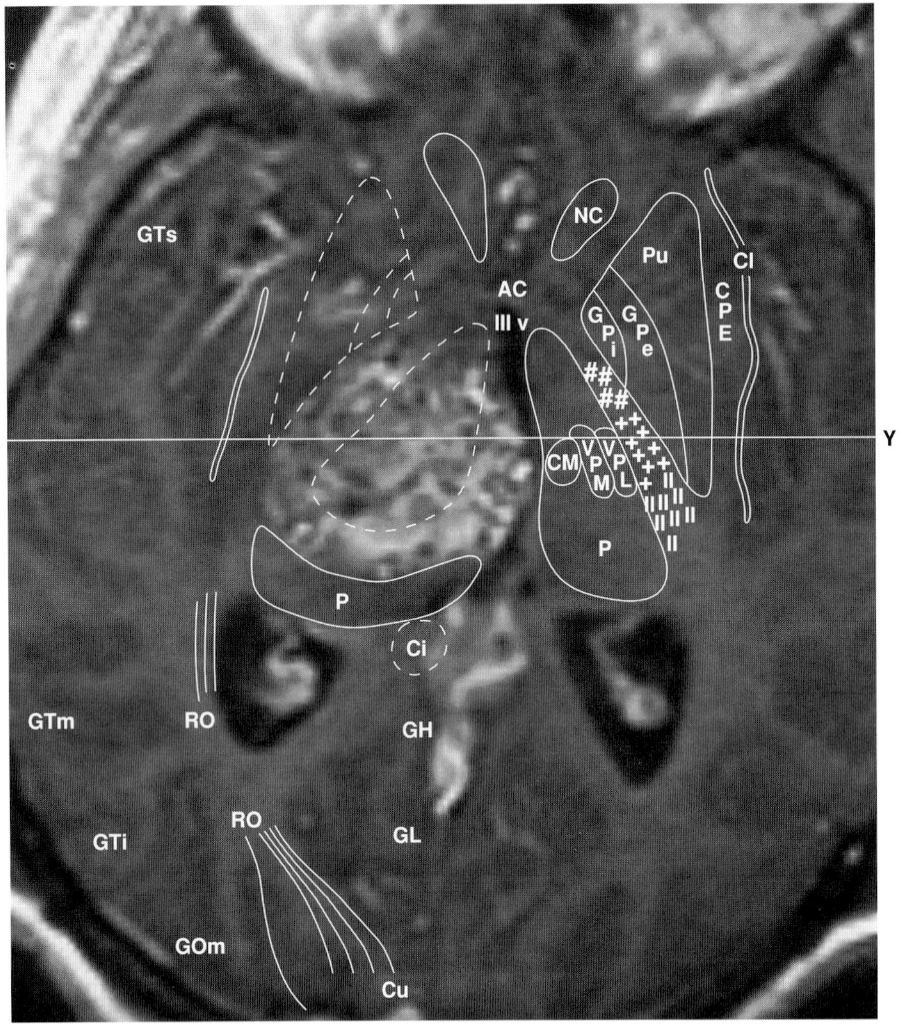
GTs
NC
Pu
Cl
AC
C
P
E
III v
G
P
i
G
P
e
Y
CM
V
P
M
V
P
L
P
P
Ci
GTm
RO
GH
RO
GTi
GL
GOm
Cu

FIG. 4-18D.

FIG. 4-19. Arteriovenous malformation of the central mid-brain tegmentum, PA and lateral stereotactic left vertebral angiogram films (**A and B**) and T_1-weighted, contrast-enhanced stereotactic axial MRIs (**C and D**) separated by 3 mm from inferior to superior. Lines Z_1 and Z_2 denote the planes of **C** and **D** on the angiographic images (**A and B**). Feeding arteries include enlarged perforating vessels from the apex of the basilar artery (BA) and from the proximal posterior cerebral arteries (PCA). These enter the AVM through the interpeduncular cistern (Cip). Venous drainage appears to traverse the right mid-brain tegmentum to course along the lateral pial surface (demonstrated best in **D**).

The compact nidus occupies the central mid-brain and extends eccentrically toward the right side, where it reaches the pial surface at the level of the aqueduct of Sylvius (Aq). The ventral AVM margin is at the crotch of the cerebral peduncles in the mid-line, where an enlarged feeding artery abuts the mammillary bodies (cm) and proximal optic tracts (TO) anteriorly, across the interpeduncular cistern. Dorsally, the nidus reaches the periaqueductal gray matter. In the transverse dimension, the AVM extends from the medial edge of the left red nucleus (NR) across the mid-line to displace or engulf a substantial portion of the right-sided red nucleus, subthalamic nucleus (CL), and spinothalamic/quintothalamic tract (STT). The more laterally located substantia nigra (SN) is spared.

Microsurgical resection of this AVM probably is not feasible. Radiosurgical treatment carries the risk of inducing visual loss (optic tracts), disorders of memory (mammillary bodies), and/or a variety of involuntary movement disorders such as rubral tremor (red nucleus) or hemiballismus (subthalamic nucleus). Injury to the right-sided spinothalamic and quintothalamic tracts also could cause contralateral hemibody and hemifacial numbness. Because the pyramidal tracts within the cerebral peduncles lie a centimeter or more lateral to the nidus, motor weakness would be an unlikely complication. However, because fibers of the oculomotor nerve (not labeled) traverse the AVM and because elements of the oculomotor/trochlear nucleus complex lie near the dorsal margin of the AVM, a variety of eye movement disorders could occur as well. In fact, radiosurgical obliteration of this AVM was accomplished without worsening this patient's mild tremor and oculomotor paresis. *(Figure continued on following pages.)*

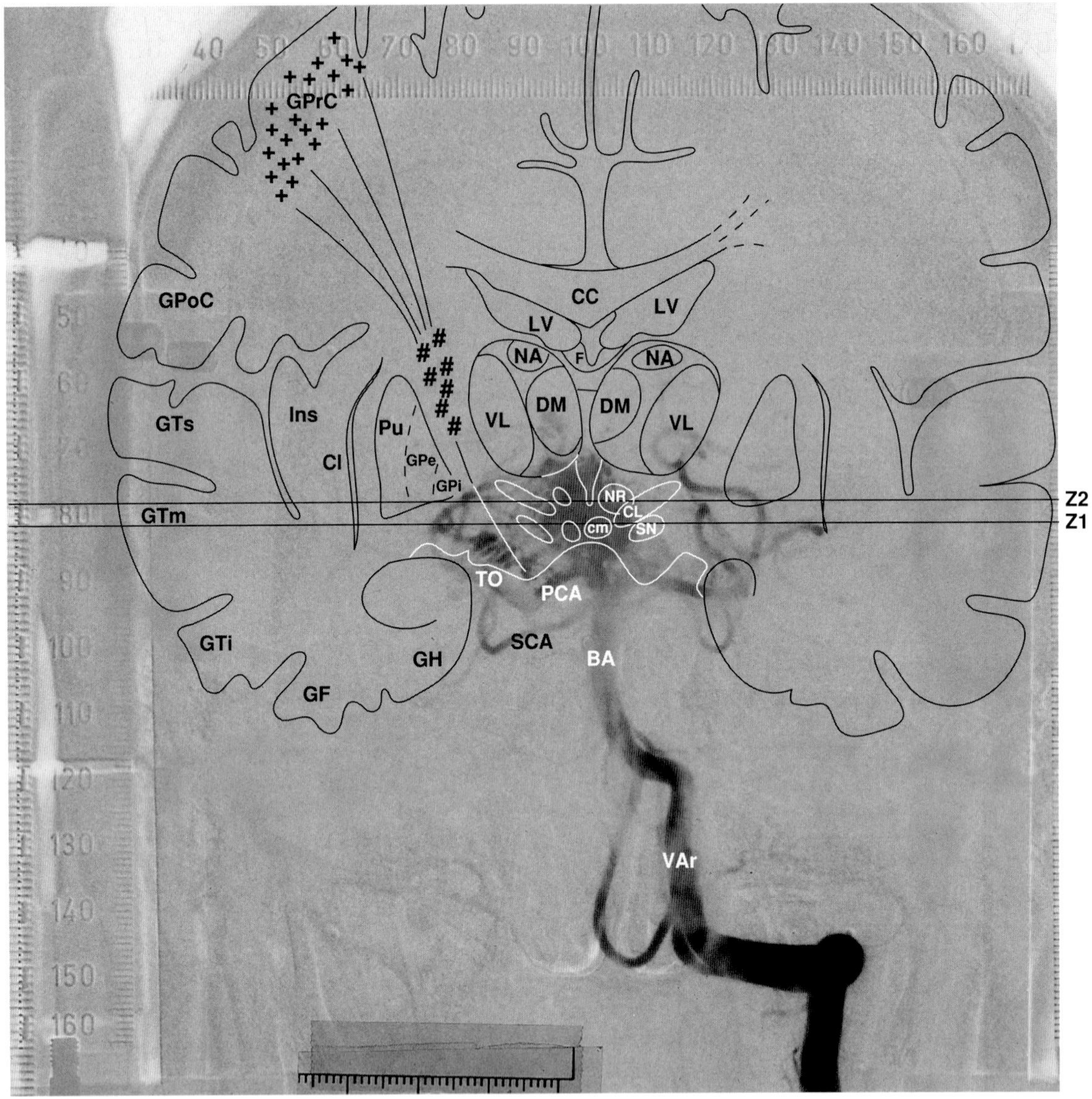
GPrC
GPoC
GTs
Ins
Cl
Pu
GPe
GPi
CC
LV
LV
NA
F
NA
VL
DM
DM
VL
NR
CL
cm
SN
Z2
Z1
GTm
TO
PCA
SCA
BA
GTi
GH
GF
VAr

FIG. 4-19A.

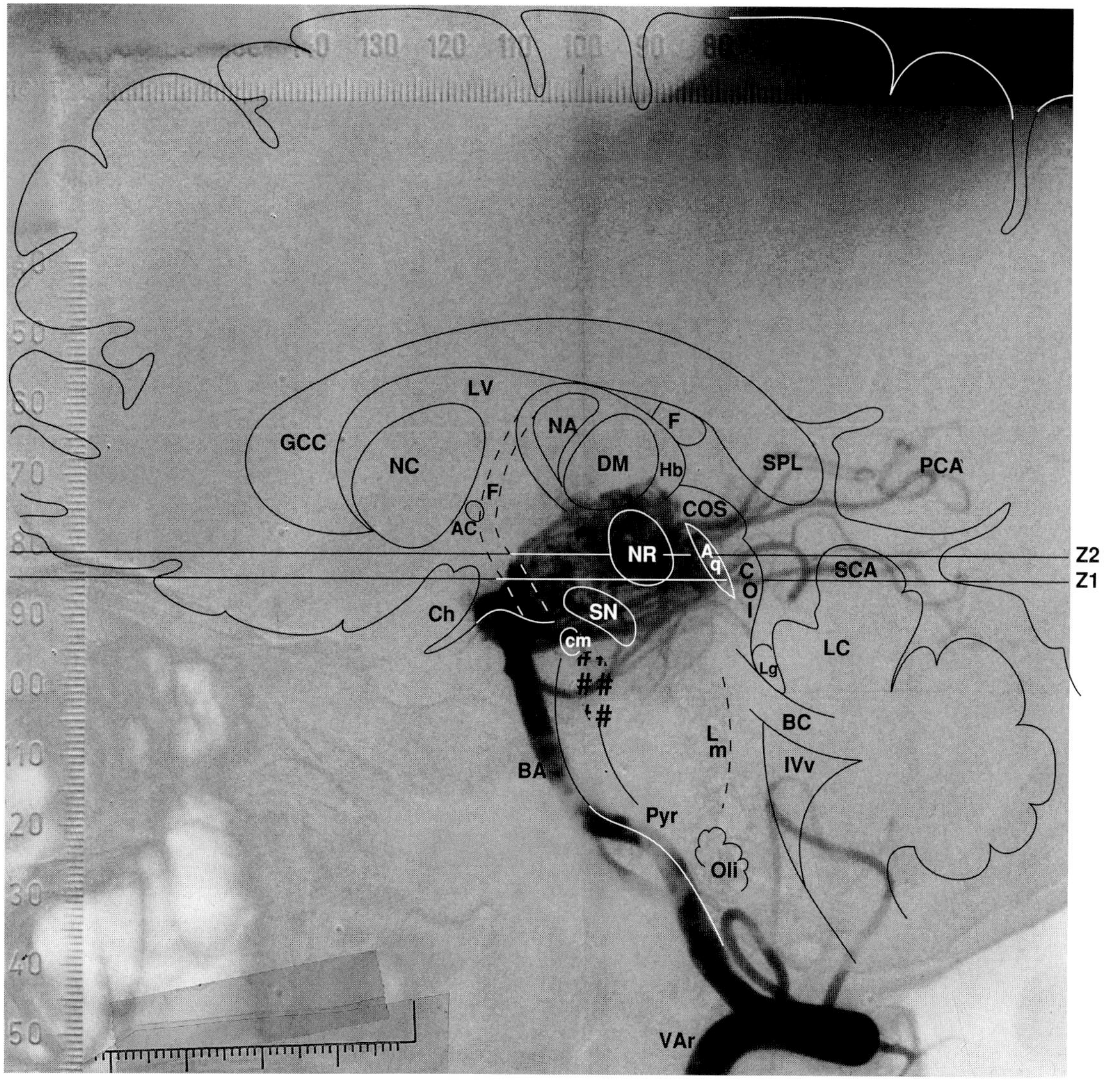

LV
GCC
NC
NA
F
DM
Hb
SPL
PCA
F
AC
COS
NR
Aq
Z2
Z1
C
O
I
SCA
Ch
SN
cm
LC
Lg
BC
L
m
IVv
BA
Pyr
Oli
VAr

FIG. 4-19B.

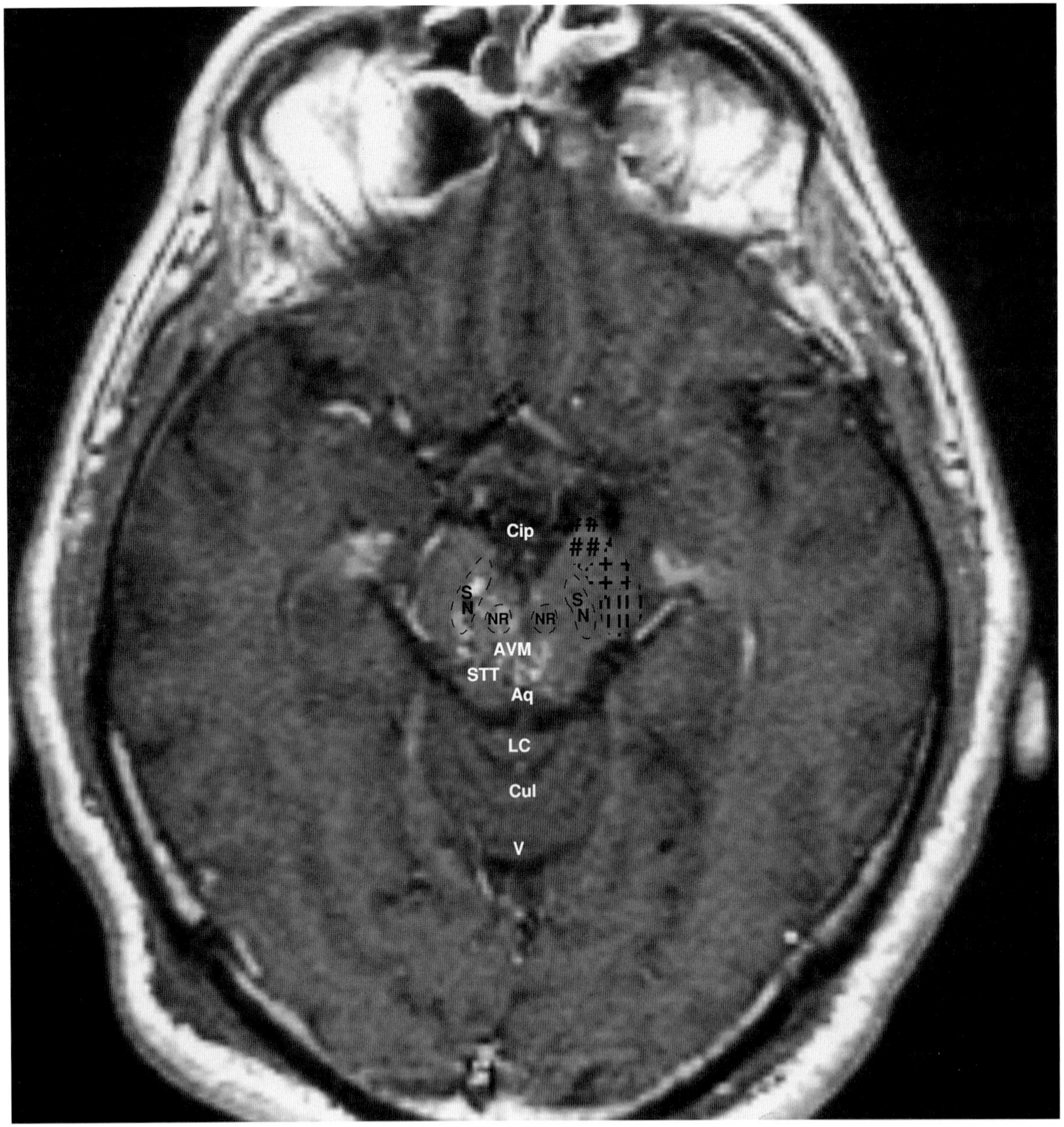

FIG. 4-19C.

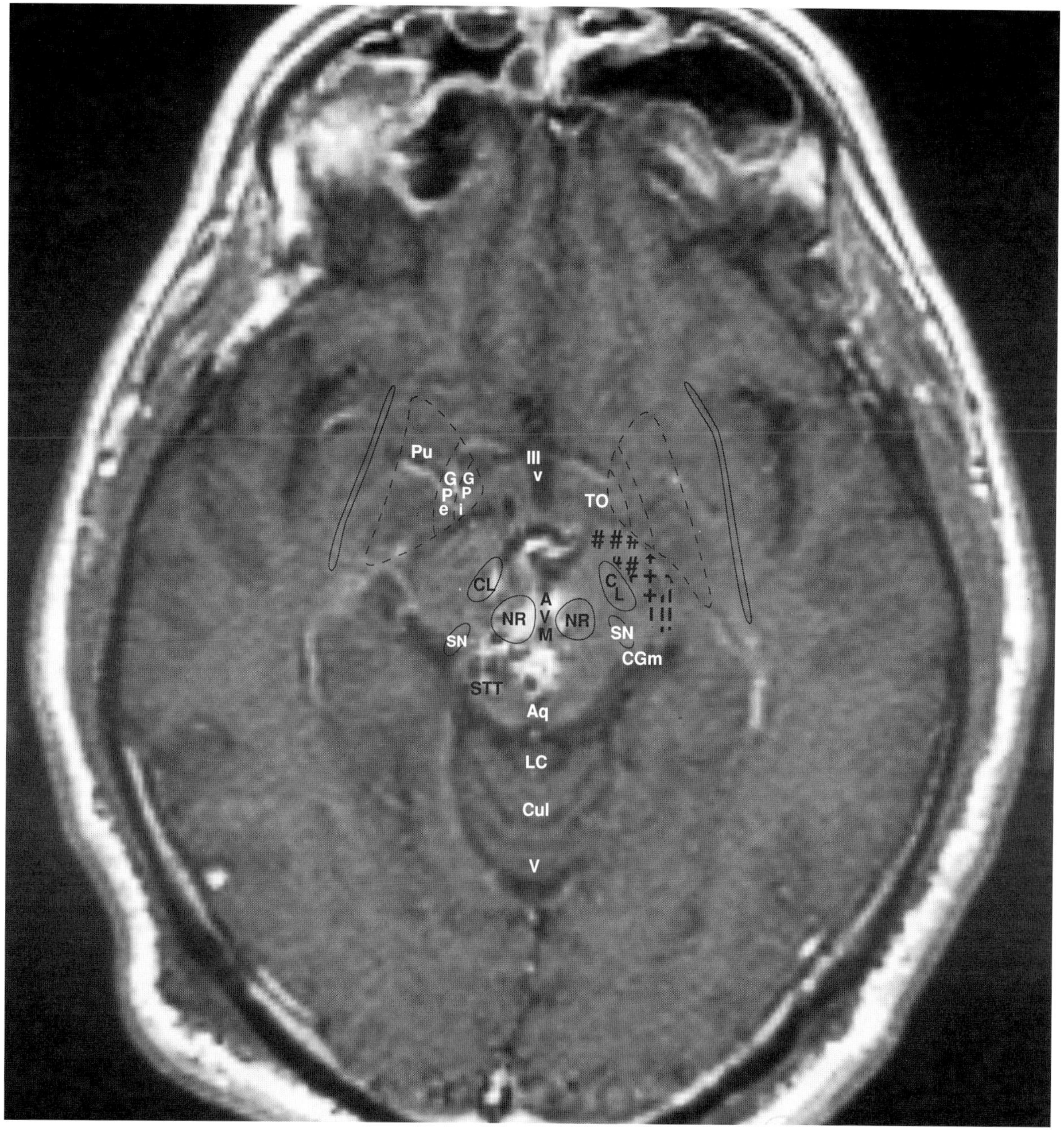

FIG. 4-19D.

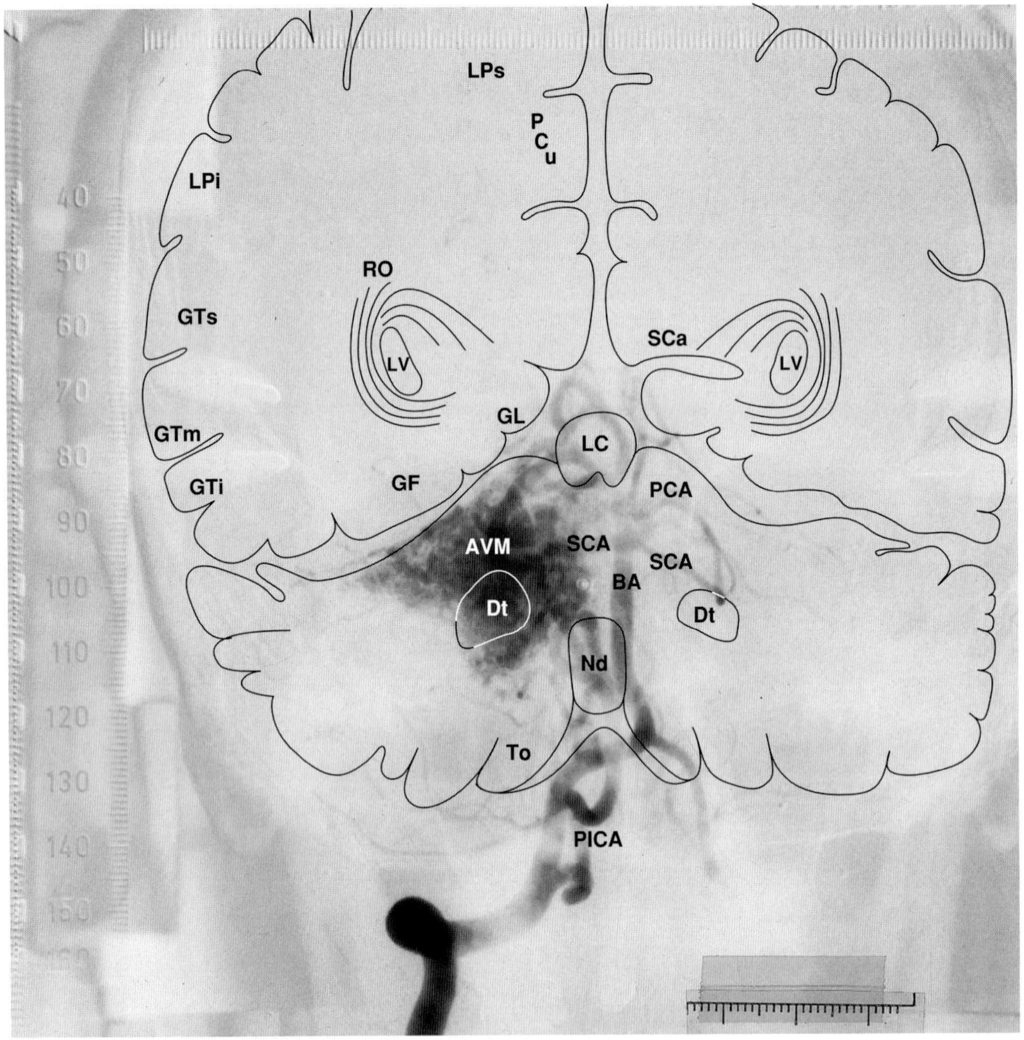
LPs
P
C
u
LPi
RO
GTs
SCa
LV
LV
GL
LC
GTm
GTi
GF
PCA
AVM
SCA
SCA
BA
Dt
Dt
Nd
To
PICA

FIG. 4-20A.

FIG. 4-20. Arteriovenous malformation of the right superior cerebellar hemisphere, PA and lateral stereotactic right vertebral angiogram films (**A and C**) and nonstereotactic coronal T_1-weighted (**B**) and axial fast spin-echo (**D**) MRIs, respectively. Line Z in **C** denotes the plane of **D**. Feeding arteries include distal segments of the right superior cerebellar (SCA) and posterior inferior cerebellar arteries (PICA). The SCA feeders appear to enter the superolateral and anterior portion of the nidus, whereas the PICA contribution enters the posteromedial portion of the AVM. Venous drainage is seen faintly in two adjacent areas of **C**. The inferior component (vvi) appears to exit the posteromedial AVM margin near the PICA and to involve the inferior vermian veins. The more superior component of the venous drainage (vvs) appears to involve bridging veins between the superior cerebellar surface and the underside of the tentorium and transverse sinus near the torcular.

The nidus itself occupies the posterior portion of the right quadrangular lobule (LQ). The superior (superficial) AVM margin fans out across the tentorial surface of the quadrangular lobule, whereas the deep margin reaches the level of the dentate nucleus (Dt) and other deep cerebellar nuclei. In the transverse dimension the AVM extends from the edge of the culmen (cul) medially to the superior portion of the semilunar lobule (LSs) laterally.

Neurologic risks associated with surgical removal or radiosurgical treatment of this AVM include ispilateral (right-sided) dysmetria and cerebellar outflow tremor from injury to the cerebellar hemisphere, deep nuclei, or their vascular supply. *(Figure continued on following pages.)*

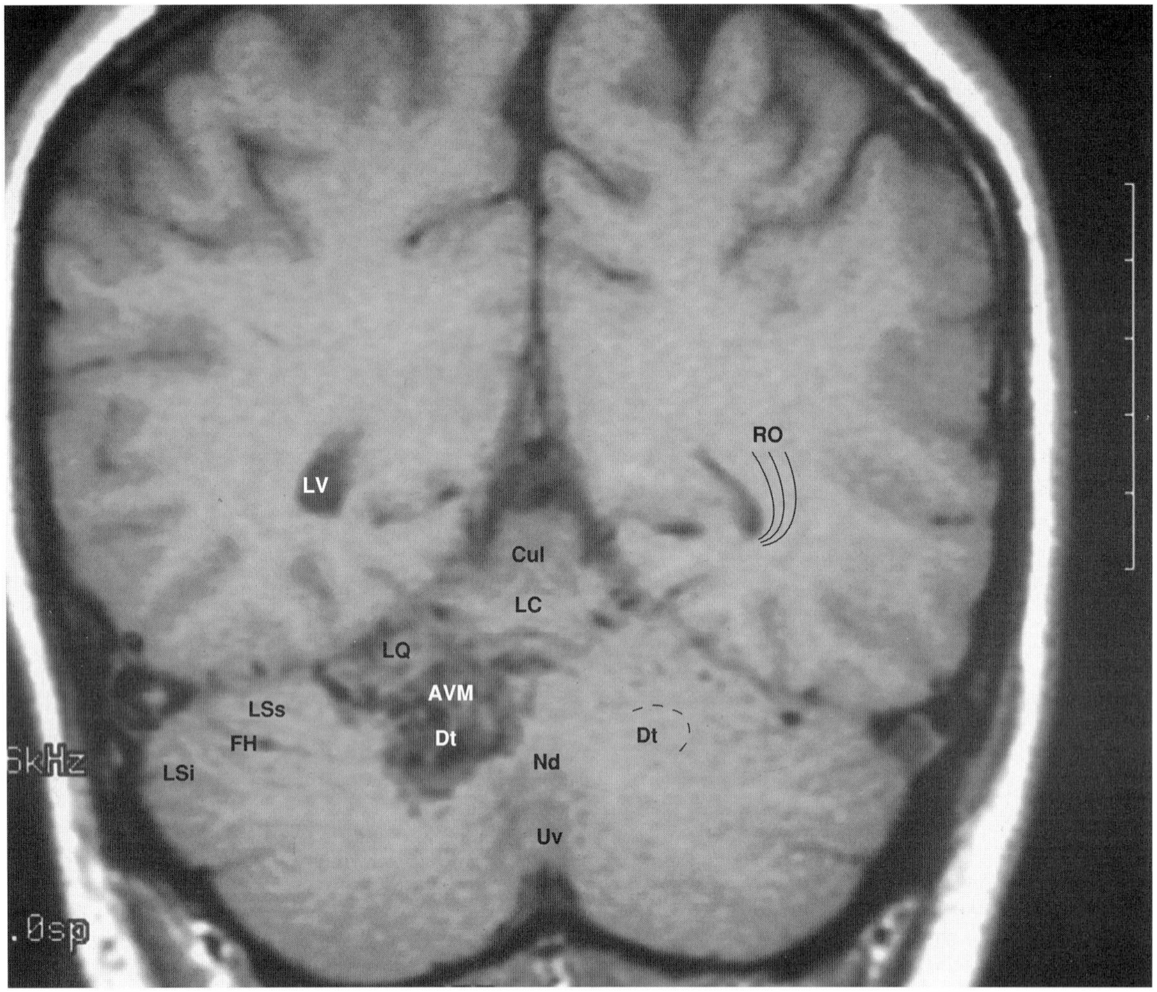

FIG. 4-20B.

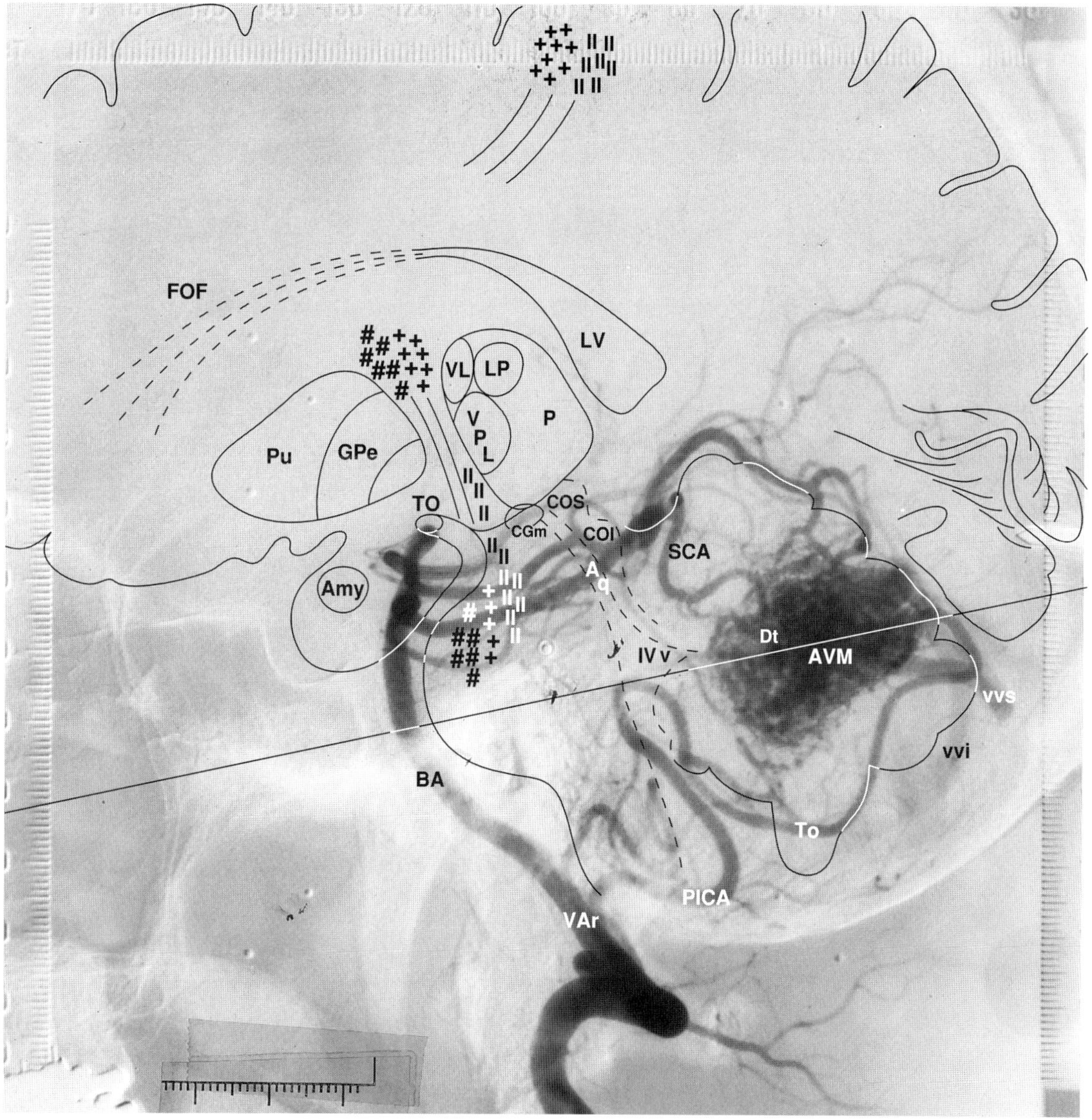

FOF
LV
VL
LP
V
P
L
P
Pu
GPe
TO
COS
CGm
COI
SCA
Amy
Aq
IV v
Dt
AVM
Z
vvs
vvi
BA
To
PICA
VAr

FIG. 4-20C.

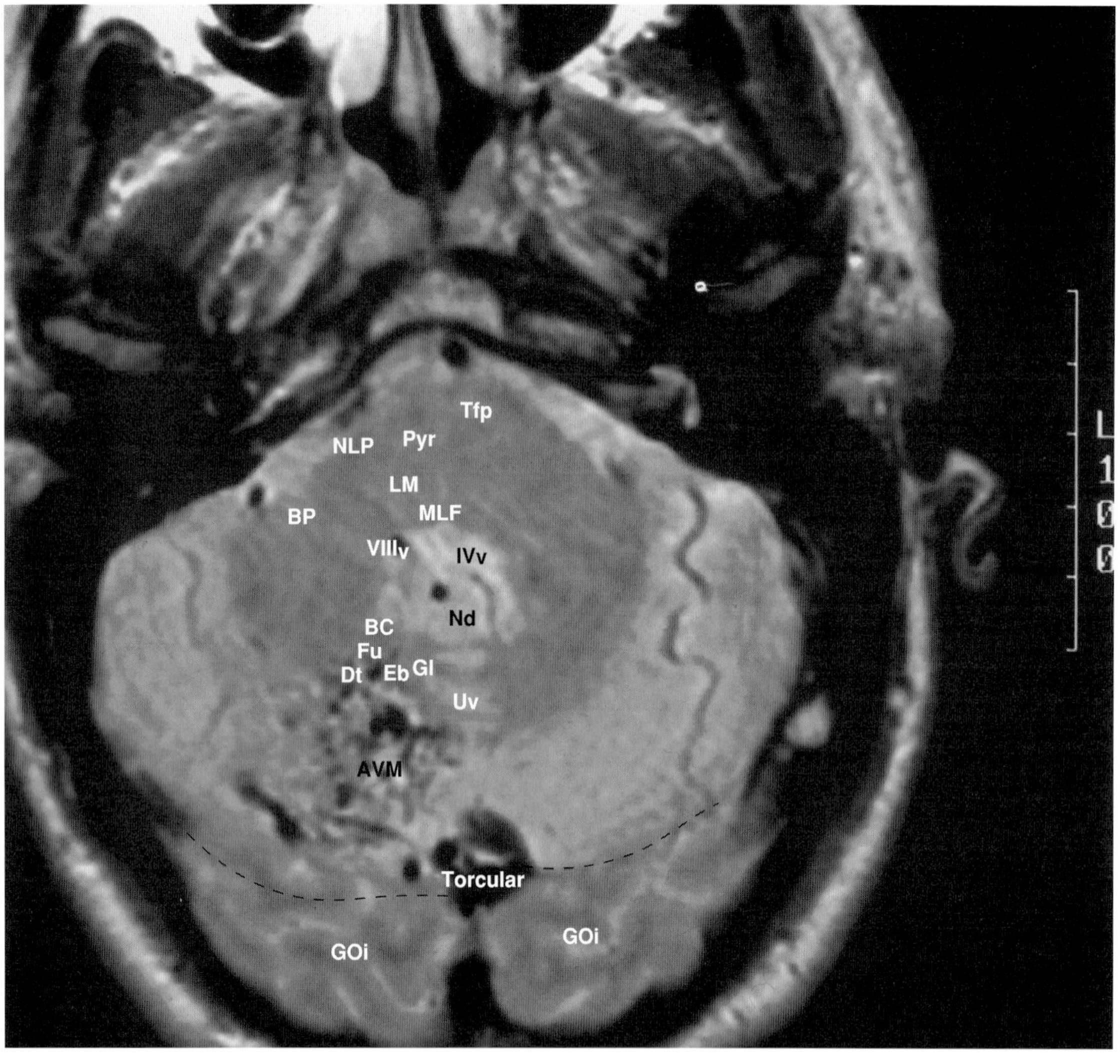

Tfp
NLP
Pyr
LM
BP
MLF
VIIIv
IVv
Nd
BC
Fu
Dt
Eb
Gl
Uv
AVM
Torcular
GOi
GOi

FIG. 4-20D.

FIG. 4-21. Previously ruptured and operated arteriovenous malformation of the left inferolateral cerebellar hemisphere, stereotactic PA and lateral left vertebral angiogram films (**A and C**), nonstereotactic coronal T_2-weighted (**B**) and sagittal T_1-weighted (**D**) MRIs. Both MRIs pass through the center of the AVM nidus, which is located immediately lateral to the surgical cavity (**B**) and occipital bone defect (labeled "surg" in **D**) that were created by removal of an acute cerebellar hematoma 1 year before these imaging studies were performed. The principal feeding artery appears to be an enlarged hemispheric branch of the left posterior inferior cerebellar artery (PICA). It enters the posterior-inferior AVM margin. Additional feeding vessels from the superior cerebellar artery (SCA) enter the AVM from the anterolateral and superior direction. A faint anterior inferior cerebellar artery (AICA) is seen in **C**, but no definite supply to the malformation can be ascertained from these films. The major draining vein (vv) exits the inferolateral margin of the nidus to turn upward along the lateral suboccipital surface of the cerebellum to enter the transverse sinus at the undersurface of the tentorium.

The nidus lies within the semilunar lobule (LS), centered in or near the horizontal fissure, and has its superior and inferior margins encroaching upon the respective portions of the semilunar lobule (LSs and LSi). The lateral margin reaches the cerebellar cortical surface, whereas the medial margin abuts the old hematoma resection cavity. The roof of the cavity lies below the dentate nucleus (Dt), and the inferomedial edge of the cavity barely reaches the tonsil (To).

This AVM probably could have been removed relatively easily by the original neurosurgeon had angiogram films been available. However, as the patient presented in extremis with a sizable cerebellar hematoma during the third trimester of pregnancy, preoperative angiography was not performed. Because of the posterolateral location of the AVM and hematoma in this case, no permanent neurologic deficit was caused by surgery and subsequent radiosurgery. *(Figure continued on following pages.)*

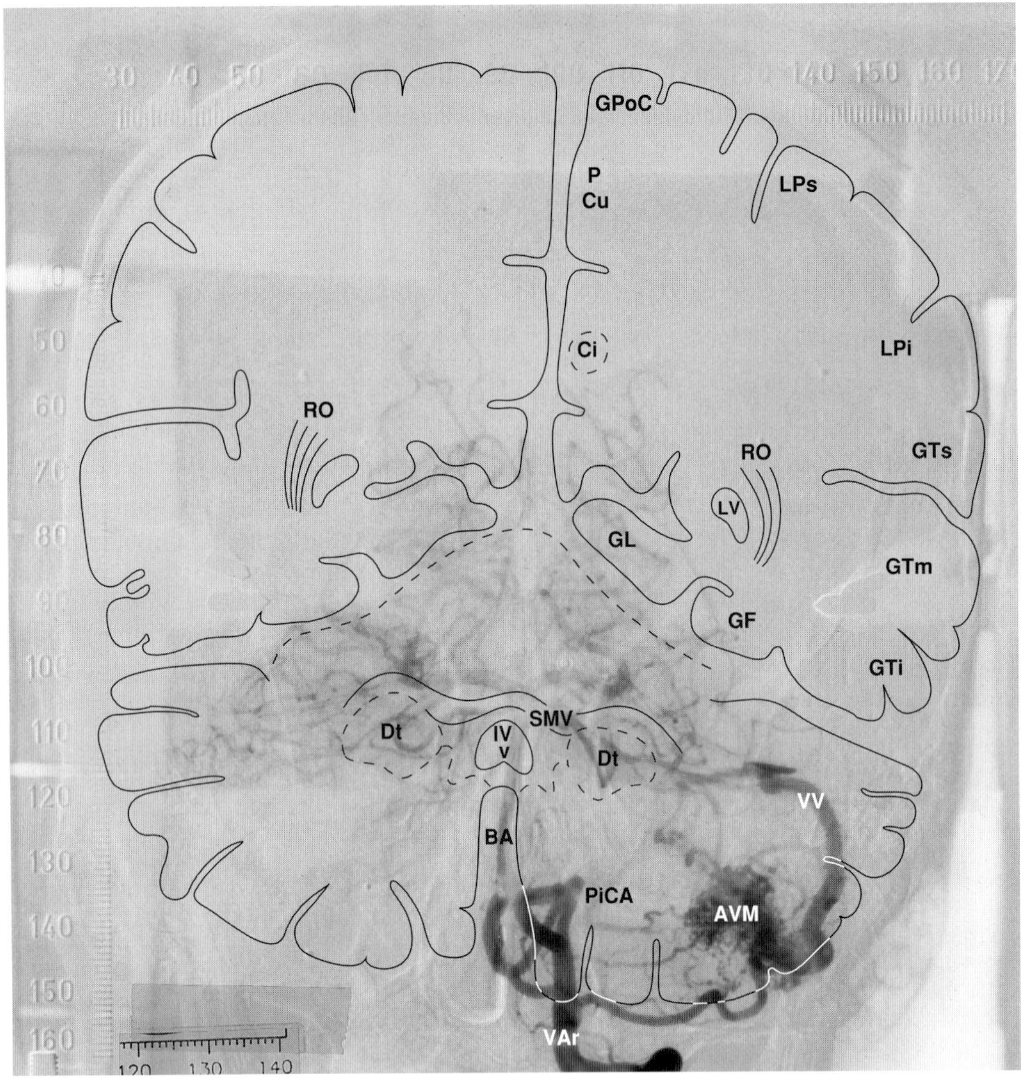
GPoC
P
Cu
LPs
Ci
LPi
RO
RO
GTs
LV
GL
GTm
GF
GTi
SMV
Dt
IV
v
Dt
VV
BA
PiCA
AVM
VAr

FIG. 4-21A.

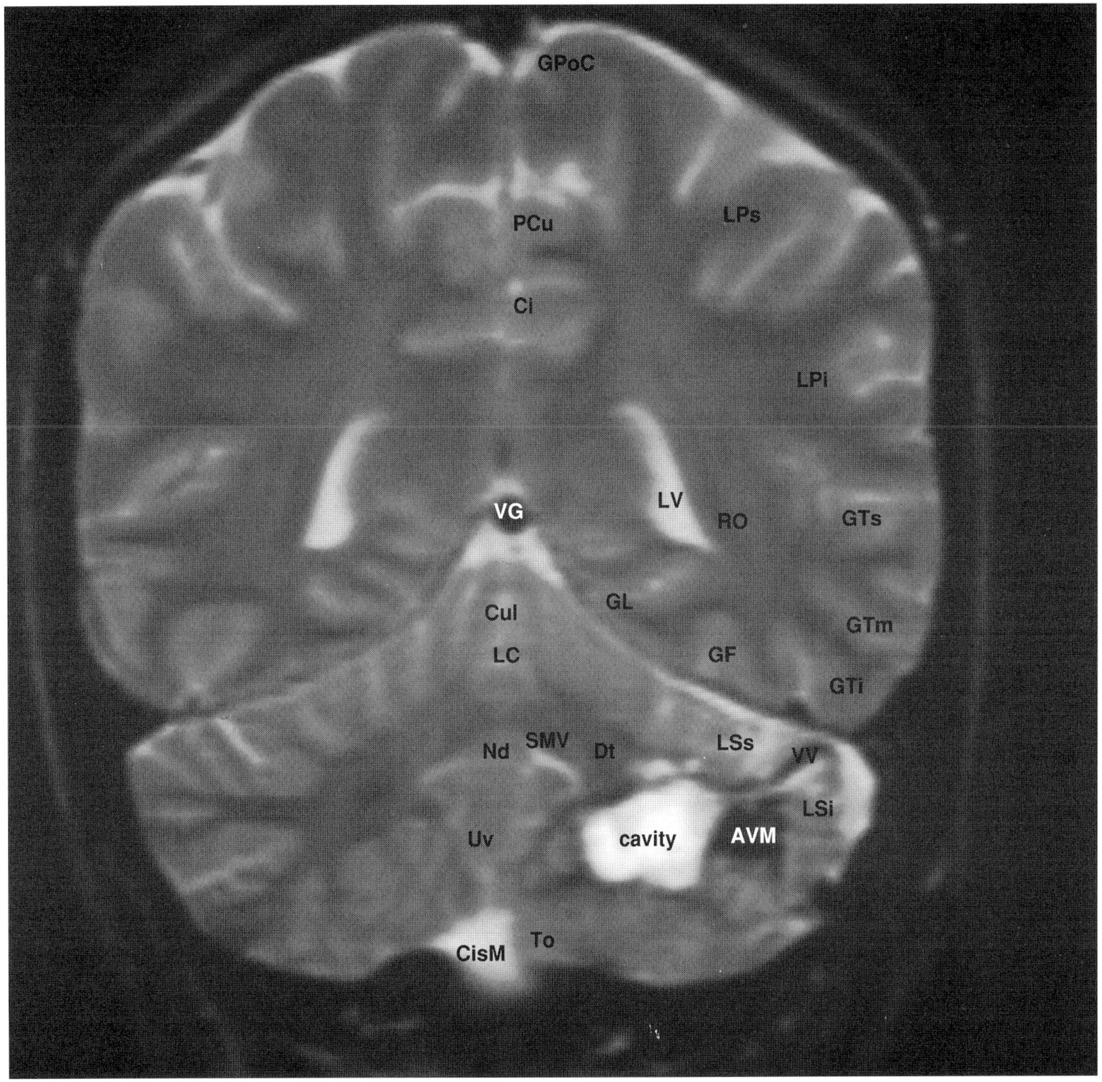
GPoC
PCu
LPs
Ci
LPi
VG
LV
RO
GTs
Cul
GL
GTm
LC
GF
GTi
Nd
SMV
Dt
LSs
VV
LSi
Uv
cavity
AVM
To
CisM

FIG. 4-21B.

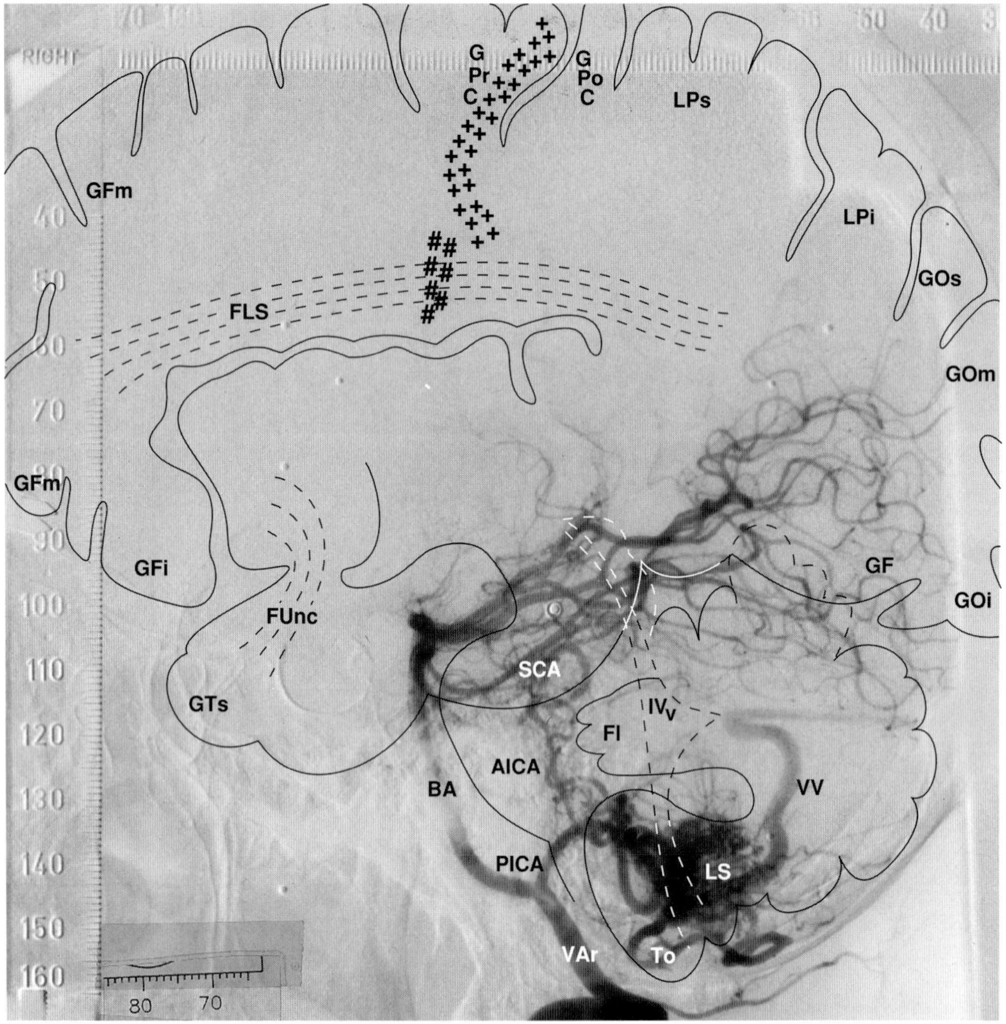
RIGHT
G
Pr
C
G
Po
C
LPs
GFm
LPi
GOs
FLS
GOm
GFm
GFi
GF
GOi
FUnc
SCA
GTs
IVv
FI
AICA
VV
BA
PICA
LS
VAr
To
80
70

FIG. 4-21C.

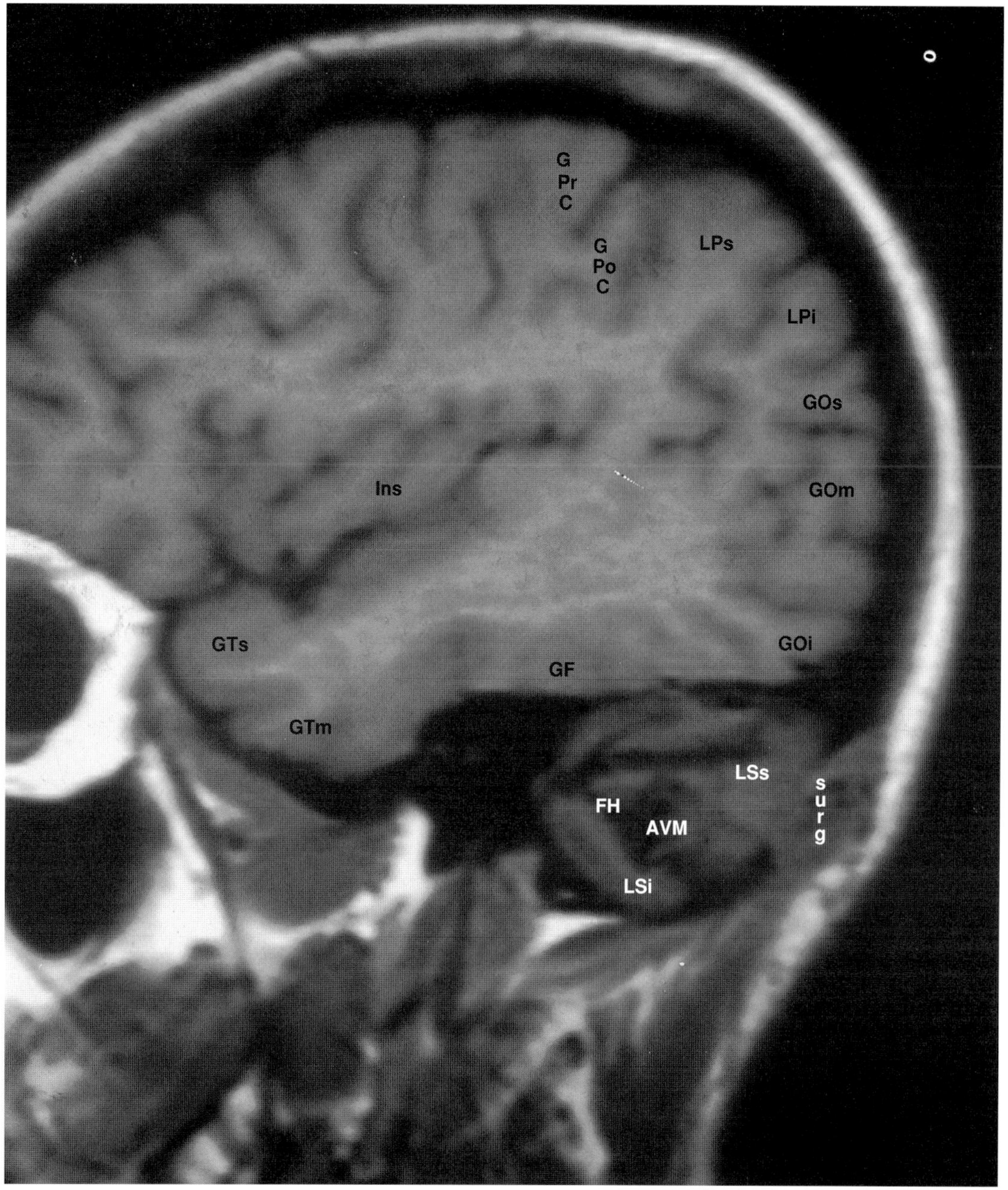

FIG. 4-21D.

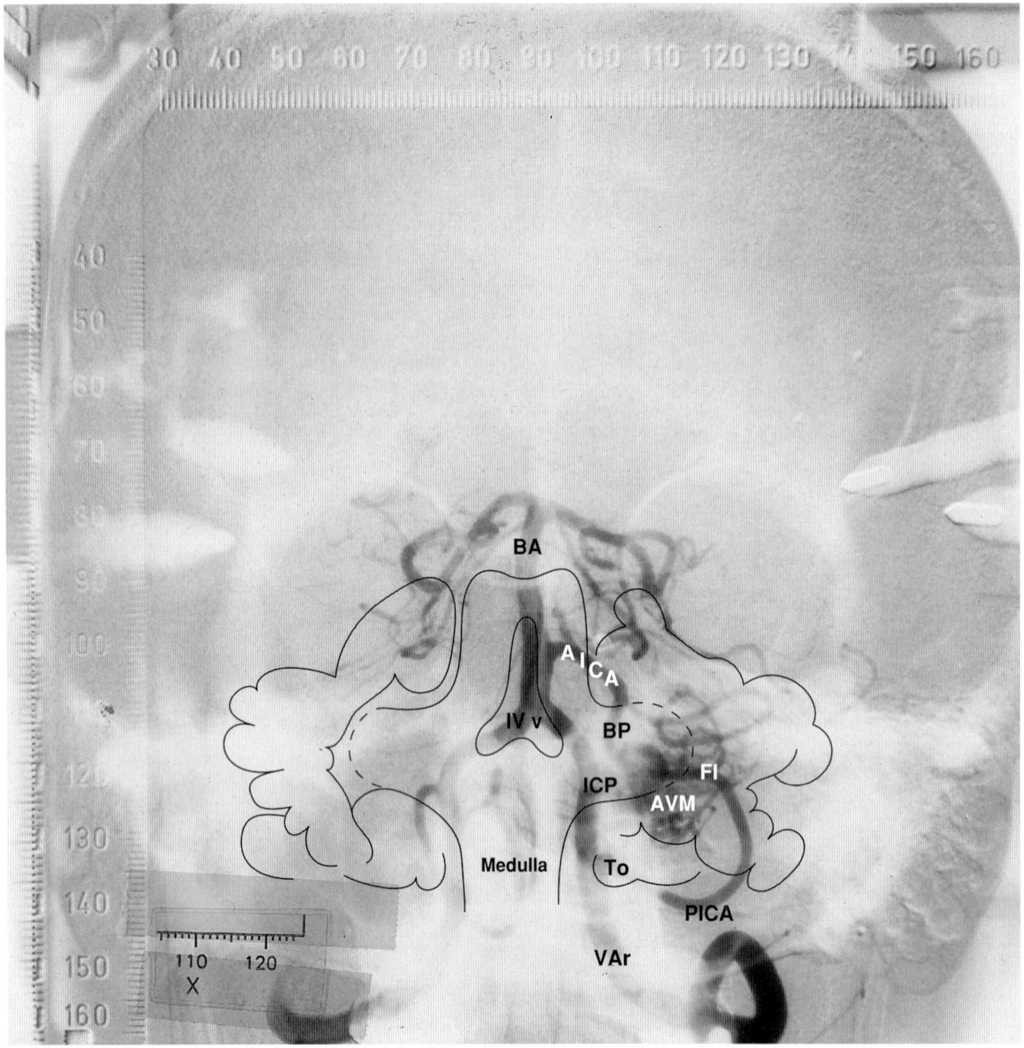

FIG. 4-22A.

FIG. 4-22. Arteriovenous malformation of the left cerebellopontine angle, PA and lateral left vertebral stereotactic angiogram films (**A and B**) and nonstereotactic T_1-weighted, contrast-enhanced axial MRIs (**C and D**) separated by 3.5 mm from inferior to superior, respectively. The MRI study was performed 8 months after the stereotactic angiogram, and is included here instead of the pretreatment study because the AVM was invisible before postradiosurgical changes in the nidus and surrounding tissues became apparent. The principal feeding vessel is the left anterior inferior cerebellar artery (AICA), which also supplies the vascular territory of the left posterior inferior cerebellar artery (PICA) in this patient. Feeding vessels enter the AVM at the medial edge of the nidus within the cerebellomedullary fissure.

The nidus resides lateral to the foramen of Luschka (FoL), partially within or just ventral to the flocculus of the cerebellum (Fl), which shows reactive contrast enhancement in **C** and **D**. The superomedial margin of the nidus reaches the inferior cerebellar peduncle (ICP, restiform body) and nearly reaches the level of the vestibulocochlear (CN VIII) and facial nerve (CN VII) complex. The caudal (inferomedial) margin of the AVM lies just dorsal to the glossopharyngeal nerve (CN IX). Other neural structures within the lateral medulla along the medial edge of the nidus (or just deep to it) include the ventral spinocerebellar tract (Tspcv), dorsal spinocerebellar tract (Tspcd), ventral cochlear nucleus (VIIIcv), descending spinal trigeminal tract and nucleus (Vst, Vsp), spinothalamic tract (STT), and inferior olive (Oli). The vestibular nuclei (VIIIv), hypoglossal (XII) and vagal nuclei (X), tectospinal tract (Ttsp), medial lemniscus (LM), and pyramidal tract (Pyr) all lie sufficiently medial and/or ventral to the AVM as to be unaffected by radiosurgical treatment.

Neurologic risks of surgery or radiosurgery in this case could include ipsilateral hearing loss (cochlear nerve or nuclei), vertigo and/or balance difficulties (vestibular nerves or nuclei, flocculus of cerebellum, spinocerebellar tracts), swallowing difficulties (vagal or glossopharyngeal nerves), ipsilateral facial sensory loss (trigeminal spinal nucleus or tract), or contralateral hemibody sensory loss (spinothalamic tract). *(Figure continued on following pages.)*

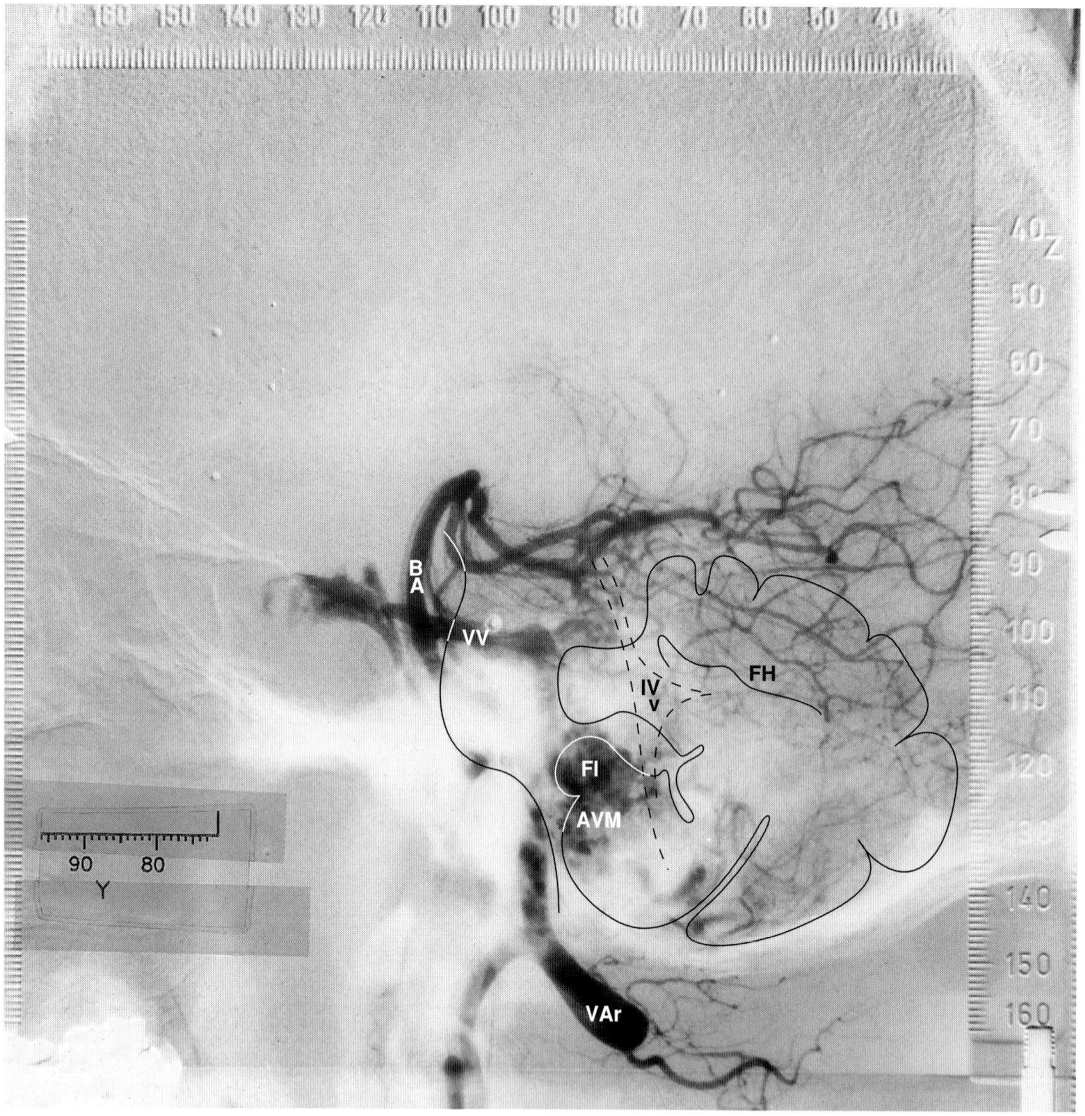

FIG. 4-22B.

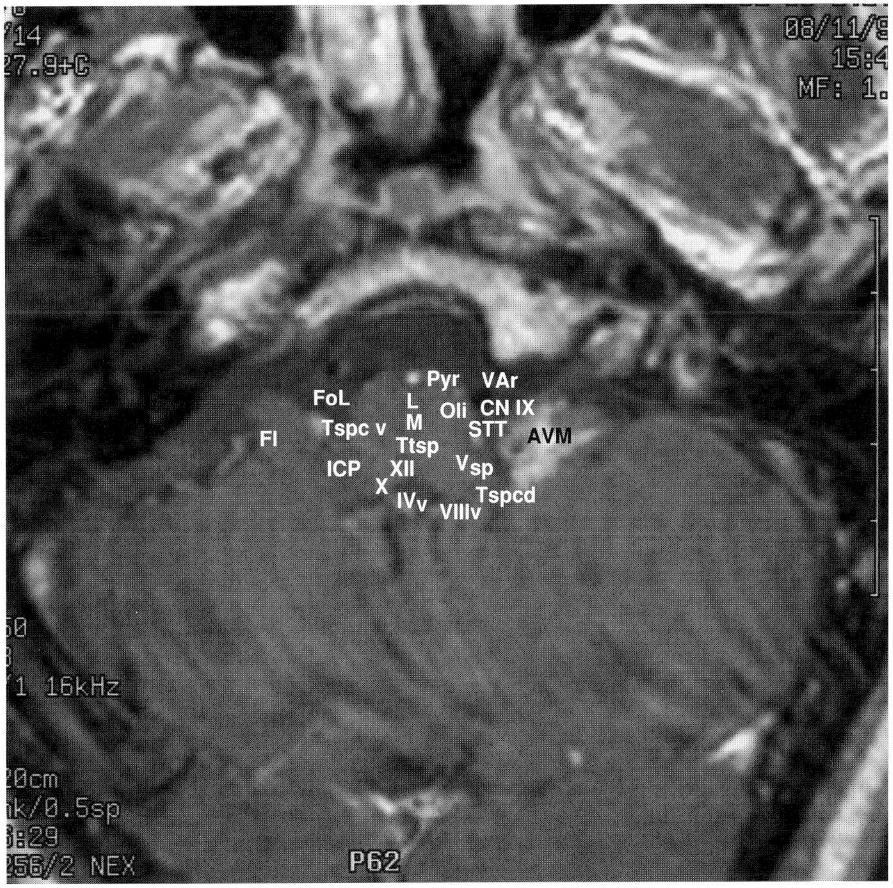
Pyr
VAr
FoL
L
Oli
CN IX
Tspc v
M
STT
AVM
Fl
Ttsp
ICP
XII
Vsp
X
Tspcd
IVv
VIIIv

FIG. 4-22C.

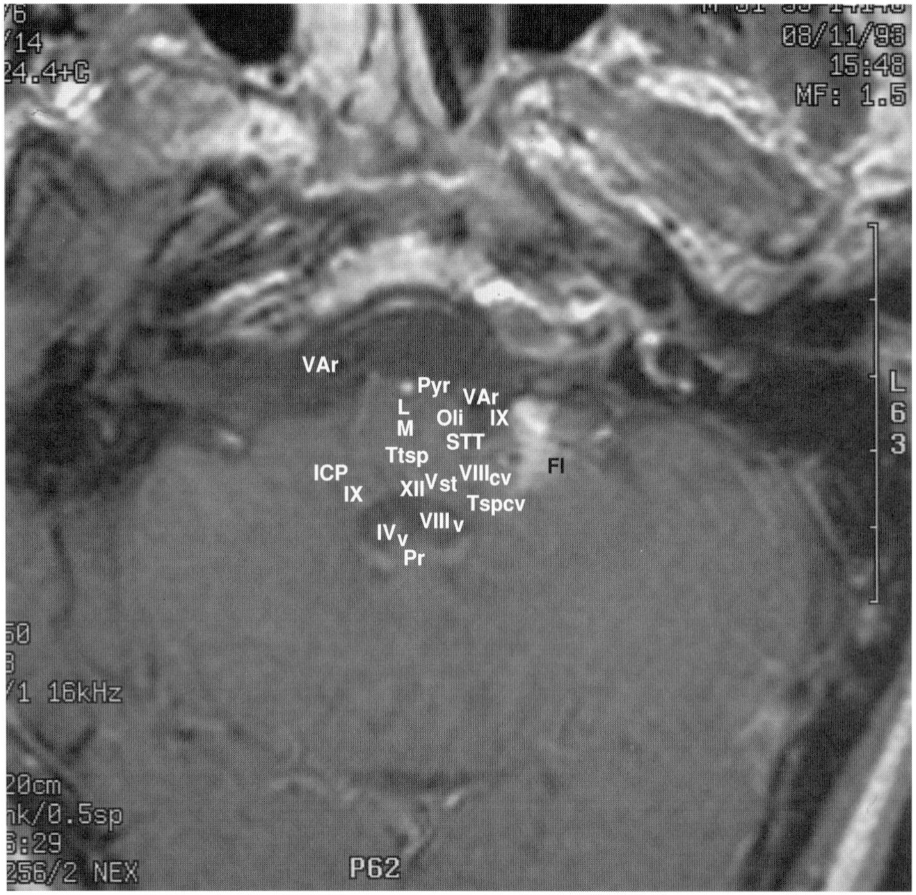
08/11/93
15:48
MF: 1.5
VAr
Pyr
VAr
L
Oli
IX
M
STT
Ttsp
ICP
VIIIcv
Fl
IX
XII
Vst
Tspcv
VIIIv
IVv
Pr
L
6
3
1 16kHz
20cm
P62
256/2 NEX

FIG. 4-22D.

References

1. Afshar F, Watkins ES, Yap JC. *Stereotaxic Atlas of the Human Brainstem and Cerebellar Nuclei.* New York: Raven; 1978.
2. Atlas SW, ed. *Magnetic Resonance Imaging of the Brain and Spine*. New York: Raven; 1991.
3. Baird RA, Spiegel EA, Wycis HT. Studies in stereoencephalotomy IX. The variability in the extent and position of the amygdala. *Confin Neurol* 1960;20:26–36.
4. Benz RA, Wycis HT, Spiegel EA. Studies in stereoencephalotomy XI. Variability studies of the nuclei ventralis lateralis thalami. *Confin Neurol* 1960;20:366–374.
5. Coffey RJ. Stereotactic atlases in printed formats. In: Gildenberg PL, Tasker RR, eds. *Textbook of Stereotactic and Functional Neurosurgery*. New York: McGraw-Hill; 1997:237–248.
6. Damasio H. *Human Brain Anatomy in Computerized Images*. New York: Oxford; 1995.
7. Schaltenbrand G, Bailey P. *Introduction to Stereotaxis With an Atlas of the Human Brain.* Stuttgart: Thieme; 1959.
8. Schaltenbrand G, Wahren W. *Atlas for Stereotaxy of the Human Brain.* Stuttgart: Thieme; 1977.
9. Schaltenbrand G, Walker AE. *Stereotaxy of the Human Brain. Anatomical, Physiological and Clinical Applications.* Stuttgart: Thieme; 1982.
10. Schnitzlein HN, Murtagh FR. *Imaging Anatomy of the Head and Spine. A Photographic Color Atlas of MRI, CT, Gross, and Microscopic Anatomy in Axial, Coronal, and Sagittal Planes.* 2d ed. Baltimore: Urban & Schwarzenberg; 1990.
11. Spiegel EA, Wycis HT. *Stereoencephalotomy, Thalamotomy and Related Procedures. Part I, Methods and Stereotaxic Atlas of the Human Brain.* New York: Grune & Stratton; 1952.
12. Spiegel EA, Wycis HT. *Stereoenchephalotomy. Part II. Clinical and Physiological Applications.* New York: Grune & Stratton; 1962.
13. Talairach J, Hecaen H, David M, Monnier M, De Ajuriaguerra J. Recherches sur la coagulation therapeutique de structures sous-corticales chez l'homme. *Rev Neurol* 1949;81:1–24.
14. Talairach J, David M, Tournoux P, Corredor H, Kvasina T. *Atlas d'Anatomie Stereotxique.* Paris: Masson & cie; 1957.
15. Talairach J, Tournoux P. *Co-Planar Stereotaxic Atlas of the Human Brain. 3-Dimensional Proportional System: An Approach to Cerebral Imaging.* Stuttgart: Georg Thieme Verlag; 1988.
16. Talairach H, Tournoux P. *Referentially Oriented Cerebral MRI Anatomy: An Atlas of Stereotaxic Anatomical Correlation for Gray and White Matter.* Stuttgart: Georg Thieme Verlag & Thieme Medical; 1993.
17. Tasker RR, Organ LW, Hawrylyshyn PA. *The Thalamus and Midbrain of Man. A Physiological Atlas Using Electrical Stimulation.* Springfield: Charles C. Thomas; 1982.
18. Truwit CL, Lempert TE. *High Resolution Atlas of Cranial Neuroanatomy.* Baltimore: Williams & Wilkins; 1994.
19. Van Buren JM, Borke RC. *Variations and Connections of the Human Thalamus.* Berlin: Springer-Verlag; 1972.
20. Yamamoto Y, Coffey RJ, Nichols DA, Shaw EG. Interim report on the radiosurgical treatment of cerebral arteriovenous malformations. The influence of size, dose, time and technical factors on obliteration rate. *J Neurosurg* 1995;83:832–837.

Subject Index

N

O

P

Q

R

S